Deep Learning in Biomedical Signal and Medical Imaging

This book offers detailed information on biomedical imaging using Deep Convolutional Neural Networks (Deep CNN). It focuses on different types of biomedical images to enable readers to understand the effectiveness and the potential. It includes topics such as disease diagnosis and image processing perspectives.

Deep Learning in Biomedical Signal and Medical Imaging discusses classification, segmentation, detection, tracking, and retrieval applications of non-invasive methods such as EEG, ECG, EMG, MRI, fMRI, CT, and X-RAY, among others. It surveys the most recent techniques and approaches in this field, with both broad coverage and enough depth to be of practical use to working professionals. It includes examples of the application of signal and image processing employing Deep CNN to Alzheimer's disease, brain tumor, skin cancer, breast cancer, and stroke prediction, as well as ECG and EEG signals. This book offers enough fundamental and technical information on these techniques, approaches, and related problems without overwhelming the reader. It presents the results of the latest investigations in the field of Deep CNN for biomedical data analysis. The techniques and approaches presented in this book deal with the most important and/or the newest topics encountered in this field. They combine the fundamental theory of artificial intelligence (AI), machine learning (ML), and Deep CNN with practical applications in biology and medicine. Certainly, the list of topics covered in this book is not exhaustive, but these topics will shed light on the implications of the presented techniques and approaches on other topics in biomedical data analysis.

The book is written for graduate students, researchers, and professionals in biomedical engineering, electrical engineering, signal process engineering, biomedical imaging, and computer science. The specific and innovative solutions covered in this book for both medical and biomedical applications are critical to scientists, researchers, practitioners, professionals, and educators who are working in the context of the topics.

Artificial Intelligence for Sustainable Engineering and Management

Sachi Nandan Mohanty
College of Eng., Pune
Deepak Gupta

Artificial intelligence is shaping the future of humanity across nearly every industry. It is already the main driver of emerging technologies like big data, robotics and IoT, and it will continue to act as a technological innovator for the foreseeable future. Artificial intelligence is the simulation of human intelligence processes by machines, especially computer systems. Specific applications of AI include expert systems, natural language processing, speech recognition and machine vision. The future of business intelligence combined with AI will see the analysis of huge quantities of contextual data in real-time. So, the tool will quickly capture customer needs and priorities and do what is needed.

AI for Climate Change and Environmental Sustainability
*Edited by Suneeta Satpathy, Satyasundara Mahapatra, Nidhi Agarwal,
and Sachi Nandan Mohanty*

Green Metaverse for Greener Economies
Edited by Sukanta Kumar Baral, Richa Goel, Tilottama Singh, and Rakesh Kumar

Healthcare Analytics and Advanced Computational Intelligence
*Edited by Sushruta Mishra, Meshal Alharbi, Hrudaya Kumar Tripathy,
Biswajit Sahoo, and Ahmed Alkhayyat*

AI in Agriculture for Sustainable and Economic Management
*Edited by Sirisha Potluri, Suneeta Satpathy, Santi Swarup Basa,
and Antonio Zuorro*

Deep Learning in Biomedical Signal and Medical Imaging
Edited by Ngangbam Herojit Singh, Utku Kose, and Sarada Prasad Gochhayat

www.routledge.com/AI-for-Sustainable-Engineering-and-Management-series/
book-series/AISEM

Deep Learning in Biomedical Signal and Medical Imaging

Edited by Ngangbam Herojit Singh, Utku Kose, and Sarada Prasad Gochhayat

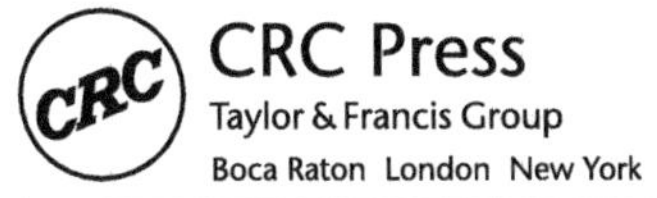

CRC Press
Taylor & Francis Group
Boca Raton London New York

CRC Press is an imprint of the
Taylor & Francis Group, an **informa** business

Designed cover image: © Shutterstock

First edition published 2025
by CRC Press
2385 NW Executive Center Drive, Suite 320, Boca Raton FL 33431

and by CRC Press
4 Park Square, Milton Park, Abingdon, Oxon, OX14 4RN

CRC Press is an imprint of Taylor & Francis Group, LLC

Library of Congress Cataloging-in-Publication Data
Names: Singh, Ngangbam Herojit, editor. | Kose, Utku, 1985– editor. | Gochhayat, Sarada Prasad, editor.
Title: Deep learning in biomedical signal and medical imaging / edited by Ngangbam Herojit Singh, Utku Kose, and Sarada Prasad Gochhayat.
Description: First edition. | Boca Raton : CRC Press, 2025. | Includes bibliographical references and index.
Identifiers: LCCN 2024009477 (print) | LCCN 2024009478 (ebook) | ISBN 9781032622606 (hardback) | ISBN 9781032635132 (paperback) | ISBN 9781032635149 (ebook)
Subjects: MESH: Diagnostic Imaging | Image Processing, Computer-Assisted | Deep Learning | Neural Networks, Computer | Medical Informatics
Classification: LCC RC78.7.D53 (print) | LCC RC78.7.D53 (ebook) | NLM WN 182 | DDC 616.07/54—dc23/eng/20240521
LC record available at https://lccn.loc.gov/2024009477
LC ebook record available at https://lccn.loc.gov/2024009478

ISBN: 978-1-032-62260-6 (hbk)
ISBN: 978-1-032-63513-2 (pbk)
ISBN: 978-1-032-63514-9 (ebk)

DOI: 10.1201/9781032635149

Typeset in Times
by Apex CoVantage, LLC

Contents

Chapter 7   Design and Development of Computer-Aided Diagnosis to
Detect Lung Cancer Disease by Using Intelligent Deep
Learning Principle 111

*Jayaraj R., Sivakamasundari N., Satyajeet Sahoo,
Niranjana S., and Ramkumar G.*

Chapter 8   Novel Methodology to Predict and Classify Liver Diseases
Based on Hybrid Deep Learning Strategy 129

*Sathesh Abraham Leo E., Rajalakshmi R., Kavitha T.,
Prathima C., and Anitha G.*

Chapter 9   Improvements in Analyzing Biomedical Signals and Medical Images Using Deep Learning 150

Manjula Nandi, Ngangbam Phalguni Singh, and Ashok Babu P.

Chapter 10   A Survey on Lung Cancer Diagnosis Using Deep Learning Techniques 169

Jiddu Krishnan O.P. and Dr. Pinki Roy

Chapter 14 Deep CNN in Healthcare... 221

*Farooq Shaik, Rajesh Y., Noman Aasif Gudur,
and Jatindra Kumar Dash*

Contents

*Jullie Josephine D.C., Sudhakar J., Helan Vidhya T.,
Anusuya R., and Ramkumar G.*

About the Editors

Dr. Ngangbam Herojit Singh is presently working as an assistant professor at NIT Agartala in the Department of Computer Science and Engineering. He received his Ph.D. degree from NIT Manipur and M.Tech and B.Tech from Anna University, Chennai. His areas of interest include machine learning, biomedical image processing, hybrid intelligent system, and mobile robotics. He has published more than 12 referred journals, including SCI and Scopus-indexed journals. Furthermore, he has published many conference papers and book chapters. Dr. Herojit has participated in many international conferences as an organizer and session chair.

Dr. Utku Kose received a B.S. degree in 2008 in computer education from Gazi University, Turkey, as a faculty valedictorian; an M.S. degree in 2010 from Afyon Kocatepe University, Turkey, in the field of computer; and a D.S./Ph. D. degree in 2017 from Selcuk University, Turkey, in the field of computer engineering. Between 2009 and 2011, he worked as a research assistant at Afyon Kocatepe University. Furthermore, he has also worked as a lecturer and vocational school vice director at Afyon Kocatepe University between 2011 and 2012, as a lecturer and research center director at Usak University between 2012 and 2017, and as an assistant professor at Suleyman Demirel University between 2017 and 2019. Currently, he is an associate professor at Suleyman Demirel University, Turkey. He has to his credit more than 200 publications, including articles, authored and edited books, proceedings, and reports. He is also on the editorial boards of many scientific journals and serves as one of the editors of the Biomedical and Robotics Healthcare (CRC Press) book series. His research interests include artificial intelligence, machine ethics, artificial intelligence safety, biomedical applications, optimization, chaos theory, distance education, e-learning, computer education, and computer science.

Dr. Sarada Prasad Gochhayat is currently working as an assistant teaching professor at Villanova University, Philadelphia, USA. He has earned his Ph.D. degree in communication engineering from IISc Bangalore, M. Tech. in signal processing from IIT Guwahati, and B. Tech. in ECE from ITER, SOA University, Bhubaneswar. He has past working experience as a faculty member at Manipal University, India, and Old Dominion University, Virginia, USA; post-doctoral research experience at the University of Padua, Italy; and Virginia Modeling, Analysis and Simulation Center, Virginia, USA. His research interests include blockchain, privacy in cloud computing, privacy-preserving data analytics, security and privacy in healthcare systems, and security in IoT and 5G networks.

Contributors

Khwairakpam Amitab
North-Eastern Hill University
Shillong, Meghalaya, India

Kausik Basak
JIS University
Kolkata, West Bengal, India

Prathima C.
Mohan Babu University
Tirupati, Andhra Pradesh, India

Palungbam Roji Chanu
National Institute of Technology
Nagaland
Dimapur, Nagaland, India

Sasirekha D
Rajalakshmi Engineering College
Chennai, Tamil Nadu, India

Jullie Josephine D.C
Kings Engineering College
Chennai, Tamil Nadu, India

Smita Das
Tripura University
Agartala, Tripura, India

Jatindra Kumar Dash
SRM University-AP
Amaravati, Andhra Pradesh, India

Sathesh Abraham Leo E
Kings Engineering College
Chennai, Tamil Nadu, India

Ramkumar G
Saveetha Institute of Medical and
Technical Sciences
Chennai, Tamil Nadu, India

Anitha G
Saveetha Institute of Medical
and Technical Sciences
Chennai, Tamil Nadu, India

Noman Aasif Gudur
SRM University-AP
Amaravati, Andhra Pradesh, India

Jogendra Haobam
National Institute of Technology
Nagaland
Dimapur, Nagaland, India

Sudhakar J
Vinayaga College of Engineering
and Technology
Chennai, Tamil Nadu, India

Valarmathi K
Vellore Institute of Technology
Chennai, Tamil Nadu, India

Tamilarasi K
Jeppiaar Institute of Technology
Chennai, Tamil Nadu, India

Nepoleon Keisham
National Institute of Technology
Nagaland
Dimapur, Nagaland, India

Piyush Kumar
National Institute of
Technology Patna
Patna, Bihar, India

Gopila M
Sona college of Technology
Salem, Tamil Nadu, India

Swanirbhar Majumder
Tripura University
Agartala, Tripura, India

Madhusudhan Mishra
NERIST
Nirjuli, Arunachal Pradesh, India

Anita Murmu
National Institute of Technology Patna
Patna, Bihar, India

Sivakamasundari N
Hindustan Institute of Technology and
    Sciences
Chennai, Tamil Nadu, India

Manjula Nandi
Koneru Lakshmaiah Education
    Foundation (K L Deemed to be
    University)
Vijayawada, Andhra Pradesh, India

Arambam Neelima
National Institute of Technology
    Nagaland
Dimapur, Nagaland, India

Jiddu Krishnan O.P
National Institute of Technology Silchar
Silchar, Assam, India

Ashok Babu P
Institute of Aeronautical Engineering
Hyderabad, Telangana, India

Neelaveni P
Rajalakshmi Engineering College
Chennai, Tamil Nadu, India

Kalpana Devi P
VelTech Rangarajan Dr. Sagunthala
    R & D Institute of Science and
    Technology
Chennai, Tamil Nadu, India

Rusha Patra
Indian Institute of Information
    Technology Guwahati
Guwahati, Assam, India

Bondita Paul
Indian Institute of Information
    Technology Guwahati
Guwahati, Assam, India

Thandaiah Prabu R
Saveetha Institute of Medical and
    Technical Sciences
Chennai, Tamil Nadu, India

Rajalakshmi R
Panimalar Engineering
    College
Chennai, Tamil Nadu, India

Jayaraj R
SRM Institute of Science and
    Technology
Chennai, Tamil Nadu, India

Anusuya R
Modern Institute of Technology
    and Research Centre
Alwar, Rajasthan, India

Pinki Roy
National Institute of Technology
    Silchar
Silchar, Assam, India

Niranjana S
Jeppiaar Institute of
    Technology
Chennai, Tamil Nadu, India

Ngangbam Phalguni Singh
Koneru Lakshmaiah Education
    Foundation, (K L Deemed to be
    University)
Vijayawada, Andhra Pradesh, India

Satyajeet Sahoo
Vignan's Foundation for Science,
    Technology and Research
Guntur, Andhra Pradesh, India

Farooq Shaik
SRM University-AP
Amaravati, Andhra Pradesh, India

Amrita Leima Singha
North-Eastern Hill University
Shillong, Meghalaya, India

Kavitha T
Vel Tech Multi Tech Dr. Gangaran
    Dr. Sakunthala Engineering College
Chennai, Tamil Nadu, India

Helan Vidhya T
Rajalakshmi Engineering College
Chennai, Tamil Nadu, India

Nancy W
Jeppiaar Institute of Technology
Chennai, Tamil Nadu, India

Gayathry S. Warrier
Christ (Deemed to be
    University)
Bangalore, Karnataka, India

Rajesh Y
SRM University-AP
Amaravati, Andhra Pradesh,
India

1 Detection of Diabetic Retinopathy from Retinal Fundus Images by Using CNN Model ResNet-50

Smita Das, Madhusudhan Mishra,
and Swanirbhar Majumder

1.1 INTRODUCTION

One of the most severe side effects of diabetes is diabetic retinopathy (DR), which damages the retina and results in blindness. It affects the blood vessels in the retinal tissue, which leads to fluid leakage and eventually irreversible vision loss. By 2030, it is predicted to affect 191 million people, making it the main factor in vision loss and permanent blindness in middle-aged and older people [1]. DR is typically asymptomatic in its early stages. If DR is identified in its early stages, vision impairment caused by it can be considerably diminished [2]. DR is made up of a distinct collection of lesions that have been seen in the retina of persons with diabetes mellitus for a number of years. The other sign of DR is the appearance of exudates on the retina, which has emerged as a crucial clinical marker for automated disease recognition and diagnosis. Due to the difficulties in spotting them when they appear in smaller sizes, early identification of DR by an ophthalmologist is more difficult [3]. Figure 1.1 depicts a DR-affected retina image [4, 5]. Deep learning algorithms can be used in a real-time automated system to identify the early symptoms of DR disease. As a result, it is simple to reduce both the likelihood of human error and the amount of effort required by the ophthalmologist. Deep learning methods are frequently employed for feature extraction from retinal fundus images in the diagnosis of diabetic retinopathy.

Due to depth in architecture, Residual connections, Pre-trained weights, and Generalization characteristics, Pretrained Convolutional Neural Network (CNN) variant ResNet-50 is proposed here to detect DR in retinal fundus images that classify fundus images by automatically extracting the features. The performance of the technique is evaluated based on different performance parameters like Sensitivity, Specificity, Precision, and Accuracy. The retinal fundus images used for this analysis are the Asia Pacific Tele-Ophthalmology Society 2019 Blindness Detection (APTOS 2019 BD) dataset. This dataset includes 3662 image samples that were compiled by India's Aravind Eye Hospital. After that, a team of medical professionals

DOI: 10.1201/9781032635149-1

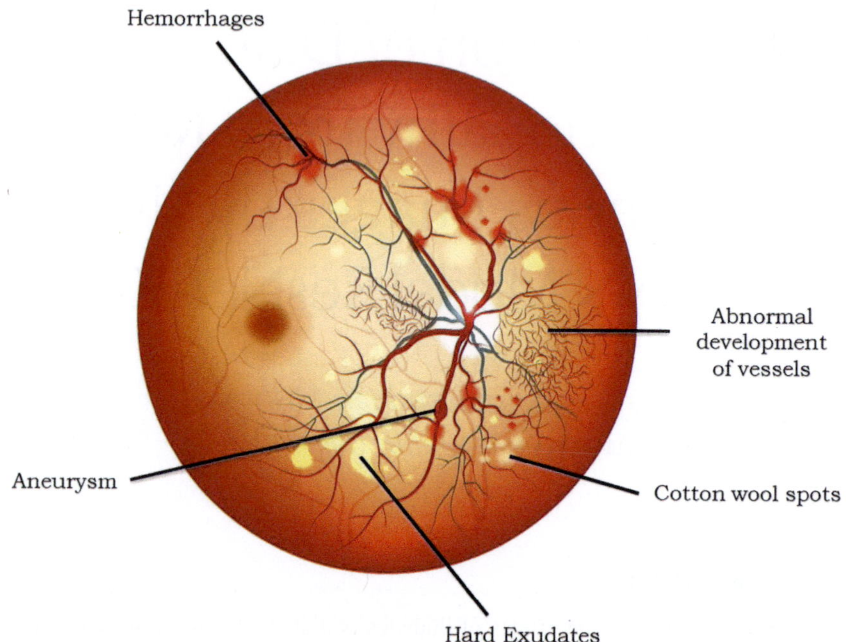

FIGURE 1.1 Diabetic retinopathy-affected retina.

evaluated and classified the samples collected using the International Clinical Diabetic Retinopathy Disease Severity Scale (ICDRSS).

So, this chapter gives a comprehensive study of the ResNet-50 model for the detection of DR and provides a short illustration of quantitative performance measures like sensitivity, specificity, and accuracy. This chapter is organized as follows: in Section 1.2, we present Related works, in Section 1.3 we present the Basic CNN model; Section 1.4 presents the proposed CNN model; Section 1.5 presents results and discussion; and in Section 1.6, we provide a conclusion and future direction.

1.2 RELATED WORKS

A thorough understanding of all the techniques currently being used for DR detection will be given to us through a review of the pertinent literature. It offers useful tools for extracting or segmenting retinal images. A literature survey determines which has the necessary statistical skills for this research area. Learn more about the statistics related to the research topic. A method to recognize microaneurysms, exudates, and haemorrhages was employed by Khojasteh et al. [1], utilizing a probabilistic CNN. Pretrained CNN was used by Mateen et al. [4] to identify exudates. Li et al. [6] introduced an approach that makes use of teaching learning-based optimization, Structured Vector Machines, and Deep CNN. Shinde et al. [7] developed the Le-Net architecture for the Region of Interest recognition and input fundus image validation. For the purpose of glaucoma diagnosis, Nawaz et al. [8] combined EfficientDet-D0 and EfficientNet-B0. Akil et al. [9] introduced a hybrid approach which combines preprocessing, postprocessing, and CNN Deep Learning Networks for feature segmentation and classification. CNN was utilized for the classification of Fundus images by Bulut et al. [10]. To discriminate between various vascular diseases and healthy controls on fundus pictures, Abitbol et al. [11] used a CNN classifier. Ajitha et al. [12] used a CNN algorithm for the autonomous diagnosis of glaucoma. For DR detection, deep transfer learning techniques were studied by Nour et al. [13], which is one of the first to use the APTOS 2019 dataset, having just been published in the second quarter of 2019. The deep transfer models used in this investigation were VGG16, VGG19, ResNet, SqueezeNet, and GoogLeNet. The study by Mushtaq et al. [14] investigates a deep learning methodology for the early identification of DR using the densely connected CNN, DenseNet-169. Qureshi et al. [15] proposed active deep learning method for the classification of fundus images. Nneji et al. [16] identified DR using the weighted fusion deep learning based on Dual-channel Fundus scans. Bilal et al. [17] proposed Artificial Intelligence based classification of DR using U-Net and deep learning. Sundaram et al. [18] used a hybrid segmentation approach for the extraction of retinal blood vessels. Albahli et al. [19] detected DR using Custom CNN to Segment the Lesions. Yazid et al. [20] proposed CNN for DR detection. Yasashvini et al. [21] proposed CNN and Hybrid Deep CNN for Diabetic Retinopathy Classification. This evaluation reveals the research's connected question's originality and significance. It points out areas to avoid repetition and highlights inconsistencies, including gaps in the literature, disagreements in earlier studies, and unanswered concerns. Making a case for the necessity of additional research using the concepts of existing literature, we plan new fresh and original research.

1.3 CNN MODEL

The CNN is the most familiar algorithm in the field of deep learning. CNN model is more familiar rather than others because it automatically recognizes the relevant features without the need for human intervention. CNN is mostly used in image recognition and classification, and it is the only use case which is used in the most advanced frameworks, especially in the field of medical imaging. CNNs were modelled after the neurons found in human and animal brains.

1.3.1 History

The world's first CNN was developed by Yann LeCun for the processing of gridlike topological data in the 1980s [22]. It was named as LeNet after Yann LeCun himself. It was primarily created between 1989 and 1998 for the purpose of handwritten digit recognition. The ImageNet (a dataset) classification task known as the "ImageNet large scale visual recognition challenge (ILSVRC)" is to be credited for the development of newer architectures of CNNs [23]. Researchers made a substantial effort to compare their machine learning and computer vision models, particularly for image classification, on a shared dataset when it was initiated in 2010. Alex Krizhevsky and Geoffrey Hinton finally developed a CNN design in 2012 that is still used today and known as AlexNet [24]. Since 2012, CNN has won the ImageNet challenge every year.

AlexNet, the first winner of the competition, was also based on CNN. In the year, 2013, ZFNet, named for its creators Zeiler and Fergus, won the ImageNet competition ILSRVC. Moving on to 2014, one of the year's most important contributions was the debut of the VGGNet, a brand-new architecture. The Visual Geometry Group (Oxford University) created an arcade architecture referred to as the VGGNet. In the ILSRVC, it was claimed that by making CNN deeper, one might address issues more effectively and get a reduced error rate. The Group's main contribution was the recognition of depth as an essential element in design. In 2014, the architecture came in second place in the ImageNet challenge. Notably, VGG-16 has 138 million parameters and a memory overhead of 48.6 MB, which is considerable [25]. VGG-19, a deeper variation, was also created. Google unveiled GoogLeNet in 2014 [26]. Once more concentrating on deeper networks, GoogLeNet sought to maximize efficiency by minimizing parameter count, memory utilization, and computation. Although it reached a depth of 22 layers, none of the layers were fully connected (FC). "Inception Module" was a newly introduced module. The ILSVRC-14 classification was won by GoogLeNet. One of the most important innovations at that time was the inception module. It was the basis for the architecture, therefore the name "Inception." The structure is also referred to as Inception-v1. Additionally, Inception versions 3 and 4 were released in 2015 and 2016, respectively. In their architecture ResNet, Kaiming He et al. [27] from Microsoft Research proposed the concept of "residual blocks," which are linked to one another through identity (skip) links. A stack of numerous residual blocks makes up a residual network. Similar to GoogLeNet, a "bottleneck" layer was utilized for deeper networks (ResNet-50+) to increase efficiency. ResNet took first place in every ILSVRC competition, and it is still a preferred option for many applications. Wide Residual Networks (WideResNet), Aggregated Residual Transformations for Deep Neural Networks (ResNeXt), Deep Networks with Stochastic Depth, and Densely Connected Convolutional Networks (DenseNets), including more recent ones like MobileNet, EfficientNet, and SENet, are just a few examples of recent architectures that extend the philosophy used [28]. The story seems to go on forever as fresh and newer architecture is introduced.

1.3.2　Basic Architecture

CNN mainly contains three types of layers, convolutional layers (CL), fully connected (FC) layers, and pooling layers. Additionally, the activation function and the dropout layer parameters are needed to create CNN. The basic CNN architecture [5] is shown in Figure 1.2.

- **Convolutional Layer:** The convolutional layer is an important component of a CNN, and its primary role is feature extraction. It convolutes the input image using convolution operators and saves the convolution results to different channels of the convolution layer.
- **Pooling Layer:** The feature maps' size is reduced by pooling layers. As a result, it reduces the number of parameters to learn as well as the amount of computation done in the network.

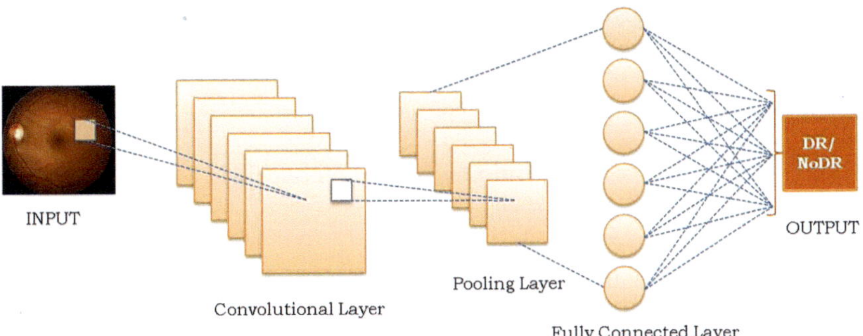

FIGURE 1.2 CNN architecture.

- **Fully Connected Layer:** Convolution and pooling layers extract features from image. Fully connected layers perform classification based on these extracted features.
- **Dropout Layer:** Adding Dropout layers to the network's architecture can prevent overfitting.
- **Activation Functions:** The goal of incorporating an activation function is to give neural networks nonlinear expression capability, allowing them to better match the results and hence enhance accuracy.

1.3.3 OPPORTUNITIES, CHALLENGES, AND APPLICATIONS

The opportunities, challenges, and applications of using CNNs over other traditional neural networks in the computer vision environment are listed as follows:

1.3.3.1 Opportunities of CNN

CNN is a network model of deep learning that learns directly from data without requiring any manual feature engineering or preprocessing. This means that they can automatically discover and adapt to the most salient characteristics of the images, such as edges, shapes, colours, textures, and objects. CNNs are especially useful for detecting patterns in images that can be used to recognize items, classifications, and categories. They can also be used for categorizing audio, time series, and signal data. The weight sharing feature, which decreases the amount of trainable network parameters and so enables the network to improve generalization and avoids overfitting, is the major reason to consider CNN. Learning the feature extraction layers and the classification layer at the same time results in a model output that is both highly organized and heavily reliant on the extracted features. CNN makes large-scale network installation much easier than other neural networks. CNN has a powerful feed-forward architecture, which is capable of learning highly abstract information and effectively recognizes objects. The idea of employing weight sharing, which significantly reduces the number of parameters that need training and improves generalization, is the primary motivation for using CNN. Fewer parameters provide a smoother training process and prevent overfitting. Both the feature extraction stage and the classification stage involve the learning process. Finally, compared to utilizing CNN, using general models of an artificial neural network (ANN) is significantly more complex to create big networks [29].

1.3.3.2 Advantages of Convolutional Neural Networks

- Don't require human supervision
- Automatic feature extraction
- Highly accurate at image recognition and classification
- Weight sharing
- Minimizes computation
- Uses the same knowledge across all image locations
- Ability to handle large datasets
- Hierarchical learning

1.3.3.3 Challenges of CNN

CNNs confront numerous problems, including overfitting, bursting gradients, and class imbalance. They take a lot of computer power and a lengthy period to train, which limits the scope of the research. CNN does not encode object location and orientation. It is inability to be spatially independent of input data. CNNs typically require large datasets to train effectively. This is because they learn to recognize patterns in data by analysing many examples of those patterns. If the dataset is too small, the CNN may not be able to learn the patterns effectively and may perform poorly on new data. The large amount of data can be costly and time-consuming to obtain and annotate. Moreover, they are prone to overfitting, which means that they can memorize the noise and details of the training data and fail to generalize to new and different data. To prevent overfitting, various regularization techniques, such as dropout, batch normalization, and data augmentation, have to be applied, which can increase the complexity and computational cost of the network. Another challenge of CNNs is that they are often considered black boxes, which means that they are hard to interpret and explain. This can pose challenges for debugging, validating, and trusting the network's decisions, especially in sensitive and critical domains, such as healthcare, security, and law.

1.3.3.4 Applications of CNN

CNNs perform a wide range of computer vision tasks, like Face detection, Facial emotion recognition, Biometric authentication, Document classification, 3D medical image segmentation, X-ray image analysis, Cancer detection, Visual question answering, Object detection, Self-driving or autonomous cars, Auto translation, Next word prediction in sentence, Handwritten character recognition and Image captioning.

1.4 THE PROPOSED CNN MODEL

In this section, the proposed technique ResNet-50 based on CNN to detect Diabetic Retinopathy is presented. Due to depth in architecture, Residual connections, Pre-trained weights, and Generalization characteristics, Pretrained CNN variant ResNet-50 is proposed here. This network provides us with high-performance output with the efficient use of computer resources along with a small increase in computational load. The image dataset APTOS-2019 BD used here for the analysis was compiled by India's Aravind Eye Hospital. The particulars of the fundus image dataset APTOS-2019 BD are shown in Table 1.1 [30].

1.4.1 ResNet-50 Architecture

ResNet, which stands for Residual Network, is an architecture made up of Residual Neural Networks. Each residual block's end is reached immediately by identity connections, which take the input. It is trained using a million images from the ImageNet collection, divided into 1000 groups. It is an important tool because it has strong generalization performance with lower error rates on recognition tasks. The ResNet-50 model's architecture comprises Rectified Linear Unit and batch normalization and is implemented by skipping connections on two to three layers. ResNet-50 outperforms in image classification and is good at extracting image features. The basic architecture of ResNet-50 model is shown in Figure 1.3 [31].

The Resnet-50 model consists of the following components:

- A convolution layer with 64 distinctive kernels, with a stride size 2, and a kernel of 7 × 7 sizes, creates one layer.
- The next layer is Max pooling with a stride size 2.
- There are three layers in the subsequent convolution: a 1 × 1, 64 kernel, a 3 × 3, 64 kernel, and finally a 1 × 1, 256 kernel. These three layers have been repeated a total of three times and create nine layers in total.

TABLE 1.1

Particulars of Images in the Dataset

Dataset	Total number of images	Training	Testing	Classes
APTOS-2019 BD	3662	80%	20%	2

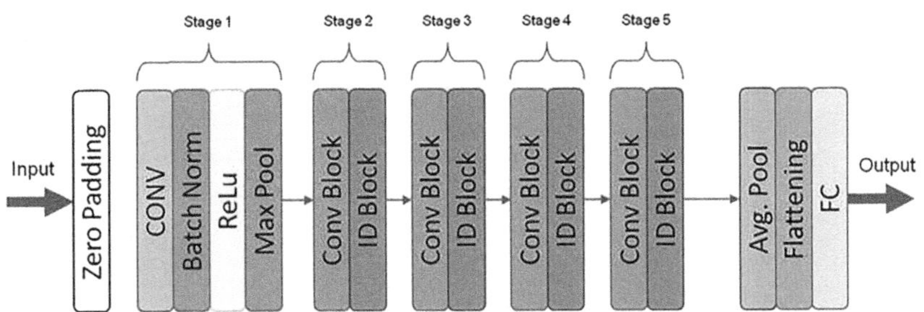

FIGURE 1.3 Basic architecture of ResNet-50 model.

- Then, a kernel of $1 \times 1, 128$ is displayed, followed by a kernel of $3 \times 3, 128$, and, finally, a kernel of $1 \times 1, 512$. We performed this procedure four times to create a total of 12 layers.
- The following kernels are $1 \times 1, 256, 3 \times 3, 256$, and $1 \times 1, 1024$, and this is done six times to create 18 layers in total.
- After that, a $1 \times 1, 512$ kernel was added, then two more $3 \times 3, 512$, and $1 \times 1, 2048$ kernels. Then this procedure was repeated three times to create nine layers in total.
- Next, an average pool with a fully connected layer and a softmax function to create one layer.

So, in total it creates 50 layers Deep CNN.

1.4.2 IMPLEMENTATION STEPS OF RESNET-50 MODEL

Figure 1.4 shows the steps of implementation of the model in our proposed Integrated Development Environment (IDE).

The Precision, Specificity, Sensitivity, and Accuracy of the confusion matrix can be calculated using the formula (1), (2), (3), and (4), respectively.

$$\text{PRECISION} = \text{TP}/(\text{TP} + \text{FP}) \tag{1}$$
$$\text{SPECIFICITY} = \text{TN}/(\text{TN} + \text{FP}) \tag{2}$$
$$\text{SENSITIVITY} = \text{TP}/(\text{TP} + \text{FN}) \tag{3}$$
$$\text{ACCURACY} = (\text{TP} + \text{TN})/(\text{TP} + \text{FP} + \text{TN} + \text{FN}) \tag{4}$$

where TP stands for True Positive, TN stands for True Negative, FP stands for False Positive, and FN stands for False Negative.

1.5 RESULTS AND DISCUSSION

The ResNet-50 model is trained first time for 5 epochs with batch size 8. The hardware configuration used for the experiments is AMD Ryzen 9 5900Hx with Radeon Graphics, NVIDIA GeForce RTX 3060 Laptop GPU GDDR6 @ 6GB(192 bits). Table 1.2 depicts the training and validation achievements like Training Loss, Training Accuracy, Validation Loss, and Validation Accuracy of the ResNet-50 model.

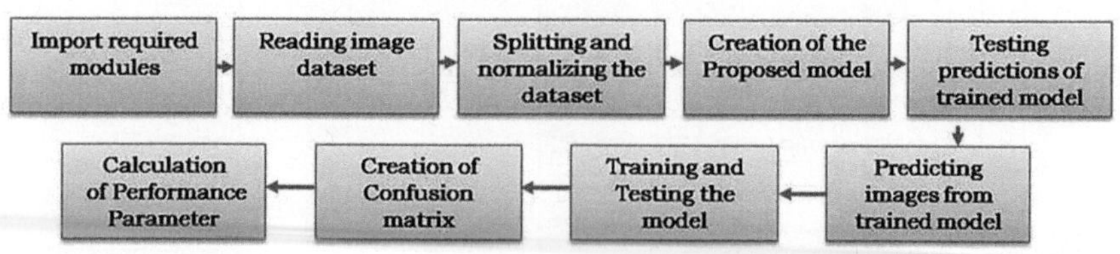

FIGURE 1.4 Steps of implementation of model.

TABLE 1.2

The Training Achievement of the ResNet-50 Model on 5 Different Epochs

EPOCH	Training Loss	Training Accuracy	Validation Loss	Validation Accuracy
1/5	1.1354	0.8412	3.6717	0.9072
2/5	0.5334	0.8774	3.0562	0.9059
3/5	0.4148	0.8867	5.1180	0.9100
4/5	0.2879	0.8914	0.2106	0.9086
5/5	0.2346	0.9024	0.2119	0.9100

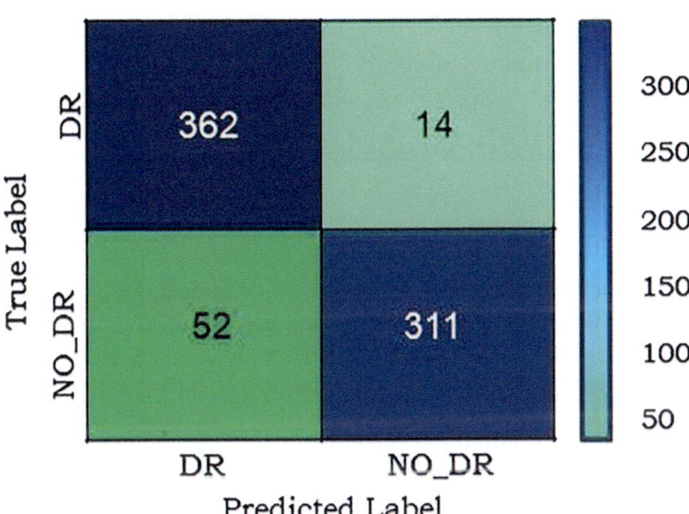

FIGURE 1.5 Confusion matrix of Resnet-50 model.

The confusion matrix of the proposed model ResNet-50 for 5 epochs is depicted in Figure 1.5.

From the results produced by the ResNet-50 model with 5 epochs, we can analyse the model's training and validation loss and accuracy. Figure 1.6 shows the Graphical analysis of the results, where Figure 1.6(a) shows Training and validation loss per epoch and Figure 1.6(b) shows Training and Validation Accuracy per epoch graph. A CNN's validation loss per epoch graph shows how the model's loss on a different validation dataset changes during the course of training. A CNN's training accuracy per epoch graph illustrates how the accuracy of the model on the training data changes throughout the period of training. In contrast, a CNN's validation accuracy

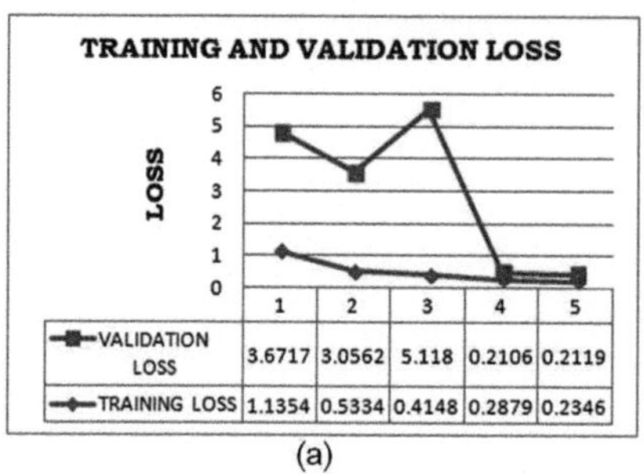

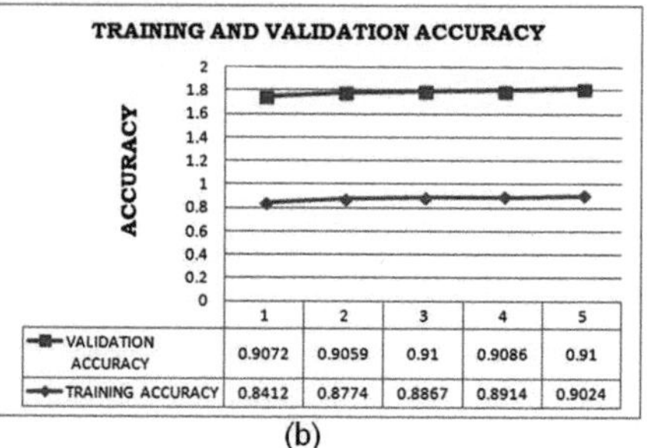

FIGURE 1.6 (a) Training and validation loss per epoch of ResNet-50 model. (b) Training and validation accuracy per epoch of ResNet-50 model.

TABLE 1.3

Performance of the Proposed Model

Model	Sensitivity	Specificity	Precision	Accuracy
Resnet50	87.5	95.58	85.35	90.99

per epoch graph shows how the model's performance on a different validation dataset evolves throughout the period of training. The validation accuracy represents how well the model is performing on fresh and untested data during each epoch of training. The x-axis of the graph represents the epochs, which refers to the number of times the model has iterated through the entire dataset during training, whereas the y-axis represents the training loss, training accuracy, validation loss, and validation accuracy, respectively. Additionally, Table 1.3 depicts the Performance of ResNet-50 model on 5 epochs.

For effectiveness analysis of the proposed model, the Sensitivity, Specificity, Precision, and Accuracy of the model have been computed. Table 1.3 shows the efficacy outcomes of the model. We can note that the ResNet-50 model has achieved Sensitivity of 87.5, Specificity of 95.58, Precision of 85.35, and accuracy of 90.99. ResNet-50 has shown to be effective in a variety of applications, but one significant problem is that it typically takes a long time to train, rendering it virtually unusable in real-world applications. There are various ResNet model versions, but we chose ResNet-50 in this case because it was featured in the tutorial on Kaggle and was already acquainted with us. Retraining roughly 40% of all the parameters is the best outcome ResNet-50 can produce. By applying identity mapping, ResNet-50 assists in solving the vanishing gradient problem. To address the declining gradient issue, the ResNet-50 model was suggested. In order to allow the model to continue training, the idea is to skip the link and transfer the residual to the subsequent layer.

1.6　CONCLUSION AND FUTURE DIRECTION

In this work, we proposed ResNet-50 model for Diabetic Retinopathy detection. A classifier is used to detect the accurate class of the input image. Without using any extra image processing operations for enhancement, the ResNet-50 method outperforms state-of-the-art approaches in examined fundus images. To evaluate the effectiveness of the model, the performance of the technique is evaluated based on different performance parameters like sensitivity, specificity, precision, and accuracy. Overall, the experiment provides valuable insights into the performance of the ResNet-50 model. Future resources will concentrate on hybrid-based strategies that will remove the drawbacks of the current methods. The method will examine online databases as well as local databases. Different performance metrics, such as sensitivity, specificity, and accuracy will be utilized to assess the suggested approach.

REFERENCES

[1] Khojasteh P, Aliahmad B, Kumar DK (2018) Fundus images analysis using deep features for detection of exudates, hemorrhages and microaneurysms. BMC Ophthalmology 18(288) pp 1–13. https://doi.org/10.1186/s12886-018-0954-4.

[2] Sugirtha K, Menaka SR (2021) Deep learning based automatic diabetic retinopathy detection using fundus images: A survey. International Research Journal of Engineering and Technology (IRJET) 8(12) pp 1128–1134.

[3] Sundharamurthy G, Kaliappan VK (2021) Cloud-based onboard prediction and diagnosis of diabetic retinopathy. Concurrency and Computation: Practice and Experience pp 1–11. https://doi.org/10.1002/cpe.6444 ("Wiley")

[4] Mateen M, Wen J, Nasrullah N, Sun S, Hayat S (2020) Exudate detection for diabetic retinopathy using pretrained convolutional neural networks. Hindawi Complexity 2020 Article ID 5801870 p 11. https://doi.org/10.1155/2020/5801870

[5] Das S, Das S, Debroy S, Mishra MS, Majumder S (2023) Automatic Detection of Diabetic Retinopathy to Avoid Blindness. CRC Press, Applied Artificial Intelligence: A Biomedical Perspective. https://doi.org/10.1201/9781003324430

[6] Li YH, Yeh NN, Chen SJ, Chung YC (2019) Computer-assisted diagnosis for diabetic retinopathy based on fundus images using deep convolutional neural network. Hindawi Mobile Information Systems 2019 Article ID 6142839 p 14. https://doi.org/10.1155/2019/6142839 pp 1–14

[7] Shinde R (2021) Glaucoma detection in retinal fundus images using U-Net and supervised machine learning algorithms. Intelligence-Based Medicine 5(2021), p 100038. https://doi.org/10.1016/j.ibmed.2021.100038

[8] Nawaz M, Nazir T, Javed A, Tariq U, Yong HS, Khan MA, Cha J (2022) An efficient deep learning approach to automatic glaucoma detection using optic disc and optic cup localization. Sensors 22(434) pp 1–18. https://doi.org/10.3390/s22020434.

[9] Akil M, Elloumi Y, Kachouri R (2020) Detection of Retinal Abnormalities in Fundus Image Using CNN Deep Learning Networks. Elsevier, State of the Art in Neural Networks, HAL Id: hal-02428351 pp 1–57

[10] Bulut B, Kalın V, Gunes BB, Khazhin R (2020) Deep learning approach for detection of retinal abnormalities based on color fundus images. 2020 Innovations in Intelligent Systems and Applications Conference (ASYU) 2020 pp 1–6. https://doi.org/10.1109/ASYU50717.2020.9259870.

[11] Abitbol E, Miere A, Excoffier JB, Mehanna CJ, Amoroso F, Kerr S, Ortala M, Souied EH (2022) Deep learning-based classification of retinal vascular diseases using ultra-widefield colour fundus photographs. BMJ Open Ophthalmology 2022(7) p e000924. https://doi.org/10.1136/bmjophth-2021–000924 pp 1–7.

[12] Ajitha S, Akkara JD, Judy MV (2021) Identification of glaucoma from fundus images using deep learning techniques. Indian Journal of Ophthalmology 69(10) pp 2702–2709. https://doi.org/10.4103/ijo.IJO_92_21

[13] Khalifa N, Loey M, Taha M, Mohamed H (2019) Deep transfer learning models for medical diabetic retinopathy detection. Acta Informatica Medica 27(5) p 327. https://doi.org/10.5455/aim.2019.27.327-332.

[14] Mushtaq G, Siddiqui F (2020) Detection of diabetic retinopathy using deep learning methodology. IOP Conference Series: Materials Science and Engineering 1070(2021) p 012049. https://doi.org/10.1088/1757-899X/1070/1/012049

[15] Qureshi I, Ma J, Abbas Q (2021) Diabetic retinopathy detection and stage classification in eye fundus images using active deep learning. Multimedia Tools and Applications 80(8) pp 11691–11721. https://doi.org/10.1007/s11042-020-10238-4.

[16] Nneji GU, Cai J, Deng J, Monday HN, Hossin MA, Nahar S (2022) Identification of diabetic retinopathy using weighted fusion deep learning based on dual-channel fundus scans. Diagnostics 12(2) p 540. https://doi.org/10.3390/diagnostics12020540.

[17] Bilal A, Zhu L, Deng A, Lu H, Wu N (2022) AI-based automatic detection and classification of diabetic retinopathy using U-Net and deep learning. Symmetry 14(7) p 1427. https://doi.org/10.3390/sym14071427.

[18] Sundaram R, Ravichandran KS, Jayaraman P, Venkatraman B (2019) Extraction of blood vessels in fundus images of retina through hybrid segmentation approach. Mathematics 7(2) p 169. https://doi.org/10.3390/math7020169.

[19] Albahli S, Nabi Ahmad Hassan Yar G. (2022) Detection of diabetic retinopathy using custom CNN to segment the lesions. Intelligent Automation & Soft Computing 33(2) pp 837–853. https://doi.org/10.32604/iasc.2022.024427.

[20] Yazid RK, Samsuryadi S (2022) Detection of diabetic retinopathy using convolutional neural network (CNN). Computer Engineering and Applications Journal 11(3) pp 203–213. https://doi.org/10.18495/comengapp.v11i3.406.

[21] Yasashvini R, Raja Sarobin MV, Panjanathan RS, Jasmine G, Anbarasi LJ (2022) Diabetic retinopathy classification using CNN and hybrid deep convolutional neural networks. Symmetry 14(1932). https://doi.org/10.3390/sym14091932

[22] LeCun Y, Bottou L, Bengio Y, Haffner P (1998) Gradient-based learning applied to document recognition. Proceedings of the IEEE 86(11) pp 2278–2324.

[23] https://machinelearningmastery.com/introduction-to-the-imagenet-large-scale-visual-recognition-challenge-ilsvrc/ accessed on 01/08/2023.

[24] Krizhevsky A, Sutskever I, Hinton GE (2017) ImageNet classification with deep convolutional neural networks. Communications of the ACM 60(6) pp 84–90.

[25] Simonyan K, Zisserman A (2014) Very deep convolutional networks for large-scale image recognition. arXiv preprint arXiv:1409.1556

[26] Szegedy C, et al (2015) Going deeper with convolutions. IEEE Conference on Computer Vision and Pattern Recognition (CVPR) 2015 pp 1–9. https://doi.org/10.1109/CVPR.2015.7298594.

[27] He K, Zhang X, Ren S, Sun J (2016) Deep residual learning for image recognition. Proceedings of the IEEE Conference on Computer Vision and Pattern Recognition, IEEE Xplore, pp. 770–778.

[28] https://medium.com/appyhigh-technology-blog/convolutional-neural-networks-a-brief-history-of-their-evolution-ee3405568597 accessed on 01/08/2023.

[29] Indolia S, Goswami AK, Mishra SP, Asopa P (2018) Conceptual understanding of convolutional neural network is a deep learning approach. Procedia Computer Science 132(2018) pp 679–688. https://doi.org/10.1016/j.procs.2018.05.069.

[30] www.kaggle.com/datasets/mariaherrerot/aptos2019

[31] https://medium.com/@nina95dan/simple-image-classification-with-resnet-50–334366e7311a

2 DNASNet-RF

Automated Deep NAS-Network with Random Forest for Classifying and Detecting Multi-Class Brain Tumor

Anita Murmu and Piyush Kumar

2.1 INTRODUCTION

Medical imaging modalities including X-rays, Computed Tomography (CT), ultrasound, and Magnetic Resonance Imaging (MRI) are currently evolving, producing larger datasets every day, while increasing popularity [1]. Moreover, analysis of medical images is also necessary to develop tools for faster diagnosis and treatment. Because of its superior soft tissue contrast and lack of radiation exposure, MRI is a widely used imaging technique to assess brain malignancies.

Brain tumors are one of the most deadly and common cancer types worldwide, according to global cancer statistics recorded in 2020 [2]. The brain is the origin of most primary brain tumors, accounting for around 90% of all cases. Depending upon the imaging method used, the price of treating brain tumors may vary significantly [3]. However, according to existing treatments, patients having brain tumors should expect to spend US\$62,602 to extend their lifespan by 16.4 months [4]. Brain tumor patients are dying more often than previously and the survival rate after five years is only 72.5% [5]. MRI provides a better image of soft tissue for characterizing the tissues, but CT scans still cannot characterize the tissue [6]. The brain tumor (FLAIR) and the tissues can be segmented using a variety of MRI imaging techniques, including T1, T1-weighted, T2-weighted, post-contrast, and fluid-attenuated reversal recovery [7]. Enhanced necrosis, edema, and tumor necrosis are the three types of tumor necrosis that can be recognized in visual results of MRI modality [8]. In clinical practice, three tumor sites are used: enhancement, necrosis, and peritumoral edema. The World Health Organization lists brain tumor types as one of the worst types of cancer that may develop anywhere in the globe. The most frequent primary brain tumors are gliomas, which develop from cell-mediated tumorigenesis in the brain and spinal cord. Non-invasive MRI provides a wide range of cell contrasts for every

   DOI: 10.1201/9781032635149-2

imaging modality and has been effectively used to identify brain cancers [9]. Since the process is laborious and time-consuming, only skilled neuroradiologists can currently classify and interpret structural MRI data of brain tumors [10, 11]. This means that the features of each scan and volume may make it difficult to track and quantify lesions. MRI is a typical noninvasive imaging procedure that provides high-quality brain images free of skull abnormalities and artifacts for the diagnosis and identification of brain malignancies [12]. Because gliomas have a very broad range of differences in size, structure, and function, making it exceedingly challenging to manually segment them accurately, automated multi-class classification makes diagnosis and treatment more accurate and easier.

Artificial intelligence (AI), a common approach for medical diagnostics, is required for brain tumor detection. It presents tools for ongoing classification and segmentation. In the initial stage of brain tumor classification, the traditional method is used most frequently. Machine learning- and deep learning-based AI systems dominated both the second- and third-place phases [13, 14]. To extract features from instances, ML and DL use several strategies. A large number of ML category algorithms are developed as independent analytical models of learning that provide accurate predictions based on the characteristics of the data. ML has been found to be advantageous for tissue characterization in applications for medical imaging [15]. Radiologists and researchers who utilize ML techniques [15] are alone in charge of selecting the qualities that are most compelling, which results in an unbalanced methodology. Farajzadeh et al. [16] have proposed to categorize and segment brain tumor MRI images into a single architecture are combined layers of attention for segmentation with a hyperbolic kernel for convolutional layers. A hybrid convolutional neural network with a feature impact control module that automatically weighs extracted features. Moreover, it analyzes the effects of several modules using ablative research to demonstrate the influence of every component on overall performance. Wozniak et al. [17] have presented a new correlation learning method for deep CNN structures, mixing CNN with conventional design. In order to determine the best files for the pooling stage and convolution layers, CNN uses a support neural network. As a result, the primary CNN classifier gains efficiency and learns more quickly. An effective method for transferring the effectiveness of a 2D classification architecture trained on images to 2D, 3D single- and multiple-modal segmentation of medical imaging techniques has been proposed by Messaoudi et al [18]. The unique architecture is based on two fundamental ideas: dimensions transfer by enlarging a 2D segmented scheme into an additional dimensional one or transfer of weight by implementing a 2D pre-trained encoder-decoder into a greater dimensional Unet.

The methods discussed previously concern several BTC and categorization models. The form and size issues on multi-class brain imaging datasets were not taken into account while testing any models; only single-class image datasets were used. The suggested technique uses a classification network using NASNetLarge-RF to supply the crucial characteristics and produce robust classification from MRI images of the brain in order to address these problems. The approach proposed in this research offers a unique BTC network that can effectively acquire representations of individual representations while handling many classes. Figure 2.1 shows the sample images of brain tumor MRI scan [20].

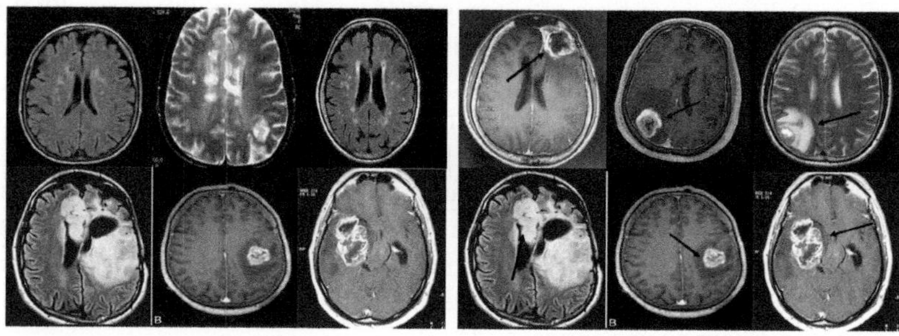

FIGURE 2.1 Brain tumor dataset sample images of pituitary adenoma, glioma, and meningioma.

2.1.1 MOTIVATION

The proposed work is to use a new modified Deep Learning (DL)-based Neural Architecture Search Network Large (NASNetLarge) model with Random Forest (RF) and a preprocessing technique for brain tumor classification and detection. A model is to address the classification problems of a higher rate of brain tumors from MRI images. The preprocessing procedures are used to improve the dataset quality and the functionality of the system.

2.1.2 PROBLEM STATEMENT

The main contributions of this chapter are as follows:

- The effective classification of brain tumors due to the tumor information can vary in size and shape, making it challenging to identify where the tumor cells are located in the brain. The proposed scheme solves these issues by using the NASNetLarge-RF technique.
- In the proposed method, a new modified Deep Learning (DL)-based NASNetLarge with RF is proposed for predicting and classifying the tumor cell locations in a brain MRI dataset. The NASNet model is more efficient and improves performance.
- Furthermore, the proposed scheme used the RF technique as a classifier rather than softmax. The RF classification approach resolves the separable problem of a nonlinear function and prevents over-fitting during training. Moreover, gaussian smoothing boundary box edge detection is used to detect and validate the edges of the infected region.
- The experimental evaluation of the proposed scheme is carried out by performance matrices, such as accuracy, recall, precision, F1-score, and MSE. The result showed that the proposed model outperforms the other existing related models.

2.1.3 APPLICATIONS OF MEDICAL IMAGING

Medical imaging is essential to contemporary healthcare because it offers non-invasive means to view the internal organs and bodily processes. Medical imaging has several uses in a variety of medical professions and fields [19]. Here are a few important examples:

a. *Orthodontic and dental care:* X-rays and CT scans assist dentists in identifying dental issues and making treatment plans, such as for dental implants and orthodontic therapies. Imaging is helpful in the diagnosis of joint problems, degenerative diseases, and bone fractures in the context of orthopedics, directing orthopedic procedures and therapies.
b. *Cancer detection:* A variety of cancer forms, including lung, breast, prostate, and brain tumors, are detected using medical imaging procedures, including X-rays, CT scans, MRIs, and PET scans.
c. *Cardiovascular disease:* Echocardiography, angiography, and MRI are imaging techniques that aid in the diagnosis of heart disorders such as coronary artery disease, heart defects, and heart failure.
d. *Neurological disorder:* Imaging techniques like MRI and CT scans help in the diagnosis of neurological disorders such as multiple sclerosis, brain tumors, and strokes.
e. *Surgical planning:* Surgeons utilize imaging to plan difficult procedures, reducing risks and increasing accuracy. Imaging gives precise anatomical information.
f. *Radiation therapy:* Radiology aids in the planning and direction of radiation therapy for the treatment of cancer, enabling focused delivery while preserving healthy tissues.

These uses illustrate the various ways that medical imaging improves patient care, facilitates early diagnosis, directs treatment choices, and aids in medical research and innovation.

2.2 EXPERIMENTAL DESIGN AND IMPLEMENTATION

The proposed modified NASNetLarge-RF model structure is shown in Figure 2.2. The proposed system is used for brain tumor, classification, detection, and boundary box of the infected region and helps to diagnose the tumor in its early stages. The architecture of the proposed scheme contains NASNet nodes, imagenet as a backbone, an activation function node, and batch normalization in downsampling. The details should be described in depth in this section, starting with the network architecture and essential network components. Furthermore, an overview of the proposed loss function and boundary box of the segmented image is provided.

2.2.1 DATASET DESCRIPTION

The brain tumor dataset is downloaded from Kaggle [20]. Moreover, this database includes meningioma, pituitary samples, and glioma with their corresponding mask image sample. The images in the dataset collection are 256 × 256 pixels in size. The datasets with complete descriptions are given in Table 2.1.

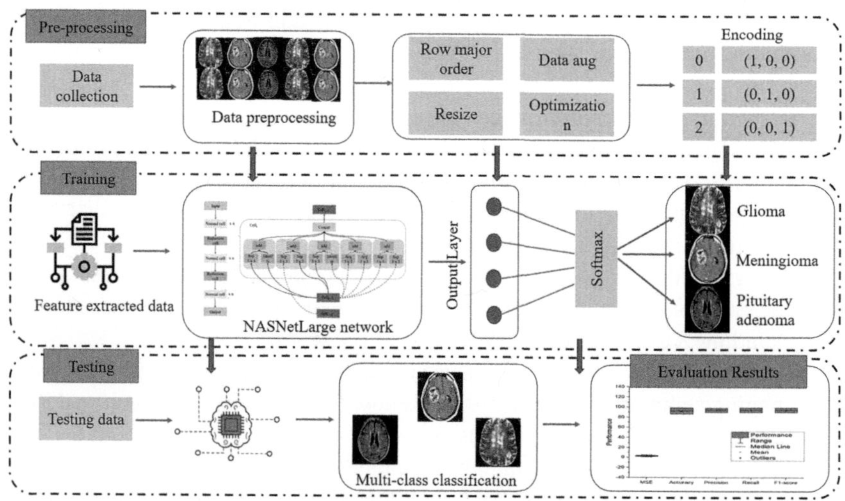

FIGURE 2.2 The proposed methodology.

TABLE 2.1

Dataset Description

Types of Tumors	No. of Images	No. of Patients	No. of Axial Samples	No. of Coronal Samples	No. of Sagittal Samples
Glioma	1426	91	494	437	495
Meningioma	708	82	209	269	231
Pituitary adenoma	930	60	291	319	320

2.2.2 ENVIRONMENTAL SETUP

An Intel Core i5 CPU operating at 2.8 GHz, 8 GB of RAM, and a Graphics Processing Unit (GPU) [21] are used to train the model. TensorFlow, the Keras library, and Python 3.8.1 are used to implement the proposed approach. The 256 × 256 pixels of the brain tumor database are publicly accessible to all researchers. The complete collection of instances is used in training sessions. The neural network is instructed to use the remaining 70% of the data from training, with just 30% of it being used for testing and validation [22].

2.2.3 DEEP LEARNING-BASED NASNETLARGE

The proposed model uses a new modified Deep Learning (DL)-based Neural Architecture Search Network Large (NASNetLarge) model with Random Forest (RF) architecture for brain tumor prediction and classification. Moreover, the complete training process is defined in Algorithm 1. The proposed method identifies the input image as either infected or noninfected with a tumor after using MRI images. The DL-based block includes convolutional units with ReLU activation function, Batch Normalization (BN), softmax, and fully connected. The input for the NASNetLarge-decoder block with NASNetLarge-encoder and upsampling would be the final softmax node of the classifier block, followed by the activation function for the output layer with the RF techniques. The functional flow diagram for the proposed work is shown in Figure 2.3. The remaining part of this section details image capture and brain tumor prediction and classification.

2.2.3.1　Preprocessing

The intensity data has been normalized between 0 and 1 using the min-max normalization method. Their size changed to 224 × 224. The three channels are generated by reproducing the greyscale values three times since MRI scans are greyscale images. The proposed system is evaluated on the MRI dataset following a five-fold cross-validation at the patient level. Five separate subsets have been generated from the whole 233-patient dataset. The separated subgroups are around the same size. One subset is selected to serve as the test set, and the remaining ones as the training set. Every subset is utilized to create the test set once after repeating this process. To prevent the data of a certain patient from appearing in the test at the same time, the dataset has been divided into training sets.

Algorithm 1: Training process of NASNetLarge with RF

Input : Let, E is epochs, w is model parameters, η is the learning rate, b is the batch size, X_{test}, X_{train} are training and testing image, and X' is NASNet dataset

Output: R_{test} test result

Initialize NASNetLarge model with parameters w

NASNetLarge:

for *local epoch e1 to E* **do**
　for $b = (n,m) \in$ *random batch from X'_i* **do**
　　Optimize model parameters
　　　$w_i \leftarrow w_i - \eta(\nabla(\iota(w_i; b)))$
　end
end

Initialize upper layers model parameters for classification θ with trained NASNetLarge model parameter w

Traning of brain tumor Classification:

$X_{train} \leftarrow preData(X_{train})$

$X_{test} \leftarrow preData(X_{test})$

while *θ has not converged* **do**
　for *local epoch e ← 1 to E* **do**
　　for *s = (n, m)∈ random batch from X_{train}* **do**
　　　Update model parameter
　　　　$\theta_i \leftarrow \theta_i - \eta(\nabla(\iota(\theta_i; b)))$
　　　Classify with RF
　　end
　end
end

With tested completed model evaluation metrices

　$R_{test} \leftarrow computeMatrics(\theta, X_{test})$

　return R_{test}

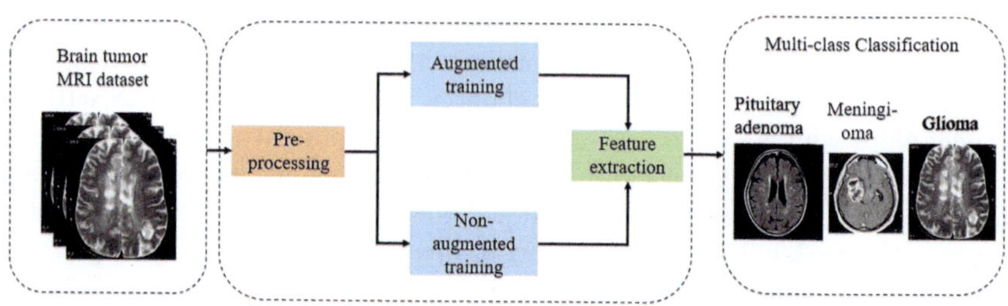

FIGURE 2.3 Training process of NASNetLarge model.

2.2.3.2 Feature Extraction

In the work proposed, a built-in feature extractor is used to demonstrate feature extraction from the model, a technique to shorten the time needed to create and train a successful Deep-CNN model. In order to gather more data for exact prediction, different characteristics are extracted at different levels, or deeper features are recovered layer by layer. After preprocessing, discrete wavelet transformations are used to extract a subset of characteristics from the medical images.

The integrated feature extractor performs the next image using a model generated for function using the Deep-CNN methodology, which is an efficient method for feature extraction. A couple of sets of layers in the Deep-CNN model ultimately opted to combine the output. The given issue for the training process depended on the Deep-CNN model weights. The model weights are retained during training to stop the Deep-CNN from altering when the new model is built.

2.2.3.3 Data Augmentation

The pre-processed skin images from the training set are then multiplied across input images by rotating at four different angles: 0°, 90°, 180°, and 270°. The proposed scheme analyzes data augmentation, used to enhance the size of the data, create additional information from the input data, and circumvent the lack of labeled images.

2.2.3.4 Training a NASNetLarge Model

The NASNet-Large classification network has an encoder and a decoder. In Figure 2.4, the architecture is displayed. The proposed NasnetLarge-decoder network decomposes images using the first 414 layers of the NasnetLarge network, which is a highly trained classification network on ImagNet [23]. Since the brain tumor dataset considerably differs from the ImageNet, that do not utilize the pre-trained weighted models in the experiment and instead retrain each layer using the collected information to fit the NasnetLarge network. Another difference is that the proposed system does not need pooling indices because the NasnetLarge network can generate comprehensive information shown in Figure 2.4.

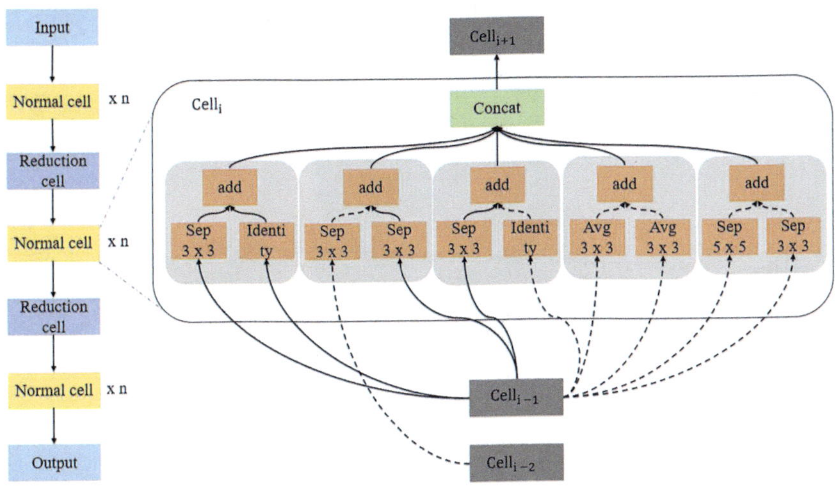

FIGURE 2.4 Working flow of NASNetLarge model.

The max-pooling layer can be used by the right decoder in the decoder network to upsample the input feature map. Figure 2.5 provides an illustration of the decoding method. The decoder contains four blocks. An upsampling layer, which can enlarge the feature map, comes first in each block and is followed by feature maps, convolution, and corrected linear units. Then, each of these maps is given a batch normalizing layer. A multi-channel feature map can be created by the first decoder, which is located closest to the final encoder. This is comparable to the Segnet, whose encoder inputs may produce a variety of sizes and channels. A trainable softmax with RF classifier receives the final output of the last decoder. And this softmax layer's output is C-channel brain images of probabilities, where C is the number of classes (two in our scenario), and the output of this layer is the output. The class C with the highest image probability at each pixel corresponds to the classification that is expected.

2.2.3.5   Random Forest for Classifying Brain Tumor

A random forest [24] is nothing more than a group of decision trees with their output combined into a single outcome. These are extremely potent models because of their capacity to restrict overfitting without noticeably raising the bias-related error. Random forests help reduce variation in one way by training on different sets of data.

2.3   RESULTS AND DISCUSSION

2.3.1   Performance Evaluation Matrices

The classification results are shown in the confusion matrix, which is separated into two sections. To highlight the amount of information included within the label's class, each result is displayed in a row. This study utilizes these parameters to assess the effectiveness of the NASNetLarge-RF model evaluation matrices, namely accuracy,

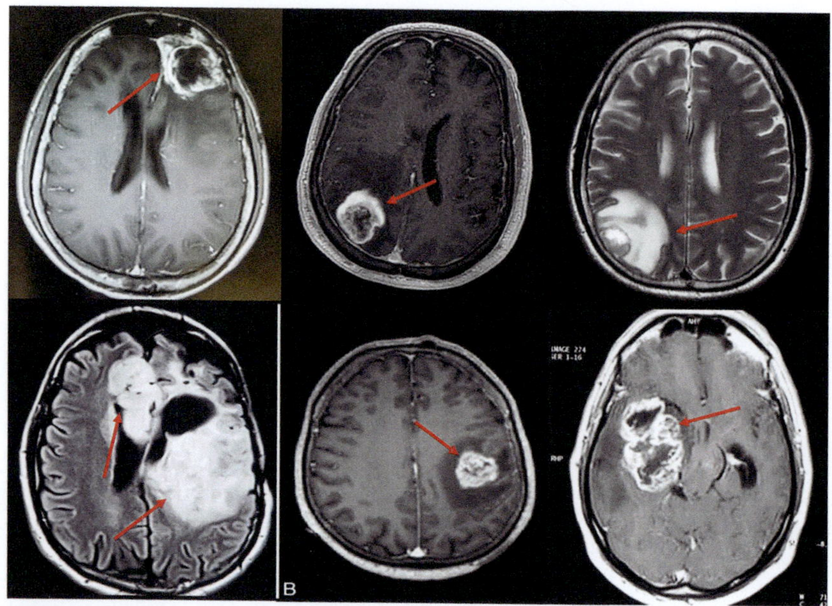

FIGURE 2.5 Performance outcome of validated brain tumor detection.

MSE, F1-score, recall, and precision using the True Positive (TP) and True Negative (TN) terms, which signify when the estimated result is positive and the actual value is positive or negative, respectively. Additionally, False Positives (FP) and false negatives (FN) refer to results that are predicted to be positive but have negative values. Results that are expected to be positive but have negative values are referred to as False Positives (FP).

2.3.2 EXPERIMENTAL RESULTS

The proposed system outcomes evaluate the performance of a NASNetLarge-RF model using a dataset of brain tumors. Deep-NASNet has been used to extract the features automatically from raw images with remarkable productivity. The cumulative distribution function of the corrected images has a pattern that is linear. Brain tumor multi-class classification is done during the process's validation, training, and testing process. Additionally, the image index values will always fall between [0, 1]. The number of overall valid predictions the model should produce using the entire set of provided data is determined by the "accuracy" parameter. All claims that the data is overfitting are refuted by the validation score of 98.97% and the training set's accuracy after 100 iterations. Finally, the test accuracy of 98.97% demonstrates that the algorithm is capable of accurately assessing and producing predictions about a range of diverse images. Figure 2.5 contrasts the proposed NASNetLarge-RF model with some of the current State-Of-The-Art (SOTA) models. The accuracy of the results is above 90%, and it is clear from Figure 2.6 that the model is very well-suited for the extremely constrained range of validation and test accuracy.

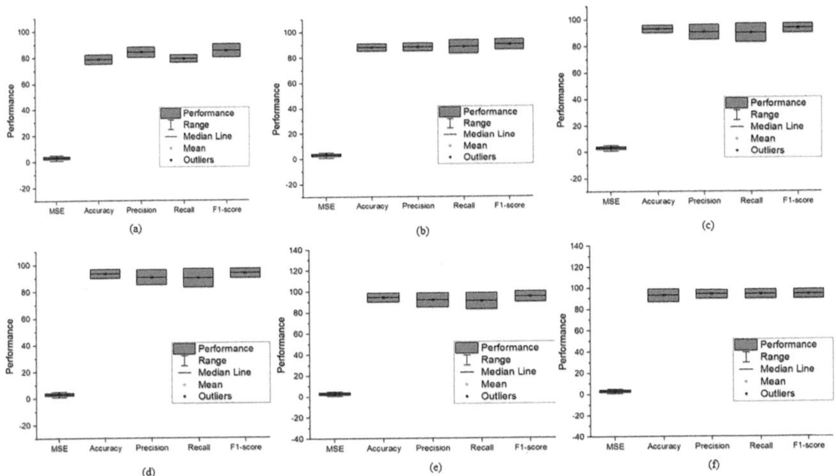

FIGURE 2.6 The graph visualization of performance outcomes (a) fold 1, (b) fold 2, (c) fold 3, (d) fold 4, (e) fold 5, and (f) fold mean.

TABLE 2.2
The Performance Outcome of the Proposed Scheme with Five-Fold Cross-Validation and Their Mean and Standard Deviation

S. No.	Performance Matrices	Fold 1	Fold 2	Fold 3	Fold 4	Fold 5	Fold Mean
1.	Accuracy	82.12 ± 0.07	90.72 ± 0.08	95.69 ± 0.08	96.69 ± 0.08	98.49 ± 0.07	98.97 ± 0.02
2.	Precision	87.91 ± 0.05	91.32 ± 0.06	96.21 ± 0.07	96.21 ± 0.07	98.61 ± 0.06	98.21 ± 0.04
3.	Recall	81.90 ± 0.08	93.72 ± 0.08	96.94 ± 0.02	96.94 ± 0.02	98.49 ± 0.05	98.72 ± 0.03
4.	F1-score	89.94 ± 0.07	93.98 ± 0.07	97.03 ± 0.03	97.03 ± 0.03	99.71 ± 0.01	99.01 ± 0.05
5.	MSE	0.0175 ± 0.03	0.0167 ± 0.02	0.0174 ± 0.02	0.0134 ± 0.02	0.0124 ± 0.01	0.0012 ± 0.01

The sample results are represented by recall, precision, F1-score, accuracy, and MSE. The proposed work's output is produced by averaging the outcomes for each tested image in each image category. Using the number of pixels in the pictures, the true positive, false positive, true negative, and false negative values are computed. The proposed approach increased classification accuracy and enhanced treatments for brain tumor detection and diagnosis. The outcomes, which are represented in Table 2.2, show that the proposed approach performs better than the most recent method in terms of medical image classification, MSE, accuracy, recall, precision, and F1-score. The proposed technique raises classification precision as well.

The image passes several processing phases, and NASNet-decoder improves classification accuracy by reducing vanishing gradient issues. A new NASNetLarge-RF with an embedded loss function with a softmax activation function. The results show improved performance when classifying brain tumor MRI images. The proposed scheme has successfully addressed the drawbacks of the current SOTA schemes. An integrated loss function, noise reduction, and cross-validation are all applied.

Additionally, the proposed methodology outperforms the findings by limiting network overfitting and removing gradient descent errors. Figure 2.6 shows that the performance outcome graphs of accuracy, MSE, F1-score, recall, and precision are display in the results. The results of the epoch are automatically used to build the performance graph. Since the results vary during the course of epochs, every parameter of the graph is changed.

2.3.3 Boundary Box Detection Using Gaussian Smoothing

The diffusion process and Gaussian smoothing are connected by the formula $\alpha = \sqrt{2D_n t}$ [25]. Here, t is the time stamp for the diffusion process, α is the standard deviation, and D_n is the diffusivity constant. In scale space, the definition of a Gaussian kernel is

$$G_{\sqrt{2D_n t}}(n, m, t) = \frac{1}{\sqrt{4D_n t}} \, exp^{\frac{-\left(n^2 + m^2\right)}{4D_n t}} \tag{2.1}$$

By using the value of $D_n = 1$ in Eq. (2.1), scale space Gaussian equivalent smoothness is produced. Now about a generalized PDE.

$$\frac{\partial^\beta}{\partial t^\beta} I_{(n, m, t)} = D_n \left(\frac{\partial^\sigma I_{n, m, t}}{\partial n^\sigma} + \frac{\partial^\sigma I_{n, m, t}}{\partial m^\sigma} \right) \tag{2.2}$$

The image functional at time t in this case is $I_{(n,m,t)}$. In the finite domains, its intensity levels are specified. T_m is a diffusion process's time stamp. The values of it are within the range of 0 to t to T_m. The initial input image function is represented by the image functional at time $t = 0$. The spatial derivative is Ω. $0 \le t \le T_m$ is the time derivative in order. D_n, frequently referred to as the diffusivity coefficient, is a positive constant. Eq. (2.2) becomes the classical energy diffusion equation for the values of $\beta = 1$ and $\sigma = 2$. Similar to this, the classical wave equation is represented by Eq. (2.2) for the values of $\beta = 2$ and $\sigma = 2$. The scenario where $10 \le \sigma \le 2$ has been taken into consideration in this equation. The super-diffusive process is represented by the Eq. (2.2) with assumed values and. The particles disperse more quickly in this procedure than in the conventional mode. The diffusive process is represented by

$$\frac{\partial}{\partial t} I_{(n, m, t)} = D_n \left(\frac{\partial^\sigma I_{n, m, t}}{\partial n^\sigma} + \frac{\partial^\sigma I_{n, m, t}}{\partial m^\sigma} \right) \tag{2.3}$$

The time derivative for Eq. (2.3) is calculated using forward difference as

$$I^n_{n, m, t} = I^n_{n, m, t} + D_n \left(\frac{\partial^\sigma I_{n, m, t}}{\partial n^\sigma} + \frac{\partial^\sigma I_{n, m, t}}{\partial m^\sigma} \right) \tag{2.4}$$

Eq. (2.4) produces diffused images, which are used in the proposed scheme to determine the Difference of Diffusion (DD) for border detection. DD may be determined using Eq. (2.5):

$$DD_{n,\,m,\,t} = D\left(I_{n,\,m,\,t}^{n+1} - I_{n,\,m,\,t}^{n}\right) \tag{2.5}$$

In the diffusion process, n and n + 1 are separate time stamps. By computing the difference between dispersed photos with various time stamps, a boundary is determined. The linear set of mesh-free radial foundation functions can be used to approximate the function $I_{n,\,m,\,t} = 0$ is used for boundary box detection as follows in Eq. (2.6) shown in Figure 2.7:

$$I_{n,\,m} = \sum_{K=1}^{N} \varnothing\left(r_K\right)\gamma \tag{2.6}$$

2.3.4 Comparison with Current SOTA Models

As a result, the proposed work on cell malaria parasite detection. The results of comparing the NASNetLarge-RF model proposed in this chapter with the most recent literature are shown in Table 2.3. Table 2.2 demonstrates that for the classification of brain tumors, the NASNetLarge-RF model has the greatest values for recall (98.72%), precision (98.21%), F1-score (99.01%), MSE (0.0012), and accuracy

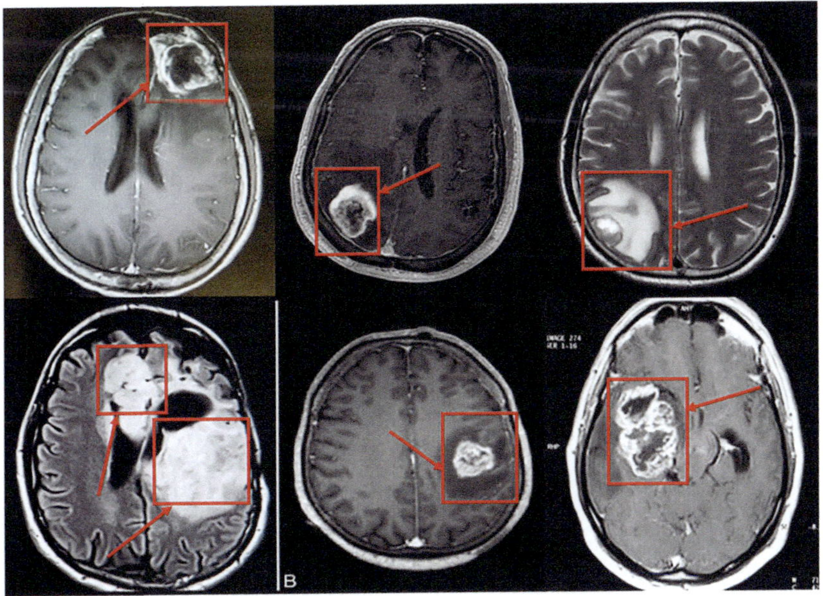

FIGURE 2.7 Boundary box detection of tumor in brain MRI image.

TABLE 2.3

Comparisons with Existing State-of-the-Model

S. No.	Methods	Accuracy	F1-score
1.	Sajjgad et al. (2019) [26]	90.67	92.10
2.	Mzoughi et al. (2020) [27]	96.49	–
3.	Siva Raja and Rani (2020) [28]	98.50	97.00
4.	Decuyper et al. (2021) [29]	90.00	91.62
5.	Isunuri and Kakarla (2022) [30]	97.52	97.26
6.	Khazaee et al. (2022) [31]	98.87	98.91
7.	Farajzadeh et al. (2023) [16]	98.81	98.81
8.	Wozniak et al. (2023) [17]	97.50	–
9.	NASNetLarge-RF (Proposed)	98.97	99.01

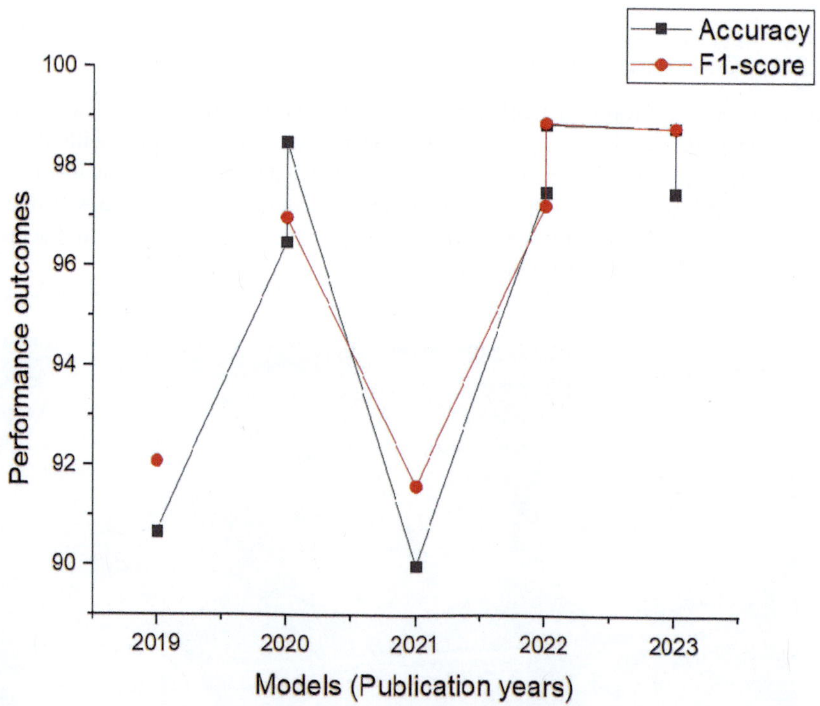

FIGURE 2.8 Comparison graph of the proposed model with current SOTA models.

(98.97%). Table 2.3 and Figure 2.8 display the experimental findings from the applications of ML algorithms using features to the analysis of medical data by Sajjgad et al. (2019) [26], Mzoughi et al. (2020) [27], Siva Raja and Rani (2020) [28], Decuyper et al. (2021) [29], Isunuri and Kakarla (2022) [30], Khazaee et al. (2022) [31], Farajzadeh et al. (2023) [16], and Wozniak et al. (2023) [17]. The accuracy is constrained by the difficulty in determining the effectiveness of the background, size, angle, and positions of key portions of an image. In addition to using the NASNetLarge advantages to extract deep features, a NASNetLarge-RF model also makes use of the RF advantages to resolve the nonlinearly separable issue. It appears in the brain tumor MRI image dataset's classification task. The combined model created by NASNetLarge-RF outperforms other models.

2.3.5 DISCUSSION

In Table 2.2, the experimental results from the brain tumor datasets are presented with a state-of-the-art comparison. Sajjgad et al. (2019) [26], Mzoughi et al. (2020) [27], Siva Raja and Rani (2020) [28], Decuyper et al. (2021) [29], Isunuri and Kakarla (2022) [30], Khazaee et al. (2022) [31], Farajzadeh et al. (2023) [16], and Wozniak et al. (2023) [17] have compared eight techniques with the proposed scheme shown in Figure 2.8, since all eight of these techniques are utilized for brain tumor MRI images. As demonstrated, the proposed system performs better than all existing models in terms of brain tumor classification.

- The qualitative analysis for performance with accuracy of 98.97%, precision of 98.21%, recall of 98.72%, F1-score of 99.01%, and MSE of 0.0012 on brain tumor MRI datasets demonstrates the greatest improvement. The proposed novel NASNetLarge-RF performs significantly better than the models proposed by Sajjgad et al. (2019), Mzoughi et al. (2020), Siva Raja and Rani (2020), Decuyper et al. (2021), Isunuri and Kakarla (2022), Khazaee et al. (2022), Farajzadeh et al. (2023), and Wozniak et al. (2023), in term of accuracy and F1-score on brain tumor medical image.
- The proposed scheme has the potential to reduce the significance of training time and increase performance because it uses the NASNet approach, which is often used to improve the performance of brain tumor classification.

Overall, the proposed scheme outperforms SOTA techniques and has comparatively minimal learning requirements.

2.4 CONCLUSION AND FUTURE WORK

The proposed NASNetLarge-RF scheme provided a scheme for segmenting polyps from colonoscopy images. The proposed NASNetLarge-encoder feature extraction is extracted from brain tumor MRI images. Furthermore, a NASNetLarge-decoder is used to handle scale variation during training and improve feature selection. Moreover, the Gaussian smoothing approach is used to detect boundary boxes of tumors. As a result, the NASNetLarge-RF learns additional specifics about the target area of tumors in the brain. In the future, different DL-based models will be tested on more medical-related tasks including secured feature detection in order to increase the effectiveness of medical image security.

REFERENCES

[1] Murmu A., Kumar P., (2023). A novel Gateaux derivatives with efficient DCNN-Resunet method for segmenting multi-class brain tumor. Medical & Biological Engineering & Computing, 1–24.

[2] Sung H., Ferlay J., Siegel R. L., Laversanne M., Soerjomataram I., Jemal A., Bray F., (2021). Global cancer statistics 2020: GLOBOCAN estimates of incidence and mortality worldwide for 36 cancers in 185 countries. CA: A Cancer Journal for Clinicians, 71(3), 209–249.

[3] Chahal P. K., Pandey S., Goel S., (2020). A survey on brain tumor detection techniques for MR images. Multimedia Tools and Applications, 79, 21771–21814.

[4] Rouse C., Gittleman H., Ostrom Q. T., Kruchko C., Barnholtz-Sloan J. S., (2016). Years of potential life lost for brain and CNS tumors relative to other cancers in adults in the United States. The Journal of Neuro-Oncology, 18(1), 70–77.

[5] NH Narayana Health, Health for all, All for health, NH CARES Brain Tumour, Types, Risk Factors, Symptoms, and Surgery. www.narayanahealth.org/brain-tumour

[6] Murmu A., Kumar P., (2021). Deep learning model-based segmentation of medical diseases from MRI and CT images. In TENCON 2021 IEEE Region 10 Conference, 608–613. IEEE.

[7] Deepak S., Ameer P. M., (2019). Brain tumor classification using deep CNN features via transfer learning. Computers in Biology and Medicine, 111, 103345.

[8] Mehnatkesh H., Jalali S. M. J., Khosravi A., Nahavandi S., (2023). An intelligent driven deep residual learning framework for brain tumor classification using MRI images. Expert Systems with Applications, 213, 119087.

[9] WHO, Cancer, (2023). www.who.int/health-topics/cancer

[10] Murmu A., Chanda C., Kumar P., (In Press). FedCNNAvg: Federated learning for preserving-privacy of multi-clients decentralized medical image classification. In International Conference on Data Science and Network Engineering (ICDSNE 2023), Springer, 21–22 July, 2023.

[11] Shaik N. S., Cherukuri T. K., (2022). Multi-level attention network: Application to brain tumor classification. Signal, Image and Video Processing, 16(3), 817–824.

[12] Zhang H., Meng Y., Zhao Y., Qiao Y., Yang X., Coupland S. E., Zheng Y., (2022). DTFD-MIL: Double-tier feature distillation multiple instance learning for histopathology whole slide image classification. In Proceedings of the IEEE/CVF Conference on Computer Vision and Pattern Recognition, IEEE Xplore, 18802–18812.

[13] Zeng Q., Xie Y., Lu Z., Xia Y., (2023). PEFAT: Boosting semi-supervised medical image classification via pseudo-loss estimation and feature adversarial training. In Proceedings of the IEEE/CVF Conference on Computer Vision and Pattern Recognition, IEEE Xplore, 15671–15680.

[14] Liu F., Tian Y., Chen Y., Liu Y., Belagiannis V., Carneiro G., (2022). ACPL: Anti-curriculum pseudo-labelling for semi-supervised medical image classification. In Proceedings of the IEEE/CVF Conference on Computer Vision and Pattern Recognition, IEEE Xplore, 20697–20706.

[15] Raghavendra U., Gudigar A., Paul A., Goutham T. S., Inamdar M. A., Hegde A., Acharya U. R., (2023). Brain tumor detection and screening using artificial intelligence techniques: Current trends and future perspectives. Computers in Biology and Medicine, 107063.

[16] Farajzadeh N., Sadeghzadeh N., Hashemzadeh M., (2023). Brain tumor segmentation and classification on MRI via deep hybrid representation learning. Expert Systems with Applications, 224, 119963.

[17] Woźniak M., Siłka J., Wieczorek M., (2023). Deep neural network correlation learning mechanism for CT brain tumor detection. Neural Computing & Applications, 35, 14611–14626.

[18] Messaoudi H., Belaid A., Salem D. B., Conze P. H., (2023). Cross-dimensional transfer learning in medical image segmentation with deep learning. Medical Image Analysis, 102868.

[19] Chen X., Wang X., Zhang K., Fung K. M., Thai T. C., Moore K., Qiu Y., (2022). Recent advances and clinical applications of deep learning in medical image analysis. Medical Image Analysis, 79, 102444.

[20] Tomar N., (2022). Brain Tumor Segmentation Dataset. www.kaggle.com/datasets/nikhilroxtomar/brain-tumor-segmentation. Accessed August 2023.

[21] Kumar P., Agrawal A., (2018). GPU-based focus-driven multi-coordinates viewing system for large volume data visualisation. International Journal of Computational Systems Engineering, 4(2–3), 86–95.

[22] Rahman M., Kumar P., (2022). 2D-CTM and DNA-based computing for medical image encryption. In International Conference on Frontiers of Intelligent Computing: Theory and Applications, Springer, 225–235.

[23] Li D., Ling H., Kim S. W., Kreis K., Fidler S., Torralba A., (2022). BigDatasetGAN: Synthesizing imagenet with pixel-wise annotations. In Proceedings of the IEEE/CVF Conference on Computer Vision and Pattern Recognition, IEEE Xplore, 21330–21340.

[24] Sangeetha M., Sugumaran V., Karthick T., Puli J., (2023). High performance cervical cancer detection using gradient boosting algorithm and Bayesian optimization. In 2023 9th International Conference on Information Technology Trends (ITT), 102–107. IEEE.

[25] Gao K., Sener O., (2022). Generalizing Gaussian smoothing for random search. In International Conference on Machine Learning, arXiv, 7077–7101.

[26] Sajjad M., Khan S., Muhammad K., Wu W., Ullah A., Baik S. W., (2019). Multi-grade brain tumor classification using deep CNN with extensive data augmentation. Journal of Computational Science, 30, 174–182.

[27] Mzoughi H., Njeh I., Wali A., Slima M. B., BenHamida A., Mhiri C., Mahfoudhe K. B., (2020). Deep multi-scale 3D convolutional neural network (CNN) for MRI gliomas brain tumor classification. Journal of Digital Imaging, 33, 903–915.

[28] Raja P. S., (2020). Brain tumor classification using a hybrid deep autoencoder with Bayesian fuzzy clustering-based segmentation approach. Biocybernetics and Biomedical Engineering, 40(1), 440–453.

[29] Decuyper M., Bonte S., Deblaere K., Van Holen R., (2021). Automated MRI based pipeline for segmentation and prediction of grade, IDH mutation and 1p19q co-deletion in glioma. Computerized Medical Imaging and Graphics, 88, 101831.

[30] Isunuri B. V., Kakarla J., (2022). Three-class brain tumor classification from magnetic resonance images using separable convolution based neural network. Concurrency and Computation: Practice and Experience, 34(1), e6541.

[31] Khazaee Z., Langarizadeh M., Ahmadabadi M. E. S., (2022). Developing an artificial intelligence model for tumor grading and classification, based on MRI sequences of human brain gliomas. International Journal of Cancer Management, 15(1).

3 Deep CNNs in Image-Guided Diagnosis of Breast and Skin Cancers

Kausik Basak and Rusha Patra

3.1 INTRODUCTION

Cancer, an insidious adversary that has plagued humanity for centuries, continues to cast a shadow over global health. Its relentless march has made it the leading cause of mortality worldwide, necessitating a relentless pursuit of innovative approaches to combat its devastating impact (Kratzer et al., 2023; Siegel et al., 2023; Giaquinto et al., 2022). As indicated by the American Cancer Society's report for 2019, an estimated 96,480 fatalities can be attributed to skin cancer, 142,670 to lung cancer, 42,260 to breast cancer, 31,620 to prostate cancer, and 17,760 to brain cancer (Cancer Facts and Figures, 2019). On a global scale, GLOBOCAN 2020 recorded approximately 19.3 million instances of cancer and 10 million cancer-related deaths. Within this comprehensive dataset, prevalent cancer types worldwide included breast cancer (2.26 million cases, accounting for 11.7%), lung cancer (2.21 million cases, constituting 11.4%), skin cancer (1.52 million cases, making up 7.9%), and different other variants (Chhikara and Parang, 2023). Amid this harrowing panorama, the clarion call for early cancer detection reverberates with urgency, a lifeline capable of saving countless lives.

Diverse imaging techniques play a crucial role in the early identification, diagnosis, and monitoring of breast and skin cancers. Mammography remains the gold standard for breast cancer (Pauwels et al., 2016), with digital mammography providing clearer, customizable images (Pisano, 2005). Ultrasound aids in real-time differentiation of solid masses and cysts (Dencks et al., 2018). Magnetic Resonance Imaging (MRI) is invaluable for assessing breast cancer extent in high-risk patients, offering detailed 3D images (Lehman and Schnall, 2005). On the other hand, Dermoscopy (Massone et al., 2005), Reflectance Confocal Microscopy (Guida et al., 2021), and Optical Coherence Tomography (OCT) (Levine et al., 2017) are pivotal in skin cancer imaging. Multispectral imaging analyses skin lesions comprehensively (Ilişanu et al., 2023). Together, these modalities enhance early detection, precise diagnosis, and effective management, improving patient outcomes.

DOI: 10.1201/9781032635149-3

The dawn of the 1980s ushered in a transformative era with the introduction of computer-aided diagnosis systems, designed to synergize human expertise with technological acumen. The crux of these systems lies in the extraction of pertinent features from medical images, enabling the application of machine learning (ML) principles to the diagnostic process. While conventional diagnostic approaches have achieved substantial success, the incorporation of artificial intelligence (AI) and deep learning (DL) techniques has unlocked a new dimension of diagnostic precision. Harnessing the capacity to autonomously acquire hierarchical features from raw data, deep convolutional neural networks (CNNs) have exhibited extraordinary efficacy in detecting and categorizing cancerous lesions. However, it's important to note that these AI systems should be used as adjuncts to human expertise, as they are tools that enhance diagnostic capabilities. This chapter thoroughly examines the application of deep CNNs in diagnosing breast and skin cancers through image analysis. It delves into the architecture and operational principles of deep CNNs. Topics include the vital role of deep CNNs in breast and skin cancer diagnosis. It explores multimodal strategies and interpretability enhancements to boost diagnostic precision. Despite progress, challenges remain in acquiring diverse datasets, interpreting CNN-generated decisions, and addressing biases. This chapter also addresses these challenges, providing insights into ongoing efforts and future prospects.

3.2   FUNDAMENTALS OF DEEP CNN

Deep CNNs constitute a fundamental pillar in the landscape of modern ML, particularly in the realm of medical image analysis. The efficacy of traditional algorithms often hinges on the quality of input data representation. Various studies have demonstrated that a skilfully constructed data representation substantially boosts performance (Rana and Bhushan, 2022; Barragán-Montero et al., 2021). Consequently, a central focus in ML research for years has been feature engineering, involving the construction of relevant features from raw data. However, this approach demands substantial human involvement. In contrast, deep CNN algorithms automate feature extraction as shown in Figure 3.1, encouraging the creation of discriminative features with minimal human intervention (Wang et al., 2021). At the heart of their effectiveness is their aptitude to autonomously derive and extract intricate features from raw pixel data using a sequence of convolutional, pooling, and activation layers. Its initial layers extract low-level features while subsequent layers capture higher-level abstractions (Yu et al., 2016). This depth allows progressive learning, making them ideal for various tasks. Illustrated in Figure 3.2, a generalized layered architecture of a deep CNN is presented next.

3.2.1   INPUT LAYER

The input layer takes the image data as a matrix of pixel values, where each pixel's intensity or colour information is represented as an input feature. For a grayscale image, the input can be described as, $I \in \mathbb{R}^{R \times C}$, where C is the width of the image, and R is the height.

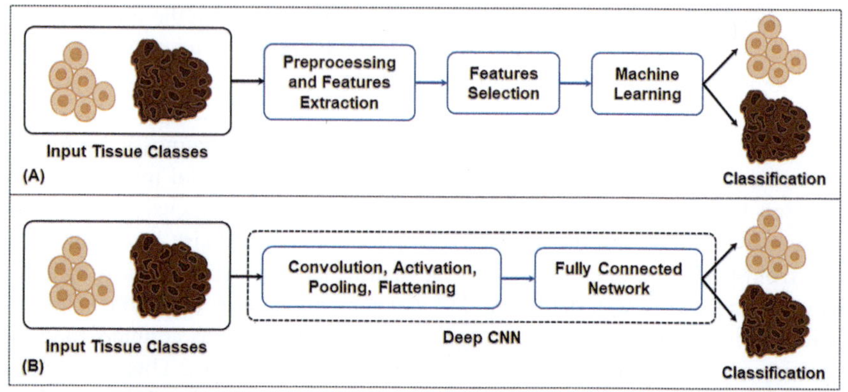

FIGURE 3.1 Distinguishing between (a) traditional ML and (b) deep CNN frameworks.

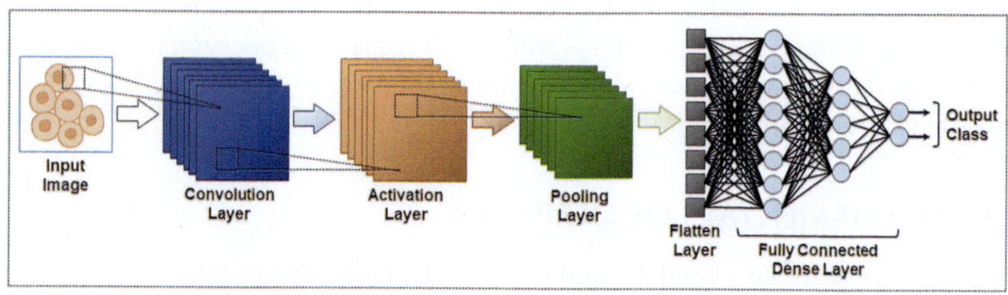

FIGURE 3.2 A generalized layered architecture of a CNN model for image classification.

3.2.2 Convolutional Layers

These layers utilize a collection of adaptable filters, or kernels, that convolve or slide over the input image. A kernel is characterized as a grid of discrete values, with each value designated as a kernel weight. Initial random assignment of weights is a precursor to CNN training. Throughout training, these weights undergo adjustments in each epoch, enabling the kernel to progressively learn to extract features. Multiple filters in each layer can extract diverse features, making convolutional layers adept at understanding the nuances of complex images. Given an input feature map X and a filter (kernel) K, the output feature map Y can be derived as:

$$Y[i,j] = \sum_m \sum_n X[i+m, j+n] \cdot K[m,n]$$

(3.1)

Convolutional layers offer key advantages stemming from two facets: (A) sparse connectivity – this translates to a limited array of weights between neighbouring layers, resulting in diminished connection and memory requirements, and (B) weight sharing – in CNNs, a singular set of weights operates across the entire input matrix, spanning all pixels. This sharing of weights markedly diminishes training time and related expenses. The absence of a need to learn specific weights for each neuron contributes to a more streamlined and proficient learning process.

3.2.3 ACTIVATION FUNCTIONS

The fundamental role of activation functions is to establish a mapping from the input to the output. It determines whether a neuron fires or remains inactive based on the weighted sum of inputs. An essential characteristic of the activation function is its differentiability, enabling the utilization of error back-propagation for network training. The activation functions commonly employed in CNNs and other deep neural networks are as follows:

ReLU: The most frequently employed function within the CNN context is rectified linear unit (ReLU). It introduces non-linearity, allowing the network to model intricate relationships within the data. The ReLU activation function is given by:

$$f(x)_{ReLU} = max(0, x) \tag{3.2}$$

Certain challenges can arise when employing ReLU. For instance, contemplate an error back-propagation algorithm where a substantial gradient courses through. When this gradient interacts with the ReLU function, weight updates could render a neuron perpetually inactive, resulting in "Dying ReLU." To address this, alternative forms of ReLU were developed.

Leaky ReLU: In contrast to ReLU, which scales down negative inputs, this activation function prevents the neglect of such inputs altogether. Mathematically, it can be expressed as:

$$f(x)_{LeakyReLU} = \begin{cases} x, & if \ x > 0 \\ mx, & x \leq 0 \end{cases} \tag{3.3}$$

In general, the leak factor m is set to a very small value, for example, 0.001.

Noisy ReLU: This introduces noise by utilizing a Gaussian distribution, allowing noisy ReLU to retain some properties of ReLU, such as addressing the vanishing gradient problem, while injecting stochasticity that can aid in optimization and prevent neurons from becoming entirely dormant. Noisy ReLU can be defined as:

$$f(x)_{NoisyReLU} = max(x + Y) \text{ with } Y \sim N(0, \sigma(x)) \tag{3.4}$$

3.2.4 POOLING LAYERS

These layers conduct down-sampling, diminishing the spatial dimensions of feature maps while preserving critical information. Commonly employed methods encompass max pooling, min pooling, and global average pooling. Max pooling, for instance, involves selecting maximum value within a pooling window, where s is the stride and f is the pooling window size.

$$Y[i,j] = max\left(X\left[(i\cdot s):(i\cdot s+f),(j\cdot s):(j\cdot s+f)\right]\right) \tag{3.5}$$

3.2.5 FLATTENING

Before feeding the data into the fully connected layers, a flattening step transforms the multidimensional feature maps into a one-dimensional vector. This can be defined as:

$$X_{flat} = flatten(X) \tag{3.6}$$

3.2.6 FULLY CONNECTED (DENSE) LAYER

This integrates the features learned in the previous layers and contributes to the final decision-making process. Given an input vector X, a fully connected layer's output Y is computed as:

$$Y = W\cdot X + b \tag{3.7}$$

where W is the weight matrix and b is the bias vector.

3.2.7 OUTPUT LAYER

The output layer generates predictions depending on the features extracted. In classification tasks, the final scores of the network are usually transformed into probabilities using the softmax function, signifying the probabilities of the input belonging to various classes. With C classes, the softmax activation function converts raw scores Z into class probabilities P:

$$P_j = \frac{e^{Z_j}}{\sum_{k=1}^{C} e^{Z_k}} \tag{3.8}$$

3.2.8 LOSS FUNCTIONS

To quantify the error incurred across training samples, specific loss functions are employed in the output layer. These functions gauge the disparity between the anticipated output and the projected outcome. Diverse loss functions are tailored to address various problem categories, some of which are elucidated next.

Euclidean Loss: Also known as mean square error, it encapsulates the essence of the squared differences between these values. Mathematically, this can be expressed as:

$$\text{Euclidean Loss} = \frac{1}{N}\sum_{i=1}^{N}(y_i - \hat{y}_i)^2 \tag{3.9}$$

where N represents the total number of data points, y_i is the actual value of the i-th data point, $\hat{y}_i$ denotes the predicted value by the model for the i-th data point. This loss function is well-suited for problems where the aim is to minimize the average squared differences.

Cross-Entropy Loss: Alternatively known as the softmax loss, it emphasizes on minimizing the negative log-likelihood of true class probabilities and imparts a robust mechanism for training models in classification tasks. This can be defined as:

$$\text{Cross} - \text{Entropy Loss} = -\frac{1}{N}\sum_{i=1}^{N}\sum_{j=1}^{C} y_{ij}\, \log(\hat{y}_{ij}) \tag{3.10}$$

where N is the total number of data points, C is the total number of classes, y_{ij} represents the binary indicator (0 or 1) if the i-th data point belongs to class j. $\hat{y}_{ij}$ denotes predicted probability by the model for the i-th data point being in class j.

Hinge Loss: This is often utilized with support vector machines, effective in establishing decision boundaries that maximize the separation between classes. This can be defined as:

$$\text{Hinge Loss} = \frac{1}{N}\sum_{i=1}^{N} max\left(0, 1 - y_i \cdot \hat{y}_i\right) \tag{3.11}$$

where y_i denotes actual class label of i-th data point, with values of -1 for the negative class and +1 for the positive class, and $\hat{y}_i$ represents the predicted class score. The core essence of the hinge loss lies in its "hinge" shape, which penalizes misclassifications.

3.2.9 REGULARIZATIONS

Deep CNNs exhibit overfitting issues—although the network excels in training data, struggles to generalize effectively novel, unseen data. Hence, regularizations are essential in mitigating overfitting and improving generalization ability. Here, we delve into different regularization techniques (Moradi et al., 2020). "L2 regularization" adds a penalty term to the loss function, proportional to the squared magnitude of weights. It discourages overly large weights and prevents the network from relying heavily on specific features. "L1 regularization" adds a penalty term to the loss function based on absolute magnitude of weights, encouraging sparsity in the network by driving some weights to zero. However, in "dropout," a randomly selected subset of neurons is dropped out with a certain probability. This prevents co-adaptation of neurons and creates an ensemble of smaller networks, improving generalization. "Data augmentation" involves artificially expanding the training dataset by applying various transformations to the original images, such as rotation, scaling, cropping, and flipping. Besides, "batch normalization" normalizes the inputs of each layer within a batch, reducing internal covariate shift and accelerating training. "DropConnect" randomly sets a fraction of connections in the weight matrix to zero during training. Applying any of these regularizations can significantly enhance the generalization, enabling them to perform well on unseen data.

3.2.10 Optimizations

Optimizing deep CNNs involves a range of techniques and strategies aimed at improving training speed, convergence, and generalization (Cong and Zhou, 2023). Let's delve into some of the most used optimization methods.

Stochastic Gradient Descent (SGD): SGD functions through iterative updates of the model's parameters, guided by gradients computed from the loss function over randomly selected mini-batches of training data. The weight update equation for SGD can be expressed as:

$$\theta_{t+1} = \theta_t - \alpha \cdot \nabla J\left(\theta_t, X_{batch}, y_{batch}\right) \tag{3.12}$$

where θ_t represents parameter vector at iteration t, α is the learning rate. $J(\theta_t, X_{batch}, Y_{batch})$ denotes the loss function computed on the input data X_{batch} with corresponding labels y_{batch}, and $\nabla J(\theta_t, X_{batch}, Y_{batch})$ represents the gradient of the loss with respect to the parameters.

Root Mean Square Propagation (RMSProp): It is built upon the SGD approach by introducing an adaptive learning rate. RMSProp adjusts the learning rate for each parameter based on the historical magnitudes of its gradients. The weight update equation can be expressed as:

$$\theta_{t+1} = \theta_t - \frac{\alpha}{\sqrt{E\left[g^2\right]_t + \epsilon}} \cdot g_t \tag{3.13}$$

where θ_t represents the parameter vector at iteration t, α is the learning rate, g_t is the gradient of the loss function with respect to the parameters at iteration t. $E[g^2]_t$ is the exponentially weighted moving average of the squared gradients up to iteration t, and a small constant θ is added to prevent division by zero.

Adaptive Gradient Descent (AdaGrad): AdaGrad enhances the standard SGD approach by adapting the learning rate for each parameter depending on the historical gradient information. The learning rate is adjusted to account for the magnitude of past gradients, allowing it to converge faster along directions with small gradients and slower along directions with large gradients. The weight update equation for AdaGrad can be expressed as:

$$\theta_{t+1} = \theta_t - \frac{\alpha}{\sqrt{G_t + \epsilon}} \cdot g_t \tag{3.14}$$

where G_t denotes the cumulative sum of squared gradients up to iteration t. However, the learning rate can become too small as G_t accumulates over time, causing slow convergence. This limitation led to the development of variants such as RMSProp.

Adaptive Moment Estimation (Adam): This popular optimization algorithm integrates the benefits of both Momentum and RMSProp by maintaining a running average of both gradients and squared gradients. This adaptive learning rate approach accelerates convergence and enhances the optimization process. The update rule for the weights can be written as:

$$\omega_t = \omega_{t-1} - \alpha m_t / \left(\sqrt{v_t} + \varepsilon \right) \tag{3.15}$$

where ω_t is the weights at time t, α is the learning rate, m_t and v_t are the first and second moments of the gradients, and θ is a small constant. The moments were computed as:

$$m_t = \beta_1 m_{t-1} + \left(1 - \beta_1 \right) g_t \tag{3.16}$$

$$v_t = \beta_2 v_{t-1} + \left(1 - \beta_2 \right) g_t^2 \tag{3.17}$$

where, g_t is the gradient at time t, and β_1 and β_2 are decay rates for the first and second moments, respectively. The general flow of a deep CNN involves stacking convolutional layers, activation functions, pooling layers, and optionally, fully connected layers, leading to the final output layer. This hierarchical architecture, characterized by its convolutional and pooling layers, enables deep CNNs to progressively capture intricate features in images. Variations of this architecture, such as different convolution and pooling layers, skip connections, and residual blocks, contribute to the adaptability and robustness of deep CNNs.

3.3 BREAST CANCER DIAGNOSIS USING DEEP CNNS

Breast cancer stands as the most prevalent and significant contributor to cancer-related fatalities in the female population (Bray et al., 2018). The World Health Organization (WHO) reports an annual incidence of breast cancer affecting 2.1 million women. Conventionally, breast tissue can be categorized into four distinct groups: healthy, benign tumour, carcinoma *in-situ*, and invasive carcinoma. Benign tumours exhibit minor structural variations in the tissue, usually posing minimal harm; however, there exists a potential for conversion to carcinoma. Carcinoma *in-situ* manifests as malignant tissue confined within the mammary gland lobules and ducts. In contrast, invasive carcinoma represents a malignant tumour with the capability to infiltrate surrounding organs. Research underscores that early-stage breast cancer detection translates to successful curative interventions, emphasizing the pivotal role of timely identification and diagnosis in effective breast cancer management.

Various medical probing modalities, viz. X-ray mammography (Moghbel et al., 2020), ultrasound (Kozegar et al., 2020), computed tomography (CT), MRI (Murtaza et al., 2020), and positron emission tomography (PET) (Domingues et al., 2020), are employed for breast cancer detection. X-ray mammography excels in early breast mass and calcification detection, relying on high-contrast local regions. However, uniformity varies with imaging conditions, mass size, and tissue characteristics, contributing to false positives. Histopathological analysis, an alternative gold standard, relies on subjective interpretation, causing time-consuming assessments and inter-observer variability due to diverse tissue structures and disease progression stages. This underscores the importance of automated image analysis systems, capable of mitigating the reliance on radiologist domain knowledge and reducing time constraints. In this context, the progress of DL has significantly improved breast cancer diagnosis. Deep CNNs now go beyond distinguishing benign and malignant tumors, engaging in multiclass classification for tumour grading. Leveraging the inherent feature extraction of deep CNNs proves more efficient than relying on manually designed features. However, training deep CNNs requires a substantial quantity of images.

3.3.1 RELATED DATABASES

Among several image datasets available for breast tissue classification, IDC dataset includes 162 images of invasive ductal carcinoma (IDC) at 400x magnification, generating 277,524 patches (50 × 50 pixels). Images are categorized into positive and negative IDC cases. BreakHis dataset comprises 7909 histopathological images of breast tumour tissue at 40x, 100x, 200x, and 400x magnifications. It includes 2480 benign and 5429 malignant samples sized 700 × 460 pixels. Besides, BACH dataset is designed for the ICIAR 2018 Grand Challenge, featuring 400 microscopic images categorized as normal, benign, *in-situ* carcinoma, and invasive carcinoma along with 30 higher-resolution whole slide images. And, BCDR dataset compiles 1010 film mammography and 724 digital mammography images annotated by radiologists. These datasets play a pivotal role in learning and validating deep CNNs. Researchers can leverage these datasets to train and assess their developed models effectively.

3.3.2 IMAGE ACQUISITION AND PRE-PROCESSING

Image pre-processing is essential in both histopathological and mammogram image analyses, involving noise and artefact removal, resizing for uniform dimensions, normalization, histogram equalization for contrast improvement, and, often, colour deconvolution for stained histopathological images. This process disentangles illumination effects and is crucial for disease progression grading. Figures 3.3 and 3.4 illustrate fundamental block diagrams for mammogram and histopathological image analysis, with explanations provided in subsequent sections.

3.3.3 IMAGE ANALYSIS

Region of Interest (ROI) Segmentation. The image is partitioned into smaller, overlapping patches that are then fed into a CNN equipped with multiple

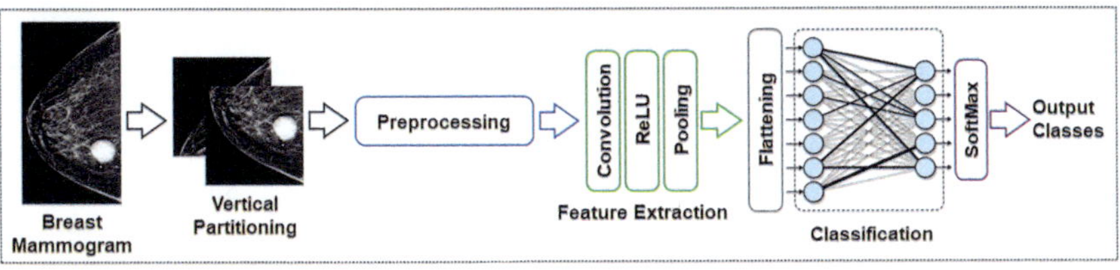

FIGURE 3.3 Block diagram of mammogram image analysis.

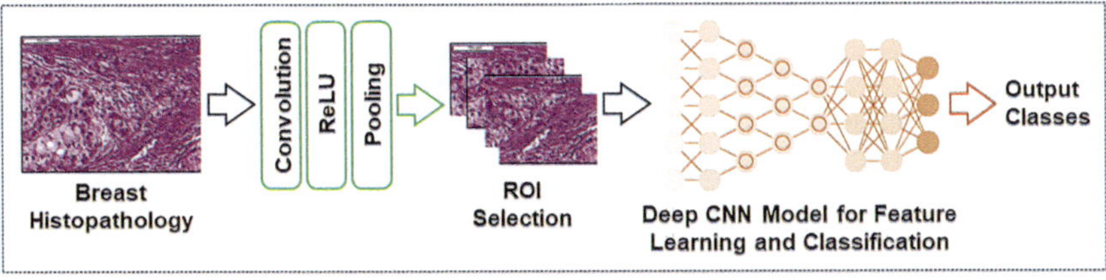

FIGURE 3.4 Block diagram of histopathological image analysis.

convolution and pooling layers, followed by fully connected and softmax layers. This configuration allows classification into two classes, namely ROI and non-ROI (Xu et al., 2016). Unlike handcrafted features such as colour, texture, or local binary patterns, the deep CNN presents an end-to-end solution that directly learns patterns from the raw image's pixel intensities.

Nucleus Segmentation: The deep CNN is trained to generate a probability map, and an iterative region merging algorithm initializes the shape. A selection-based dictionary learning creates a shape dictionary that informs the final segmentation (Xing et al., 2015). Another strategy focuses on reducing background information via sparse representation, followed by the use of a deep CNN cascade to segment the nucleus. Subsequently, morphological processes are applied to enhance segmentation (Pan et al., 2017).

Cancer Grading: Detecting mitosis is pivotal for cancer prognosis and provides valuable diagnostic details for breast cancer grading. Utilizing a deep CNN, the model extracts intrinsic feature maps using an array of filter kernels. These extracted feature maps, combined with manually engineered features, are fed into the fully connected layers to differentiate between mitotic and non-mitotic instances. This approach holds the potential to offer a more profound understanding of breast cancer grading (Saha et al., 2018).

Transfer Learning: In transfer learning, a network is initially trained for one task and then repurposed for another. Two primary strategies exist for transfer learning. The first method involves fine-tuning all the trainable parameters to align with the demands of the new task. The second approach utilizes the pre-trained network as a feature extractor, employing the extracted features to train a new classifier. Notably, architectures like VGG16, VGG19, and ResNet50 are widely employed due to their comprehensive architecture.

Computer-Aided Detection Systems: Extracted features can originate from either manual curation or automated extraction. Manual curation involves applying diverse image processing algorithms, whereas automated features are obtained using deep CNN models. Following feature extraction, they are input into classifiers. Guided by annotations, images are categorized into two or more distinct classes. In specific instances, images are divided into smaller patches and processed individually, rather than considering the entire image as a cohesive entity.

3.3.4 MULTIMODAL APPROACHES AND FUSION TECHNIQUES

Although X-ray mammography emerges as a prominent probing technique, its susceptibility to producing high false positive rates results in unnecessary biopsy interventions. To mitigate this issue, the fusion of various imaging modalities is explored. Full-field digital mammography, ultrasound, and dynamic contrast-enhanced magnetic resonance imaging are harnessed to characterize breast lesions (Antropova et al., 2017). A pre-trained VGG19 network serves for feature extraction. Pooled features from each max-pool layer are combined to characterize lesions using a support vector machine. In another way, ultrasound elastography and B-mode ultrasound are combined to assess lesions based on tissue stiffness and other properties (Adel et al., 2019). Features are extracted from B-mode ultrasound using pre-trained deep CNNs. The elastography image is used to compute the region of the lowest strain. Besides, thermography resurfaces with the integration of ML and computer-aided diagnosis (Allugunti, 2022). It detects physiological tissue changes due to angiogenesis and vasodilation. Distinguishing the causes of tissue heating poses challenges, leading to low sensitivity. The training of deep CNNs with thermography images enhances early breast lesion detection due to physiological changes occurring at the disease's onset. The utilization of deep CNNs alongside emerging or fusion imaging modalities promises to revolutionize breast cancer diagnosis and prognosis.

3.4 SKIN CANCER DIAGNOSIS WITH DEEP CNNS

Skin, a multi-layered protective barrier, sustains body homeostasis. Monitoring disruptions, acute or chronic, reveals disease dynamics for tailored treatments. Studying the progressive changes in tissue morphology and functionality aids in refining treatment approaches (Gefen, 2009). As per reports, skin cancer has affected over 3 million people globally, with nearly 1.5 million cases of melanoma skin cancer recorded in 2020 alone, displaying a compound annual growth rate of 14% (Skin Cancer Statistics, 2022). This global concern is prevalent in around 30% of infants and adolescents, particularly in low- and middle-income countries' rural and urban slum areas (Ahmed et al., 2013). The lack of awareness regarding these conditions and a limited understanding of the disease are emerging as pressing public health issues. In general, dermatologists employ invasive methods for comprehensive disease biology studies, involving tissue biopsy and histological examination. While insightful, it's invasive, time-intensive, and can cause psychological distress, impeding healing. The delayed clinical reporting exacerbates the situation, depriving patients of timely care, particularly in rural areas, impacting overall well-being and social dynamics (Hay et al., 2006; Joseph et al., 2014). In this context, AI, particularly deep CNNs, has revolutionized skin disease diagnosis by excelling in analysing dermatological images. Their multiple layers enable automatic feature extraction at different levels, discriminating between benign and malignant lesions. The success lies in their ability to adapt to diverse conditions and provide rapid, reliable preliminary assessments, reducing the need for invasive biopsies. Integrated into mobile apps, they empower individuals for early detection and prompt medical attention.

3.4.1 RELATED DATABASES

Among various standard databases, the ISIC (International Skin Imaging Collaboration) database encompasses an extensive repository of high-quality dermoscopic images, curated and annotated by dermatologists. It covers a wide range of skin types, ethnicities, ages, and regions, making it a valuable resource for understanding the global variation in skin lesions. On the other hand, HAM10000 database contains a substantial collection of dermascopic images, encompassing a wide variety of skin lesions, including melanoma, nevi (moles), and seborrheic keratosis. PH^2 database offers images of common pigmented lesions, including melanoma and nevi. The SD-198 dataset comprises dermoscopic images of melanoma, nevi, and basal cell carcinoma. And DermQuest provides an extensive collection of clinical images for various dermatological conditions, including skin cancers. Nevertheless, while these databases offer valuable material, it's crucial to ensure data quality, diversity, and annotations to bolster the trustworthiness and applicability of the resulting models. These databases continue to evolve, offering an ever-growing resource to combat this prevalent disease.

3.4.2 DERMOSCOPY IMAGE ANALYSIS

Dermoscopy involves examining the skin using a specialized magnifying tool that reveals detailed patterns and structures not visible to the naked eye (Campos-do-Carmo and Ramos-e-Silva, 2008). Deep CNNs have revolutionized the interpretation of dermoscopic images, enabling automated and accurate detection, classification, and segmentation of various skin lesions. A generalized architecture, describing the key aspects of dermoscopy image analysis, is given in Figure 3.5 and illustrated next.

Data Acquisition and Preprocessing: Initially, these images undergo various transformations to standardize the data. Techniques such as resizing images to a consistent dimension, normalizing pixel values to a common range, and applying data augmentation to generate variations of the images (Vocaturo et al., 2018). For example, normalization is often done by:

$$X_{normalized} = \frac{X - \mu}{\sigma} \tag{3.18}$$

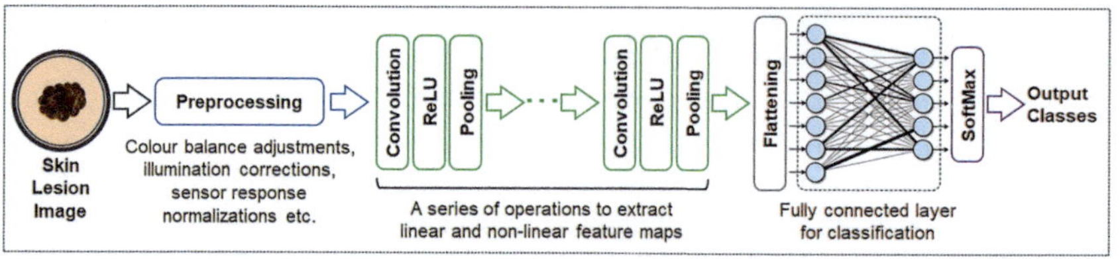

FIGURE 3.5 A generalized architecture of dermoscopy image analysis using deep CNN.

where $X_{normalized}$ is the normalized image, X is the original image, μ is the mean of pixel values, and σ is the standard deviation of pixel values. Normalization is crucial for mitigating discrepancies in illumination, camera systems, and skin lesion counts. Image processing algorithms, including colour balance adjustments and sensor response normalizations, address diversities. Compensation for skin colour variation is vital to prevent misclassification errors when distinguishing between normal and abnormal conditions.

Feature Extraction: In deep CNNs convolution layers act as specialized filters that slide over the input image, detecting patterns like edges, textures, and shapes. The hierarchical learning process enables deep CNN to capture the unique dermoscopic criteria associated with different lesions (Gajera et al., 2023). The output feature map F is computed by:

$$F(i,j) = \sum_m \sum_n X(i-m, j-n) \cdot W(m, n) \tag{3.19}$$

where $X(i, j)$ is the input image pixel, and $W(m, n)$ is the filter weight. Following this, element-wise activation functions like ReLU introduce non-linearity, capturing complex data relationships. Pooling layers, such as max pooling, decrease spatial dimensions while retaining vital information, introducing translational invariance (details in Section 3.1). Deep CNNs train on labelled datasets, refining weights and filters to minimize the gap between predicted and actual labels. Through iterative optimization, the network learns distinguishing features, achieving high accuracy and contributing to dermatology advancement (Gajera et al., 2023).

Segmentation and Boundary Detection: These processes enable the accurate identification of ROI within dermoscopic images and the precise delineation of lesion boundaries. Among numerous segmentation procedures, semantic segmentation pertains to categorizing individual pixels within an image into predefined classes. Deep CNNs can be trained to perform semantic segmentation by utilizing a fully convolutional architecture, where the final output is a pixel-wise classification map (Thanh et al., 2021). A segmentation map S is generated using:

$$S(i,j) = CNN(X(i,j)) \tag{3.20}$$

where $S(i,j)$ represents the pixel-wise segmentation output for the pixel at location (i,j) in the image X, and CNN is the trained convolutional neural network. Besides, boundary detection is concerned with accurately outlining the boundaries of skin lesions. To achieve this, instance segmentation is employed, generating a binary mask that outlines the lesion's boundary. The network's output for boundary detection (B) can be expressed as:

$$B(i,j) = CNN\left(X(i,j)\right)$$

(3.21)

where, $S(i,j)$ represents the pixel-wise boundary detection output for the pixel at location (i,j) in the image X. When training a deep CNN for semantic segmentation, an appropriate loss function is employed to assess the concordance between the predicted segmentation map and the ground truth. Dice coefficient and Jaccard index are common choices for such tasks (Thanh et al., 2021). The Dice coefficient is given by:

$$Dice = \frac{2 \cdot |A \cap B|}{|A| + |B|}$$

(3.22)

where A is the predicted segmentation mask and B is the ground truth mask.

Classification of Benign and Malignant Skin Lesions: A deep CNN classifies data by learning intricate features from input images, processed through convolutional and pooling layers. After traversing these layers, the feature maps are reshaped into a vector and input into fully connected layers, facilitating linear transformations and intricate feature amalgamations. The final output layer generates probabilities for distinct categories, with the softmax activation converting raw scores into a probabilistic distribution (details in Section 3.1). The synaptic weights are adjusted using backpropagation algorithm (Rojas, 1996). Subsequently, these weights are updated using an optimizer, aligning with the direction that minimizes the loss. The algorithm can be represented as:

Output error: $\qquad \delta_o = \left(y_{true} - y_o\right)f'\left(s_o\right)$ (3.23)

Backward pass: $\qquad \delta_j = f'\left(s_o\right)\sum_{k=1}^{p} w_{kj}\delta_k$ (3.24)

where δ_o is the output error, δ_j is the error of neurons at layer j, $f'\left(s_o\right)$ stands for the derivative of activation function, and p represents the number of output layer neurons. w_{ij} represents the weight of the connection between neurons at layers i and j. Among the notable optimization algorithms discussed in Section 3.2.10, ADAM stands out as a commonly employed choice. In SGD, batches of random samples are used to seek minimal values iteratively until convergence, often requiring more epochs. AdaGrad dynamically adjusts learning rates, but its adaptations can be aggressive, potentially affecting model precision. RMSPROP penalizes features for misclassification. ADAM, countering RMSPROP limitations, uses exponentially weighted gradient averages for efficient training, considering both first- and second-gradient moments.

3.4.3 RELATED WORKS

The integration of AI-based algorithms for automated inference of skin pathologies has propelled significant advancements. Masood et al. (2015) introduced a self-advised semi-supervised learning system for melanoma detection. It integrated deep belief networks with two SA-SVMs, trained using distinct datasets and kernels. Demyanov et al. (2016) employed stochastic gradient descent to train a CNN model for detecting network and globule patterns. Yu et al. (2016) introduced a fully convolutional residual network by integrating residual blocks into FCN's convolutional layers for classification. Later, a CNN was employed for melanoma detection, yielding sensitivity and specificity rates of 0.81 and 0.80, respectively. Moreover, Pomponiu et al. (2016) utilized 399 images captured using a standard camera to discern between benign nevi and melanoma. Their approach encircled extraction of high-level attributes from skin samples using pre-trained CNN and AlexNet models. The classification of lesions was carried out using the K-nearest neighbour algorithm. Remarkably, their findings demonstrated an accuracy of 93.62%. Building on this, researchers developed a CNN-based approach for skin tumor detection, training the model on 129,450 clinical images and benchmarking it against assessments by 21 dermatologists (Esteva et al., 2017). The attained AUC for melanomas and carcinomas stood at 0.96. The domain's complexity was addressed by Han et al. (2018), who employed Microsoft ResNet-152 to identify skin conditions, including basal cell carcinoma, squamous cell carcinoma, intraepithelial carcinoma, and melanoma.

The ISIC 2016 challenge dataset was employed to classify lesions using a CNN model and ANN (Rehman et al., 2018). They initiated the process with image segmentation via intensity thresholding, followed by CNN for feature extraction. Remarkably, they achieved an accuracy of 98.32%. A SkinNet CNN was employed for skin cancer segmentation and detection (Vesal et al., 2018). They introduced a modified U-net CNN variant. Their achievements included an average dice coefficient of 85.10% and a Jaccard index of 76.67% when implemented on the 2017 ISBI challenge dataset. The subsequent year, Fujisawa et al. (2019) introduced a deep CNN to categorize skin cancer as benign or malignant, utilizing 4867 clinically acquired images from 1842 patients. Comparative assessments against 13 dermatologists revealed the model's high sensitivity (96.3%) and specificity (89.5%). Walker et al. (2019) employed DL for skin lesion diagnosis in laboratory retrospective study (LABS) (482 biopsies) and observational study (OBS) (63 biopsies). The model, trained on 3954 data, utilized sonification, achieving ROCs of 0.976 (LABS) and 0.819 (OBS). In India, diverse demographic and environmental factors influence skin diseases. Challenges include the absence of a comprehensive database and limited access to dermatologists in remote areas. Pangti et al. (2021) addressed these gaps by integrating a deep learning algorithm with a mobile app to characterize 40 skin conditions using clinical images from the Indian population.

However, the approach lacked consideration for patients' medical histories and overlooked demographic factors influencing treatment. Bridging these gaps is crucial for effective AI-driven dermatological diagnosis in India, considering local nuances.

3.4.4 Computer-Aided Diagnosis of Skin Conditions—A Case Study

In our previous work, we developed a computational model based on deep CNN with the aim of characterizing various skin abnormalities (Sheet et al., 2019; Agrawal et al., 2016). The algorithm's training and validation involved the utilization of the ISIC database, as depicted in Figure 3.6. This database encompasses a diverse array of skin disorders, including Lentigo, Keratosis, Scar, Nevus, Basal Cell Carcinoma, and Melanoma, among others. A schematic diagram of the computational model is depicted in Figure 3.7. A series of preprocessing techniques were systematically applied. These techniques were instrumental in rectifying issues related to intensity variations, brightness disparities, and adjustments of skin colour. By addressing these concerns, the images were suitably formatted for subsequent analysis. Roughly 80% of these processed images were allocated for training. Remaining 20% were set aside for algorithmic testing, enabling a thorough evaluation of the model's performance and precision.

Within the architecture, distinct kernels such as convolution, max pooling, and ReLU were effectively deployed to encapsulate inherent attributes in images. In

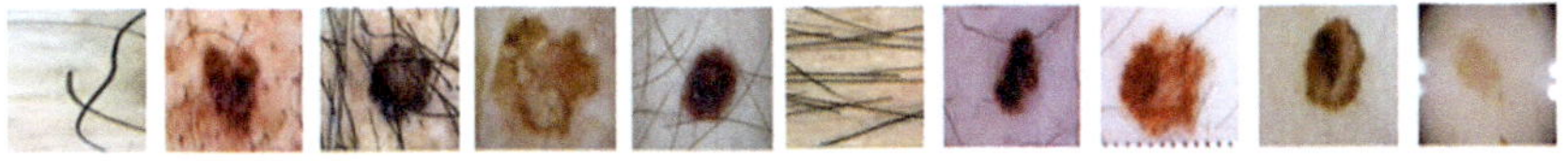

FIGURE 3.6 Sample images (from ISIC database) on which the DL framework was trained.

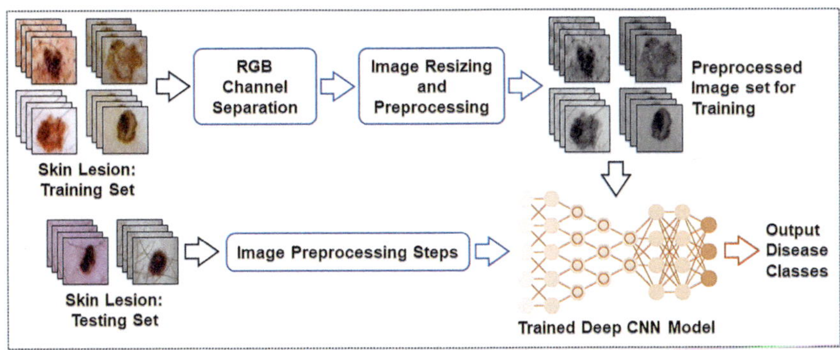

FIGURE 3.7 Process schematic of the deep CNN-based model.

TABLE 3.1

Classification Levels of Various Dermatoses (based on ISIC database)

		Normal Skin				
Abnormal skin	Cosmetic abnormality	Lentigo	Level 3A			
		Keratosis				
		Scar				
	Tumour	Benign	Level 3B	Firm Type	Level 4A	
				Nevus		
				Fibroma		
				Angioma		
		Malignant		Basal cell carcinoma	Level 4B	
				Melanoma		
				Squamous cell carcinoma		
Level 1	**Level 2**	**Level 3**		**Level 4**		

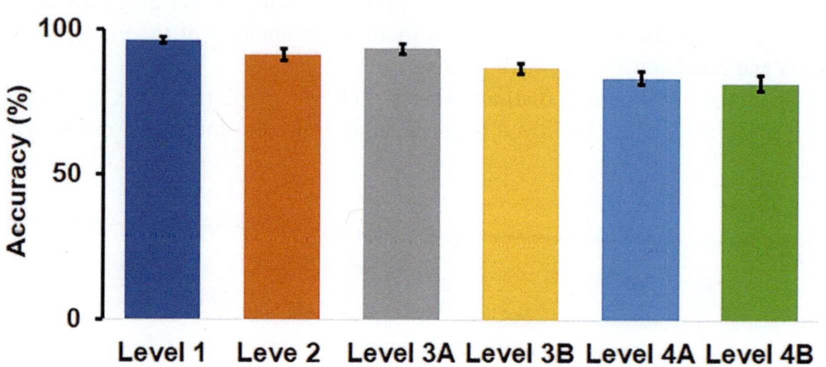

FIGURE 3.8 Performance analysis of the DL model at different classification levels.

the ultimate stratum, a soft-max function was applied. It generated probabilistic scores for individual disease classes. For comprehensive elucidation, the classification of skin diseases and their corresponding levels can be perused in Table 3.1. The model's performances, illustrated in Figure 3.8, exhibited a notable level of accuracy in adeptly characterizing the skin conditions. At level 1, the model exhibited an average accuracy of 96.4 ± 1.26%, underscoring its adeptness in precisely discerning the broader categories. At level 2, the model maintained 91.4 ± 2.13% accuracy, showcasing its prowess in distinguishing between distinct subcategories. Advancing to level 3A, the model showcased an average accuracy of 93.63 ± 1.84%. Similarly, at level 3B, the model yielded an average accuracy of 86.99 ± 1.79%, underscoring its efficiency in identifying additional subtleties. At level 4A, there was a slight decline in accuracy to 83.64 ± 2.08%. This drop signified the model's adeptness in distinguishing closely related subtypes. Finally, at level 4B, the model's accuracy reached 81.78 ± 2.77%, highlighting its finesse in identifying even the most nuanced disparities within the skin disorders. The notable accuracy achieved across diverse classification levels reinforces the computational model's robustness in precisely characterizing varied skin conditions based on the scrutinized features.

3.5 INTERPRETABILITY AND EXPLAINABILITY IN DEEP CNNS

Interpretability and explainability aspects not only empower medical professionals to trust and validate the AI's findings but also enable them to collaborate effectively with AI systems, leading to improved patient care and more accurate diagnoses. However, they possess distinct differences—(A) Complex AI models can be challenging to interpret, whereas explainability focuses on clarifying decisions. (B) Interpretability serves AI experts in comprehending model's behaviour. On the other hand, explainability is centred on conveying model decisions to end users. Primary challenges include complexity of CNNs, high-dimensional abstraction, their "black box" nature, determining influential regions in images, potential exploitation of noise, lack of clinical context consideration, and ethical concerns. Addressing these challenges requires interdisciplinary collaboration for developing techniques, ranging from visualization methods to generating explanations, ensuring AI in clinical practice. This section will reveal a few methods that aim to make deep CNNs more interpretable and explainable, focusing on their applications in breast and skin cancer diagnosis.

3.5.1 GRADIENT-WEIGHTED CLASS ACTIVATION MAPPING (GRAD-CAM)

The core concept of Grad-CAM involves leveraging the gradients of the target class score in relation to the feature maps originating from the final convolutional layer (Neal Joshua et al., 2021). Let I be the input image and y be the target class index. The deep CNN processes I through its layers, producing a class score s_y. Then a gradient, $\partial s_y / \partial A^k$, of the class score s_y is computed with respect to the feature maps A^k of the last convolutional layer. The importance of each feature map is calculated by global average pooling:

$$L^k_{Grad-CAM} = \sum_i \sum_j \frac{\partial s_y}{\partial A^k_{ij}} \qquad (3.25)$$

where, i and j iterate over the spatial dimensions of the feature maps. Following this, the weighted sum of the feature maps is obtained using the calculated importance values:

$$L_{Grad-CAM} = ReLU\left(\sum_k \alpha_k A^k \right) \qquad (3.26)$$

Here, α_k is the importance of the k-th feature map and is proportional to the corresponding $L^k_{Grad-CAM}$. Then, we up-sample the obtained $L_{Grad-CAM}$ to the size of I, resulting in a heatmap that highlights regions crucial for the prediction. The Grad-CAM heat map can be overlaid on the original image to visualize the regions that influenced the deep CNN's decision.

3.5.2 SALIENCY MAPS AND SENSITIVITY ANALYSIS

Saliency maps assist in visualizing the regions within an input image that hold the greatest influence over the CNN's prediction for a specific class. One approach involves calculating the gradients of the class score with respect to the input image (Kumari and Bhatia, 2023). This helps identify areas where small perturbations in pixel values would most affect the prediction. Let, I be the input image and y be the target class. The deep CNN processes I and produces a class score s_y. A gradient of the class score, $\delta s_y / \delta I$, is calculated with respect to the input image I. The absolute value of the gradients, S, can be found by:

$$S = \left| \frac{\partial s_y}{\partial I} \right| \tag{3.27}$$

Following this, normalization of the absolute gradients is performed:

$$S_{normalized} = \frac{S - min(S)}{max(S) - min(S)} \tag{3.28}$$

The normalized saliency map $S_{normalized}$ is overlayed on the input image I to visualize the areas of interest that contributed most to the decision.

Sensitivity analysis involves perturbing the input image and observing the alteration in the deep CNN's output. Here, a small perturbation is introduced to I by adding a noise vector N scaled by a perturbation factor ϵ:

$$I' = I + \epsilon \cdot N \tag{3.29}$$

Then, the perturbed image I' is processed through the deep CNN to obtain the new class score s'_y and the change in the class score is measured using:

$$S_{sensitivity} = \frac{s'_y - s_y}{\epsilon} \tag{3.30}$$

Finally, this sensitivity map $S_{sensitivity}$ is overlayed on the input image I to identify regions with high sensitivity. While saliency maps directly highlight important regions in the original image, sensitivity analysis investigates the response to perturbations, shedding light on sensitivity to local changes.

3.5.3 LIME AND SHAP

Local interpretable model-agnostic explanation (LIME) creates a locally faithful model around a specific prediction and approximates the original model's behaviour within that local region (Bhandari et al., 2023). At first, the specific instance (data point) is selected for which we need an explanation. Next, perturbations around the chosen instance are generated by introducing small random changes to its features, followed by obtaining the predictions for each perturbed instance from the original model. Finally, an interpretable model (e.g., linear regression) is fitted on the perturbed instances, using the model predictions as the target.

Shapley (SHAP) is based on cooperative game theory and ensures that each feature gets credit in proportion to its actual contribution to the prediction (Bhandari et al., 2023). Initially, a reference baseline is chosen and the prediction for this baseline is computed. In this manner, every conceivable subset of features is taken into account, and their contributions to the prediction are amalgamated. Following this, Shapley values are computed for each feature by considering all possible orderings in which features contribute:

$$\phi_i = \frac{1}{N!} \sum_{S \subseteq N \setminus \{i\}} \left| \binom{N-1}{|S|} \sum_{T \subseteq S} (-1)^{|T|} \cdot prediction\left(x_{T \cup \{i\}}\right) \right| \tag{3.31}$$

Here, N is the total number of features, S is a subset of features excluding feature i, and T is a subset of S including feature i. The Shapley value of each feature represents its average contribution to predictions across all possible feature combinations.

3.5.4 Concept Activation Vectors

Concept activation vectors (CAVs) aim to quantify a model's sensitivity to changes in a particular concept. The process involves training binary classifiers for the chosen concept against the remaining data using a linear model like logistic regression. This unveils how alterations in the concept influence model predictions, enhancing interpretability. The CAV calculation begins by selecting a concept, creating a binary classification dataset with positive and negative classes, and employing a binary classifier. The trained classifier's weights represent the CAV associated with the chosen concept, providing insights into how changes in the concept affect the model's predictions. This method aids in understanding the impact of specific concepts on model behaviour (Sadeghi et al., 2023). This can be calculated using the chain rule of calculus:

$$CAV_{concept} = \frac{\partial P(positive\ class)}{\partial activations} \tag{3.32}$$

Here, $P(positive\ class)$ is the probability assigned by the binary classifier to the positive class. Positive values of the CAV indicate that the concept positively influences the prediction, while negative values indicate a negative influence. This approach enhances the interpretability and transparency of deep neural networks, especially in scenarios where high-level concepts are crucial for decision-making.

3.5.5 Integrated Gradients

This calculates the contribution of each feature by integrating the gradients of the output with respect to the input attributes along a path from a baseline (usually a reference input) to the actual input (Imouokhome et al., 2023). Let's consider a deep CNN f that takes an input x and produces an output y. The goal of integrated gradients is to measure how changes in each input feature x_i contribute to the change in the output y. This can be achieved using:

$$\text{Integrated Gradients}_{x_i}(x) = \left(x_i - x_i'\right) \times \int_{\alpha=0}^{1} \frac{\partial f\left(x' + \alpha \times \left(x - x'\right)\right)}{\partial x_i} \, d\alpha \qquad (3.33)$$

Here, x is the actual input, x' is the baseline input, x_i is the value of the i-th feature in the actual input. $\dfrac{\partial f\left(x' + \alpha \times \left(x - x'\right)\right)}{\partial x_i}$ is the gradient of the output f with respect to the i-th feature at an interpolated input point $x' + \alpha \times \left(x - x'\right)$. α ranges from 0 to 1, representing the path from the baseline to the actual input. By integrating the gradients along a path, it captures how each feature's contribution changes as input transitions from the baseline to the actual input. Positive values denote that augmenting the feature value leads to heightened output, whereas negative values signify the converse.

3.6 FUTURE SCOPES

In the realm of image-guided diagnosis for breast and skin cancers, deep CNNs have opened up a remarkable chapter in medical science. The strides taken so far have laid a strong foundation, but the journey is far from over. Several compelling avenues beckon researchers and clinicians to continue advancing the field. One path involves personalizing cancer care to an unprecedented level. CNNs can be harnessed to mine not just anatomical data but also genetic and molecular information. Multimodal integration is another frontier ripe for exploration. Fusing insights from various imaging modalities like MRI, CT, ultrasound, and molecular imaging can yield a comprehensive assessment of cancer. Interpretable and explainable AI is a paramount concern. CNNs' opaque decision-making processes pose challenges to clinical adoption. Besides, collaborative efforts involving healthcare institutions and research bodies can facilitate the creation of large-scale, annotated datasets representative of varied patient populations. As CNNs become integrated into clinical practice, ethical considerations and regulatory frameworks must be solidified. In parallel with this, researchers need to engage in conversations about data privacy, bias mitigation, informed patient consent, and the establishment of guidelines for responsible AI deployment in healthcare contexts.

3.7 CONCLUSION

The integration of deep CNNs has emerged as a transformative force, revolutionizing the landscape of breast and skin cancer detection. The culmination of this chapter underscores the immense potential of Deep CNNs in augmenting the diagnostic process for breast and skin cancers. These intelligent networks have transcended conventional methods, demonstrating their prowess in feature extraction, classification, segmentation, and even interpretability. Through the incorporation of rich anatomical, textural, and contextual information, CNNs have manifested as adept diagnosticians, offering insights into intricate tissue patterns, lesion characteristics, and disease manifestations that elude the human eye.

The application of Deep CNNs in breast cancer diagnosis has unveiled a new era of precision medicine. From mammography to histopathology, CNNs have exhibited their ability to unravel intricate subtleties, enhancing the detection of malignancies at early stages. The utilization of transfer learning and pre-trained networks has leveraged the inherent knowledge captured from diverse datasets. This has been pivotal in bridging diagnostic gaps, improving detection rates, and minimizing the potential for misdiagnosis. Similarly, in the domain of skin cancer, the integration of deep CNNs has propelled the field of dermatology into a new paradigm of accuracy and efficiency. From lesion segmentation to classification, CNNs have demonstrated an unparalleled aptitude for understanding diverse lesion types, thereby assisting clinicians in making well-informed decisions. The fusion of computational intelligence with dermatological expertise has not only expedited diagnosis but has also created an avenue for telemedicine and remote patient care, transcending geographical barriers. As we embrace the ongoing evolution of AI-driven medical diagnostics, deep CNNs stand as beacons of hope, illuminating a path towards enhanced patient outcomes and reduced healthcare burdens worldwide.

REFERENCES

Adel M, Kotb A, Farag O, Darweesh MS, Mostafa H. Breast cancer diagnosis using image processing and machine learning for elastography images. In 2019 8th International Conference on Modern Circuits and Systems Technologies (MOCAST) 2019 May 13 (pp. 1–4). IEEE.

Agrawal S, Karri SPK, Basak K, Ojha T, Sheet D. Quantitative Dermatopathology of 11 Skin Conditions through Transfer Learning of Tissue Photon Interaction Statistical Physics, 2nd Indian Workshop on Machine Learning, Springer, 2016.

Ahmed A, Leon A, Butler DC, Reichenberg J. Quality-of-life effects of common dermatological diseases. Seminars in Cutaneous Medicine and Surgery. 2013 Jun 1;32(2):101–9.

Allugunti VR. Breast cancer detection based on thermographic images using machine learning and deep learning algorithms. International Journal of Engineering in Computer Science. 2022;4(1):49–56.

Antropova N, Huynh BQ, Giger ML. A deep feature fusion methodology for breast cancer diagnosis demonstrated on three imaging modality datasets. Medical Physics. 2017 Oct;44(10):5162–71.

Barragán-Montero A, Javaid U, Valdés G, Nguyen D, Desbordes P, Macq B, Willems S, Vandewinckele L, Holmström M, Löfman F, Michiels S. Artificial intelligence and machine learning for medical imaging: A technology review. Physica Medica. 2021 Mar 1;83:242–56.

Bhandari M, Yogarajah P, Kavitha MS, Condell J. Exploring the capabilities of a lightweight CNN model in accurately identifying renal abnormalities: Cysts, stones, and tumors, using LIME and SHAP. Applied Sciences. 2023 Feb 28;13(5):3125.

Bray F, Ferlay J, Soerjomataram I, Siegel RL, Torre LA, Jemal A. Global cancer statistics 2018: GLOBOCAN estimates of incidence and mortality worldwide for 36 cancers in 185 countries. CA: A Cancer Journal for Clinicians. 2018 Nov;68(6):394–424.

Campos-do-Carmo G, Ramos-e-Silva M. Dermoscopy: Basic concepts. International Journal of Dermatology. 2008 Jul;47(7):712–9.

Cancer Facts and Figures 2019. American Cancer Society, 2019. www.cancer.org/content/dam/cancer-org/research/cancer-facts-and-statistics/annual-cancer-facts-and-figures/2019/cancer-facts-and-figures-2019.pdf

Chhikara BS, Parang K. Global cancer statistics 2022: The trends projection analysis. Chemical Biology Letters. 2023;10(1):451–66.

Cong S, Zhou Y. A review of convolutional neural network architectures and their optimizations. Artificial Intelligence Review. 2023 Mar;56(3):1905–69.

Demyanov S, Chakravorty R, Abedini M, Halpern A, Garnavi R. Classification of dermoscopy patterns using deep convolutional neural networks. In 2016 IEEE 13th International Symposium on Biomedical Imaging (ISBI) 2016 Apr 13 (pp. 364–68). IEEE.

Dencks S, Piepenbrock M, Opacic T, Krauspe B, Stickeler E, Kiessling F, Schmitz G. Clinical pilot application of super-resolution US imaging in breast cancer. IEEE Transactions on Ultrasonics, Ferroelectrics, and Frequency Control. 2018 Sep 23;66(3):517–26.

Domingues I, Pereira G, Martins P, Duarte H, Santos J, Abreu PH. Using deep learning techniques in medical imaging: A systematic review of applications on CT and PET. Artificial Intelligence Review. 2020 Aug;53:4093–160.

Esteva A, Kuprel B, Novoa RA, Ko J, Swetter SM, Blau HM, Thrun S. Dermatologist-level classification of skin cancer with deep neural networks. Nature. 2017 Feb;542(7639):115–8.

Fujisawa Y, Otomo Y, Ogata Y, et al. Deep-learning-based, computer-aided classifier developed with a small dataset of clinical images surpasses board-certified dermatologists in skin tumour diagnosis. British Journal of Dermatology. 2019 Feb 1;180(2):373–81.

Gajera HK, Nayak DR, Zaveri MA. A comprehensive analysis of dermoscopy images for melanoma detection via deep CNN features. Biomedical Signal Processing and Control. 2023 Jan 1;79:104186.

Gefen A, editor. Bioengineering Research of Chronic Wounds: A Multidisciplinary Study Approach. Science & Business Media, 2009.

Giaquinto AN, Sung H, Miller KD, Kramer JL, Newman LA, Minihan A, Jemal A, Siegel RL. Breast cancer statistics, 2022. CA: A Cancer Journal for Clinicians. 2022 Nov;72(6):524–41.

Guida S, Pellacani G, Ciardo S, Longo C. Reflectance confocal microscopy of aging skin and skin cancer. Dermatology Practical & Conceptual. 2021 Jul;11(3).

Han SS, Kim MS, Lim W, Park GH, Park I, Chang SE. Classification of the clinical images for benign and malignant cutaneous tumors using a deep learning algorithm. Journal of Investigative Dermatology. 2018 Jul 1;138(7):1529–38.

Hay R, Bendeck SE, Chen S, Estrada R, Haddix A, McLeod T, Mahé A. Skin diseases. In Disease Control Priorities in Developing Countries, 2nd edition, Oxford University Press, 2006.

Ilişanu MA, Moldoveanu F, Moldoveanu A. Multispectral imaging for skin diseases assessment—State of the art and perspectives. Sensors. 2023 Apr 11;23(8):3888.

Imouokhome FA, Ehimiyein OG, Chete FO. Diagnosis and interpretation of breast cancer using explainable artificial intelligence. Journal of Science and Technology Research. 2023 Jun 7;5(2).

Joseph N, Kumar GS, Nelliyanil M. Skin diseases and conditions among students of a medical college in southern India. Indian Dermatology Online Journal. 2014;5(1):19–24.

Kozegar E, Soryani M, Behnam H, Salamati M, Tan T. Computer aided detection in automated 3-D breast ultrasound images: A survey. Artificial Intelligence Review. 2020 Mar;53:1919–41.

Kratzer TB, Jemal A, Miller KD, Nash S, Wiggins C, Redwood D, Smith R, Siegel RL. Cancer statistics for American Indian and Alaska Native individuals, 2022: Including increasing disparities in early onset colorectal cancer. CA: A Cancer Journal for Clinicians. 2023 Mar;73(2):120–46.

Kumari N, Bhatia R. Saliency map and deep learning based efficient facial emotion recognition technique for facial images. Multimedia Tools and Applications. 2023 Jul 18:1–24.

Lehman CD, Schnall MD. Imaging in breast cancer: Magnetic resonance imaging. Breast Cancer Research. 2005 Oct;7(5):1–5.

Levine A, Wang K, Markowitz O. Optical coherence tomography in the diagnosis of skin cancer. Dermatologic Clinics. 2017 Oct 1;35(4):465–88.

Masood A, Al-Jumaily A, Anam K. Self-supervised learning model for skin cancer diagnosis. In 2015 7th International IEEE/EMBS Conference on Neural Engineering (NER) 2015 Apr 22 (pp. 1012–1015). IEEE.

Massone C, Di Stefani A, Soyer HP. Dermoscopy for skin cancer detection. Current Opinion in Oncology. 2005 Mar 1;17(2):147–53.

Moghbel M, Ooi CY, Ismail N, Hau YW, Memari N. A review of breast boundary and pectoral muscle segmentation methods in computer-aided detection/diagnosis of breast mammography. Artificial Intelligence Review. 2020 Mar;53:1873–918.

Moradi R, Berangi R, Minaei B. A survey of regularization strategies for deep models. Artificial Intelligence Review. 2020 Aug;53:3947–86.

Murtaza G, Shuib L, Abdul Wahab AW, et al. Deep learning-based breast cancer classification through medical imaging modalities: State of the art and research challenges. Artificial Intelligence Review. 2020 Mar;53:1655–720.

Neal Joshua ES, Bhattacharyya D, Chakkravarthy M, Byun YC. 3D CNN with visual insights for early detection of lung cancer using gradient-weighted class activation. Journal of Healthcare Engineering. 2021 Mar 11;2021:1.

Pan X, Li L, Yang H, Liu Z, Yang J, Zhao L, Fan Y. Accurate segmentation of nuclei in pathological images via sparse reconstruction and deep convolutional networks. Neurocomputing. 2017 Mar 15;229:88–99.

Pangti R, Mathur J, Chouhan V, et al. A machine learning-based, decision support, mobile phone application for diagnosis of common dermatological diseases. Journal of the European Academy of Dermatology and Venereology. 2021 Feb;35(2):536–45.

Pauwels EK, Foray N, Bourguignon MH. Breast cancer induced by X-ray mammography screening? A review based on recent understanding of low-dose radiobiology. Medical Principles and Practice. 2016 Nov 16;25(2):101–9.

Pisano ED, Yaffe MJ. Digital mammography. Radiology. 2005 Feb;234(2):353–62.

Pomponiu V, Nejati H, Cheung NM. Deepmole: Deep neural networks for skin mole lesion classification. In 2016 IEEE International Conference on Image Processing (ICIP) 2016 Sep 25 (pp. 2623–2627). IEEE.

Rana M, Bhushan M. Machine learning and deep learning approach for medical image analysis: Diagnosis to detection. Multimedia Tools and Applications. 2022 Dec 24:1–39.

Rehman M, Khan SH, Rizvi SD, Abbas Z, Zafar A. Classification of skin lesion by interference of segmentation and convolution neural network. In 2018 2nd International Conference on Engineering Innovation (ICEI) 2018 Jul 5 (pp. 81–85). IEEE.

Rojas R. The backpropagation algorithm. Neural Networks: A Systematic Introduction. 1996:149–82.

Sadeghi Z, Alizadehsani R, Cifci MA, Kausar S, Rehman R, Mahanta P, Bora PK, Almasri A, Alkhawaldeh RS, Hussain S, Alatas B. A brief review of explainable artificial intelligence in healthcare. arXiv preprint arXiv:2304.01543. 2023 Apr 4.

Saha M, Chakraborty C, Racoceanu D. Efficient deep learning model for mitosis detection using breast histopathology images. Computerized Medical Imaging and Graphics. 2018 Mar 1;64:29–40.

Sheet D, Basak K, Ojha T, Karri SPK. Multispectral optical imaging device and computational techniques for contactless functional imaging. Patent No. IN201731022695, Jan 2019.

Siegel RL, Miller KD, Wagle NS, Jemal A. Cancer statistics, 2023. CA: A Cancer Journal for Clinicians. 2023 Jan 1;73(1):17–48.

Skin Cancer Statistics. World Cancer Research Fund International, 2022. www.wcrf.org/cancer-trends/skin-cancer-statistics/

Thanh DN, Hai NH, Tiwari P, Prasath VS. Skin lesion segmentation method for dermoscopic images with convolutional neural networks and semantic segmentation. Компьютерная оптика. 2021;45(1):122–9.

Vesal S, Ravikumar N, Maier A. SkinNet: A deep learning framework for skin lesion segmentation. In 2018 IEEE Nuclear Science Symposium and Medical Imaging Conference Proceedings (NSS/MIC) 2018 Nov 10 (pp. 1–3). IEEE.

Vocaturo E, Zumpano E, Veltri P. Image pre-processing in computer vision systems for melanoma detection. In 2018 IEEE International Conference on Bioinformatics and Biomedicine (BIBM) 2018 Dec 3 (pp. 2117–2124). IEEE.

Walker BN, Rehg JM, Kalra A, et al. Dermoscopy diagnosis of cancerous lesions utilizing dual deep learning algorithms via visual and audio (sonification) outputs: Laboratory and prospective observational studies. EBioMedicine. 2019 Feb 1;40:176–83.

Wang J, Zhu H, Wang SH, Zhang YD. A review of deep learning on medical image analysis. Mobile Networks and Applications. 2021 Feb;26:351–80.

Xing F, Xie Y, Yang L. An automatic learning-based framework for robust nucleus segmentation. IEEE Transactions on Medical Imaging. 2015 Sep 23;35(2):550–66.

Xu J, Luo X, Wang G, Gilmore H, Madabhushi A. A deep convolutional neural network for segmenting and classifying epithelial and stromal regions in histopathological images. Neurocomputing. 2016 May 26;191:214–23.

Yu L, Chen H, Dou Q, Qin J, Heng PA. Automated melanoma recognition in dermoscopy images via very deep residual networks. IEEE Transactions on Medical Imaging. 2016 Dec 21;36(4):994–1004.

4 Robust Learning Principle Design to Detect Diabetic Retinopathy Disease in Early Stages with Skilled Feature Extraction Policy

Sasirekha D., Kalpana Devi P., Nancy W., Valarmathi K., and Anitha G.

4.1 INTRODUCTION

In the medical sector, early detection of illnesses is essential for the most efficient therapy. Diabetes is characterized by a rise in blood glucose levels due to inadequate production of insulin. In all, 425 million individuals are afflicted with it. Affected organs by diabetes include the kidneys, heart, nerves, and retina. Diabetic retinopathy (DR) is the leading cause of blindness and visual impairment in persons aged 20 to 74 and is one of the most prevalent diabetic consequences.

There were 422 million diabetes people in 2014, and 35% of them acquired retinopathy due to cumulative damage to tiny blood vessels in the retina, as reported by the World Health Organization (WHO). Particular patient populations have a much greater incidence of DR. During the course of DR's slow progression, vision loss can take on a variety of forms. Non-proliferative DR (NPDR) is the first stage of DR and is defined by vitreous/pre-retinal bleeding or neovascularization. Proliferative DR (PDR) is the second stage and is characterized by neovascularization or advanced NPDR. Ten percent of diabetic individuals without DR will acquire NPDR every year, and 75% of those with severe NPDR will progress to PDR within a year. It usually takes a long time for the condition to go from normal status (no visible abnormalities in the retina) to PDR [1]. Therefore, NPDR is typically classified into three stages: mild, moderate, and severe. The two most common types of diabetes were type 1 and type 2. Nevertheless, type 2 diabetes is the most common form of the disease, affecting 90% to 95% of diabetics. Type 1 diabetes is also known as insulin-dependent diabetes mellitus. This disease was once known as juvenile-onset diabetes since it usually first appears in children. Autoimmune diseases like type 1 diabetes are brought on by the body's antibodies turning against the pancreas. Additionally, a person with type 1 diabetes will have pancreatic damage and be unable to produce

DOI: 10.1201/9781032635149-4

"

insulin. This kind of diabetes may have its origins in inherited traits from both parents. The failure of the pancreatic beta cells to generate insulin might potentially play a role. Treatment for type 1 diabetes comprises insulin, which is administered by injection into subcutaneous fat.

Type 2 diabetes, which often affects adults, is associated with childhood obesity. This kind of diabetes is more common among adolescents nowadays. In medical terms, type 2 diabetes is more severe than type 1 diabetes and was once known as non-insulin-dependent diabetes. In addition, it can cause some organs to malfunction, especially those dependent on the tiniest blood arteries for survival, such as the nerves of the kidneys and the eyes. After that, it can have an effect on the pancreas, which is responsible for producing insulin, resulting in either insufficient insulin production or cell resistance to insulin [2]. People who are obese and much shorter than their optimum height are at increased risk of developing type 2 diabetes due to insulin resistance. Nevertheless, those who get regular exercise, eat healthily, and keep their weight in check are less likely to develop type 2 diabetes. However, type 2 diabetes frequently worsens and requires the use of diabetic drugs. The presence of broken blood vessels behind the retina is diagnostic of DR. Leaving this problem unchecked can lead to major consequences, including blindness, and should be avoided at all costs. The severity of DR is now evaluated by a manual examination of fundus pictures of the eye by specialists. This takes up a lot of time, and there aren't enough doctors to treat everyone who needs them. Many people wait too long to see a doctor because of these issues. The example DR picture is displayed in Figure 4.1. Doctors may recommend annual fundus examinations for their diabetic patients, but many instances go undiagnosed until they are well advanced. Therefore, an automated approach to aid in the diagnosis of diabetic retinopathy is preferable.

Ophthalmologists, who are specialists in the field, capture high-resolution digital images of the retina of a human eye using a device called a fundus camera. Different types of DR retinal lesions can be detected via the fundus, allowing for accurate

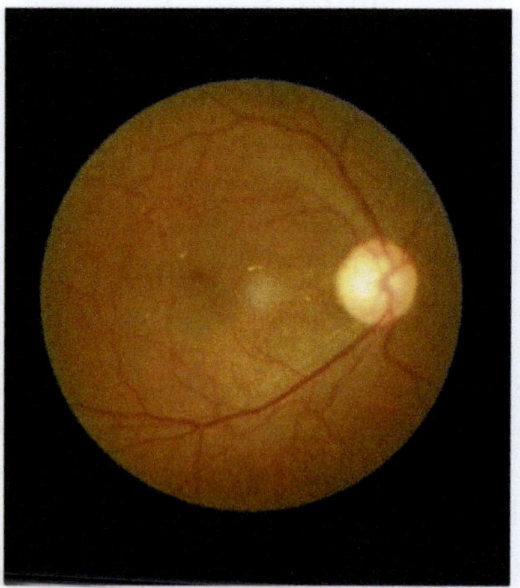

FIGURE 4.1 Sample image.

picture annotation and subsequent treatment. Physical diagnosis is time-consuming, and there is a lack of available treatment options, so spotting DR early might be difficult. Therefore, cutting-edge methods of diagnosis and therapy are required for such a medical condition [3]. Expert systems employing Deep Learning (DL) for analysis and in-depth examination of DR characteristics from fundus pictures have been offered as a solution to the difficulties of manual DR identification. When compared to conventional approaches, intelligent systems excel in areas where time is of the essence, such as feature extraction, mistake identification, and early diagnosis and treatment.

Therefore, DL-based intelligent systems are presented as a feasible early and scalable option for DR detection. Because of their inherent shallowness, traditional ML models and data analysis methodologies have failed to demonstrate improved analysis and interpretation when presented with bigger datasets, including complex non-linear properties. Inherent quality from hierarchical structures in such models improves model learning, allowing for optimal performance at the cutting edge [4]. When it comes to DR diagnosis, the feature extraction and classification capabilities of various DL designs have varied. However, it is not possible to accurately evaluate the efficacy of a whole DL model in a single experimental setting.

One of the most popular deep learning models for medical image detection, prediction, and classification is the convolutional neural network (CNN). In this study, we provide DGFM (Deep Neural Networks, Genetic Algorithms, and Firefly Algorithms), a revolutionary and powerful learning concept. The idea is to improve upon the learning process by combining the strengths of Deep Neural Networks (DNNs), Genetic Algorithms (GAs), and Firefly Algorithms (FAs). The input dataset is normalized using the Standard Scalar method in order to get it ready for modeling. This normalization method guarantees that all features are on an equal playing field, eliminating the possibility of learning bias. The next step is to use a genetic algorithm to pick out the most pertinent details from the data set [5]. The genetic algorithm aids in dimensionality reduction and better model performance by honing in on the most useful traits via repeatedly choosing and merging features based on their relevance to the target variable. The Firefly Algorithm is employed for both feature selection and dimensionality reduction. Inspired by the dazzling antics of fireflies, the Firefly Algorithm is a method for optimizing data. It aids in determining a minimal collection of characteristics that adequately captures the relevant data with little computing overhead. This study presents a complete strategy for robust learning by including DNNs, GAs, and FAs inside the DGFM framework. By combining them, we may enhance model performance and interpretability through careful feature selection and dimensionality reduction.

4.2 RELATED WORKS

Faster, more precise, and less intrusive technologies have recently been introduced, ushering in a new age in medical imaging. One of the most prevalent serious effects of diabetes is damage to the retina. Carelessness with it can cause blindness. With the use of a computer-aided diagnosis (CAD) system, retinal lesions caused by diabetes may be found and pinpointed with greater accuracy. For retinal image recognition and segmentation, several methods are used. These include image modification, machine learning, and deep learning. In the context of retinal illness identification and prognosis, deep neural networks can be of great assistance. In order to get retinal information, imaging techniques such as fundus photography, Optical Coherence Tomography (OCT), and OCT Angiography are utilized. Depending on the degree of damage caused by the illness, diabetic retinopathy may be represented in the retinal pictures in a number of distinct ways. In the case of retinal illnesses, this multi-label categorization can aid clinicians in making accurate diagnoses. In order to categorize diseases into mild, moderate, severe, and proliferative categories, the author [6] examines and analyses a number of deep neural networks.

The researchers want to compare the retinal thickness of those with and without diabetes by taking readings at several locations on the retina. In the past, it was believed that hyperglycemia as well as the metabolic pathways it activates produced DR predominantly through the direct effects on the retinal microvascular system. However, new research shows that retinal neurodegeneration, caused by an uneven ratio of neurotoxic to neuroprotective components, begins long before the onset of clinically evident microvascular damage. DR is a degeneration of the retina that occurs in long-term diabetics. Retinal abnormal blood vessel development is a hallmark of DR. Diabetes causes damage to the ocular circulatory system. Additionally, there may be no warning signs at first, but vision problems might develop with time. One of the most pressing problems in bioengineering is the accurate assessment of the physiological alterations occurring in the human body. Finding anomalies in the human eye is difficult because of the many factors at play. Diseases in retinal images are often diagnosed by a labor-intensive manual process. These methods perform less well because of the high error rate associated with human observation. Researchers [7] created the EfficientNet-B7 model, a deep learning technology, to automatically diagnose diabetic retinopathy. The best settings were found by adjusting hyperparameters. In order to lessen the likelihood of overfitting, we compared the Efficientnet-B7 model with and without an augmentation technique. The purpose of this study is to improve classification accuracy and examine the effectiveness of the suggested algorithmic effort.

Typically, ophthalmologists have numerous sorts of lesions to work with when diagnosing diabetic retinopathy (DR) in a patient's fundus imaging. Recognizing and correctly classifying DR fundus pictures, as well as identifying all types of lesions on them, is of utmost importance. For the purpose of DR classification and automated region-based lesion localization, the author [8] suggested a deep learning-based multi-label classification model using Gradient-weighted Class Activation Mapping (Grad-CAM). As a novel approach to eliminating manual annotation and increasing labeling efficiency, this research recasts lesion detection as image categorization and treats distinct types of lesions as separate labels for a fundus picture. Three thousand two hundred and twenty-eight photographs of the fundus were gathered, and five labels were pre-defined, to create our model. Our deep learning model's architecture is custom-built on top of the ResNet basis. This technique improved its DR classification sensitivity to 93.9% and specificity to 94.4% by experimental testing on the test pictures. The DR fundus pictures also showed relatively well-defined borders around the areas where lesions were located.

A recent poll by the World Health Organization found that one in four people has diabetes. Many factors, such as diet, environment, and genetics, might contribute to this condition. Over time, a person with diabetes will face increasing dangers. Diabetic retinopathy is an example of a danger to eyesight that arises as a microvascular complication of diabetes mellitus. Diabetic retinopathy now affects 93 million individuals worldwide. There has been a dearth of research on the frequency and causes of diabetic eye disease. Diabetic retinopathy is a potentially blinding eye disease that is more common in people with diabetes. If you have diabetes, you should get a dilated eye exam once a year at the very least. Researchers [9] have taken a single picture of the human fundus and utilized deep learning to determine the severity of diabetic retinopathy. Similar datasets with different labeling have been used in our proposed multistage transfer learning approach. On the APTOS 2019 dataset for detecting blindness (13,000 pictures), the suggested technique has a sensitivity and specificity of 0.99, making it suitable for early detection of diabetic retinopathy

DR is a potentially fatal eye illness that affects persons with diabetes. DR causes pain in the retina and, over time, can cause blindness. Detection of DR (DRD) using state-of-the-art Profound Proficiency methods. Using deep Convolutional Neural Network (CNN) frameworks, we apply their command to the finalization of eye fundus pictures, which has shown progressive advancements in many fields of computer vision, including therapeutic imaging. The three-part structure presented by the author [10] is a hybrid of these two. The fundus image is first subjected to a normalized approach and an enhanced method for pre-processing. Second, a point vector is extracted from the pre-processed image by feeding it into the various building blocks of the CNN architecture. Third, DRD evaluation is guided by a categorization system.

4.3 METHODOLOGY

Methods for processing retinal fundus pictures are offered for early diagnosis and severity assessment of DR. To do this, we employ a deep learning model that incorporates transfer learning to examine a set of preprocessed photos and draw conclusions on the presence of diabetic retinopathy. An intriguing and potent strategy for solving difficult optimization and search issues is to combine the powers of Deep Neural Networks (DNNs) with Genetic Algorithms (GAs). The suggested model's architecture is depicted in Figure 4.2.

4.4 IMAGE PREPROCESSING

Kaggle [11] is mined for data. Diabetic retinopathy (DR) photographs must be pre-processed before they can be used in a computer-aided diagnostic system. DR is an eye disease that can cause blindness if not diagnosed and treated in time. With proper preprocessing, retinal pictures can have noise reduced, key characteristics highlighted, and overall quality improved for better analysis and diagnosis. In order to decrease computational complexity and assure uniformity across the dataset, the first step is to resize the photographs to a standard resolution. Cropping photos to zero in on the area of interest (the retina) might be useful in some situations. When photos are normalized, the effects of lighting differences are mitigated. Remove unwanted noise from the photos using denoising methods like Gaussian or median filtering. Obtaining reliable outcomes from feature extraction relies heavily on noise reduction. Image before any processing is shown in Figure 4.3.

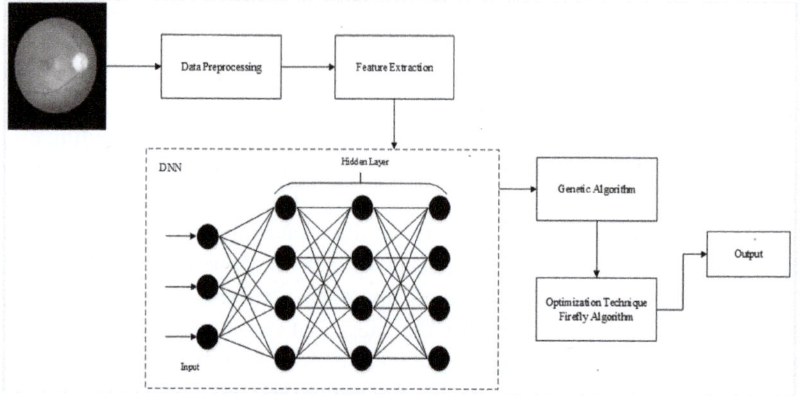

FIGURE 4.2 Architecture of proposed model.

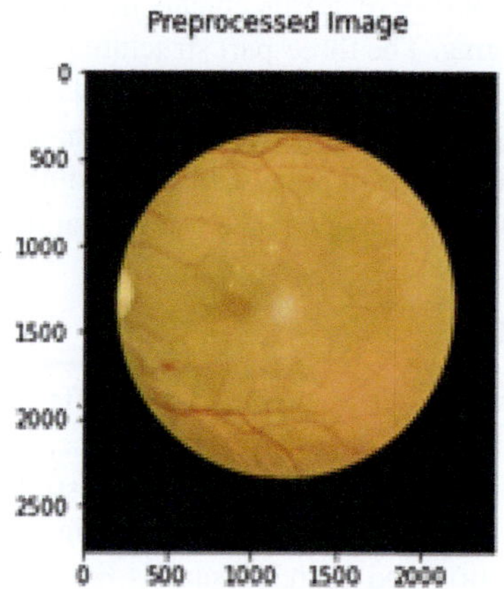

FIGURE 4.3 Preprocessed image.

4.5 DATA AUGMENTATION

The quality of the training data and the DNN's resilience may be improved with both the help of genetic algorithms' optimization of data augmentation and preprocessing procedures. Through natural selection, the GA oversees a population of potential methods for augmenting or preparing data in order to improve model performance. An intriguing and novel way to autonomously generate augmented data for machine learning tasks is the use of Genetic Algorithms (GAs). Machine learning models, and DNNs in particular, can benefit from increased generalization and resilience when trained on larger and more diverse training datasets, which is where data augmentation comes in. Figure 4.4 depicts DR in both its healthy and pathological states.

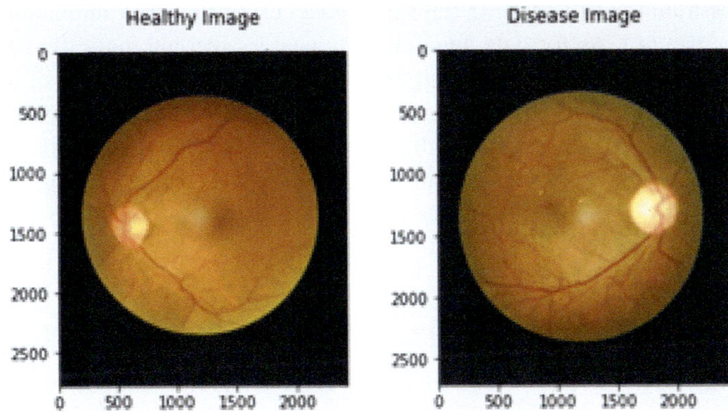

FIGURE 4.4 Healthy and disease image.

Applying a series of specified modifications (such as rotation, scaling, flipping, or cropping) to the original data to generate additional samples is the classic approach to data augmentation. Nevertheless, the range of possible modifications that might improve the model's performance may be too broad for manual creation of data augmentation techniques.

Here's how Genetic Algorithms may help with data enhancement:

The first step is to specify the GA's representation of the transformations used for data augmentation. The members of the GA population each stand in for a unique method of augmenting data. An individual's genome has instructions for a variety of transformations—rotation, translation, scaling, flipping, color modifications, and so on. The GA begins by generating a pool of candidates for data augmentation techniques. The people are produced arbitrarily or given a beginning state that includes certain predetermined augmentation processes. A DNN model is built using the original training dataset, with the modifications defined by the person, to assess the efficacy of each data augmentation technique. A person's fitness is measured by how well their model performs on a validation dataset or through cross-validation. The fitness score improves, for instance, when the validation accuracy or validation loss is increased, respectively. Normal genetic processes including selection, crossover, and mutation are used in the GA. Those with better fitness ratings are more likely to be chosen as reproductive parents. The augmentation operations of two parents can be combined through crossover to produce offspring with enhanced features, and mutation can add random alterations to the augmentation operations of offspring to keep the population genetically diverse. The GA cycles through generations, with each generation improving upon the last. When a stopping requirement is reached, for as when performance has stabilized or there has been no meaningful progress over numerous iterations, the process stops.

In order to maximize the DNN model's improvement in performance on the validation dataset, the GA eventually settles on an augmented dataset and a sequence of augmentation processes. Finally, the DNN's generalization skills may be enhanced by training it on the full original training dataset using the final augmentation technique. The use of GAs for data augmentation enables the automatic finding of efficient augmentation solutions that might not have been visible or contemplated in a hand-crafted design. It offers a more data-driven strategy for data augmentation, one that can be adjusted depending on the nature of the task and the available dataset. Effective augmentation tactics require a balance between investigating and exploiting, but this must be achieved with careful consideration of computational resources as well as hyperparameter choices.

4.6 IMAGE SEGMENTATION

The complexity of pictures, presence of noise or occlusions, and desired end results all play a role in determining the best approach to the difficult work of image segmentation. Due to their capacity to acquire complicated and hierarchical representations from the data, deep learning-based segmentation algorithms, notably those employing fully convolutional networks, have shown excellent performance across a wide range of picture segmentation applications. In cases where computing speed or interpretability are paramount, however, classic segmentation algorithms continue to find use. Image segmentation for diabetic retinopathy relies on high-quality input pictures, well-chosen segmentation methods, and readily available labeled data for training and evaluating the segmentation results. Enhanced accuracy and reliability in assessing diabetic retinopathy can be achieved via the use of multi-segmentation methodologies that are integrated with other analysis techniques including feature extraction and classification. The area of medical image analysis is expanding fast; therefore, researchers are always looking for ways to better segment and diagnose diabetic retinopathy using cutting-edge methods like deep learning.

4.7 DEEP NEURAL NETWORKS

Artificial neural networks (ANNs) with several layers of linked nodes (neurons) are known as Deep Neural Networks (DNNs). They take their cue from the intricate wiring of the human brain, namely the way in which individual neurons communicate with one another. Artificial neurons, often called nodes or units, are the DNN's basic building components. Learnable parameters, sometimes referred to as weights and biases, are associated with every layer in the network with the exception of the input layer.

In order for the network to produce reliable predictions, its trainer must discover the best settings for these weights and biases. During training, an optimization technique like stochastic gradient descent (SGD) or its variations is used to decrease the value of a loss or cost function that quantifies how far off the actual output is from the desired one. The structure and operation of a Deep Neural Network are described in great depth next.

1. Input Layer: The network's input layer acts as its foundation by taking in data from other sources. The dimensionality of the input data is reflected in

the amount of neurons in the input layer, with each neuron standing in for a feature or input characteristic.

2. Hidden Layers: Underneath the input as well as output layers is where you'll find the hidden layers. The activations of their neurons are concealed from view in the input and output, thus the name "hidden." Every neuron in a hidden layer receives inputs from all the neurons in the preceding layer, processes those inputs, and then passes along its processed output to the neurons in the next layer.

3. Output Layer: The network's last layer, the output layer, is in charge of making the network's ultimate predictions, or outputs. The challenge at hand determines the optimal size of the output layer's network of neurons. One possible neuron's output in a binary classification task is a probability value between 0 and 1.

4. Neuron Activation: In the hidden and output layers, the input data from the preceding layer is enlarged by the relevant weights and added to create the biases, and this result is then fed into an activation function by every neuron.

5. Forward Propagation: Forward propagation refers to the act of feeding input data into a network in order to generate predictions. In forward propagation, the input is processed by each layer in turn, with activations being calculated between each iteration, until the final output is produced.

6. Loss Function: The loss function evaluates how far off the model was from the actual results. Mean squared error (MSE) is a typical instance of a loss function used in regression, whereas cross-entropy loss is used for categorization.

7. Backpropagation: When the network has completed the forward propagation stage, it uses the loss function to evaluate how well its predictions match the actual target values. The gradients of the loss relative to the network's weights and biases are then computed via backpropagation. The gradients show the optimal adjustments to the weights and biases.

4.8   HYBRID DGFM

When applied to machine learning, optimization, and search problems, a hybrid of Deep Neural Networks (DNNs) and Genetic Algorithms (GAs) is a potent method that combines the advantages of both approaches. The hybridization may be accomplished in several ways depending on the nature of the challenge and the desired outcomes. The DNN-GA hybrid method has found widespread use in the field of architectural search. Finding the best neural network design for a given job can be a complex and time-consuming ordeal. Efficiently searching the space of potential designs is achievable with the help of Genetic Algorithms. Every member of the population represents a unique network setup, and the GA oversees the whole population. High-performing designs are converged upon by the GA through selection, crossover, and mutation.

Hyperparameters, or tuning options, for DNNs include learning rate, batch size, and number of layers, among many more. It can be difficult to fine-tune these hyperparameters by hand. To find the best possible hyperparameter settings, Genetic

Algorithms might be used. The GA controls a population of hyperparameter values and gradually improves DNN performance by selecting values that have worked in the past.

The most popular approach for improving DNN weights, classical backpropagation, can become trapped in local optima, especially for complicated loss surfaces. Direct optimization of the neural network's weights through Genetic Algorithms is possible. The fitness function compares each member of the GA population to a target weight distribution based on how well they performed a given job. The GA improves its performance by shifting its weight distribution throughout successive generations. To improve prediction accuracy, ensemble learning pools the information from numerous models (base learners). With the help of GAs, we may assemble neural network ensembles that are both varied and effective. Through a process of selection and combining, the GA maintains a population of diverse neural network configurations to build ensembles that outperform individual models.

Optimizing the knowledge transfer using one neural network to another (transfer learning) and selecting relevant features from high-dimensional data (feature selection) are two applications of Genetic Algorithms. In order to improve DNNs' generalization potential on a given task, the GA might evolve transfer learning techniques or feature selection subsets. When DNNs and GAs are combined, performance, convergence, and generalization may all be increased, even for difficult jobs. It is important to note, nevertheless, that this hybrid strategy may be more computationally costly and call for fine-tuning of parameters to attain best results. The success of the hybrid method additionally hinges on the problem's specifics and the skillful combination of DNNs and GAs to supplement one another.

4.9 FIREFLY ALGORITHMS

Optimization methods inspired by firefly behavior in attracting a mate are known as Firefly Algorithms (FA). Several medical optimization issues, such as diabetic retinopathy diagnosis and therapy, have benefited from the use of these techniques. Accurate diagnosis of diabetic retinopathy is aided by FA's ability to help identify the most important characteristics from retinal pictures. The approach aids in the enhancement of categorization model performance by optimizing feature selection. Variables of prediction models used to foretell the development of diabetic retinopathy in patients can be optimized using Firefly Algorithms. This allows doctors to foresee the progression of the disease and make necessary adjustments to treatment. Diabetic retinopathy may be diagnosed from retinal pictures, and FA can help optimize the variables of machine learning or deep learning models. FA improves the precision and consistency of a model by adjusting its parameters.

4.10 RESULTS AND DISCUSSION

Here, we'll go over the measures that were utilized to verify and assess the efficiency of the proposed network. To provide robust and reliable performance evaluation of the network, a five-fold cross-validation approach was used. The dataset was split in half, with each half having 950 photos, for five-fold cross-validation purposes. To reduce bias and overfitting, the dataset has been split into five groups for analysis. The model is trained and then tested repeatedly on new configurations of folds. Several measures were used to analyze the effectiveness of the proposed network. Each of these indicators sheds light on a unique facet of the model's efficiency. Area under the receiver operating characteristic curve (AUC-ROC), accuracy, precision, recall, and F1-score are frequently employed as assessment measures. Accuracy quantifies the rate at which occurrences are accurately labeled. Precision measures how successfully a model avoids false positives by quantifying the fraction of real positive predictions among all positive predictions. The research guarantees a thorough evaluation of the proposed network's performance on a wide variety of data subsets by using these evaluation criteria in conjunction with five-fold cross-validation. This method verifies the network's efficiency and applicability in picture classification. This leads to the following definition of validation precision:

$$Accuracy = \frac{TP_{os} + TN_{eg}}{TP_{os} + FP_{os} + TN_{eg} + FN_{eg}}$$

Within the bounds of a certain class C:

True Positive (TP_{os}): This stands for all occurrences where a picture from category C is accurately labeled as belonging to that category.

False Positive (FP_{os}): This describes situations where a picture does not fit in category C but is yet given that label.

True Negative (TN_{eg}): In these cases, the classification of a non-C picture as non-C was accurate.

False Negative (FN_{eg}): This represents situations in which a picture that belongs in category C was mistakenly assigned to another category.

$$Sensitivity = \frac{TP_{os}}{TP_{os} + FN_{eg}}$$

$$Specificity = \frac{TN_{eg}}{TN_{eg} + FP_{os}}$$

Class-specific sensitivity and specificity are averaged out to determine the classifier's overall performance. Using a confusion matrix displayed in tabular form, the suggested classifier's performance is assessed. Images with those expected labels in each row and those with those actual labels in each column have been tabulated in this matrix. Images where the predicted label matches the actual label are tallied and shown in a table. The ability of the classifier to distinguish between classes is often assessed by drawing a receiver operating characteristic (ROC) curve. The trade-off between sensitivity and specificity (how often a test detects genuine positives) for a given range of threshold values is graphically represented by this curve.

Determine the classifier's discriminatory power using its area under the receiver operating characteristic (AUC). The AUC of a better classifier is an indicator of its capacity to differentiate between different types of sickness. A variety of criteria, such as sensitivity, specificity, and the ability to distinguish between groups, are crucial for accurate disease classification, and all of the aforementioned may be evaluated.

4.11 EXPERIMENTAL RESULTS

The learning rate was set to 10–3, and the proposed model was trained on the Kaggle dataset for 10 epochs, as described earlier. The dataset was split into five folds before the model training so that five-fold cross-validation could be utilized to check the accuracy of the trained model. Subsequently, 64 fundus pictures were grouped together in each of these folds. The computational complexity of training procedures was reduced by splitting the work into batches. Rather than using gradient descent on the complete training set, we used stochastic gradient descent (SGD) to train the model over the batches. The suggested model was trained with an excellent accuracy of 98.14%. Confusion matrix results from using five-fold cross-validation are depicted in Table 4.1 and Figure 4.5. What this means is that the classifier can tell the difference between subjects in classes when the labels vary greatly. These methods of training and verifying the model's accuracy in categorization and suitability for clinical use provide evidence for the model's efficacy and resilience.

Table 4.2 summarizes the results of several different models on a categorization job. Accuracy, sensitivity, precision, and F1-score are compared among models in Figures 4.6, 4.7, 4.8, and 4.9. With an accuracy of 0.91, AlexNet's forecasts are highly accurate. A recall (sensitivity) of 0.89 indicates that true positives are being effectively identified. The positive predictions made with a precision of 0.92 are likely to be accurate. With an F1-score of 0.90, accuracy and recall are both optimal. GoogLeNet achieves a fair degree of correctness with an accuracy of 0.89. With a sensitivity of 0.88, accurate identification has been achieved. The rate of accuracy in making correct positive predictions is 0.88. The 0.89 F1-score represents an optimal balance between accuracy and recall. With an accuracy of 0.90, ANN (Artificial Neural Network) shows impressive precision. The sensitivity is as high as 0.91, indicating accurate positive identification. When the precision is 0.91, it's safe to make optimistic forecasts. The F1-score of 0.90 represents a good compromise between accuracy and recall. With an overall accuracy of 0.91, CNN (Convolutional Neural Network) performs admirably. A sensitivity of 0.90 indicates that correct identifications have

---

TABLE 4.1

The Effects of Five-Fold Cross-Validation on the Confusion Matrix

	No DR	Severe DR
No DR	479	7
Severe DR	4	378

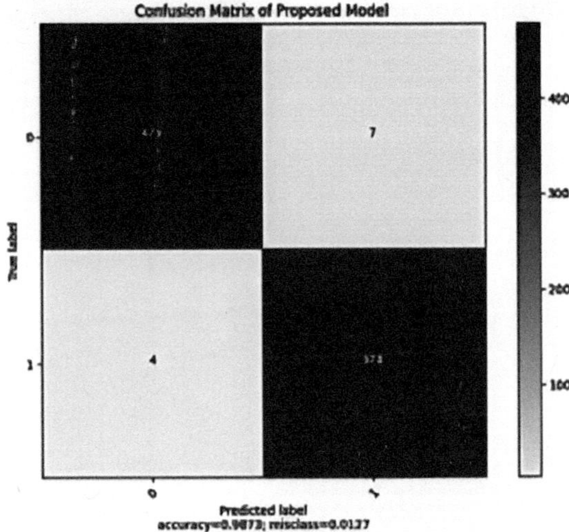

FIGURE 4.5 Confusion matrix of proposed model.

TABLE 4.2

Model Comparisons for Overall Performance

Model	Accuracy	Sensitivity	Precision	F1-Score
AlexNet	0.91	0.89	0.92	0.90
GoogLeNet	0.89	0.88	0.88	0.89
ANN	0.90	0.91	0.91	0.90
CNN	0.91	0.90	0.90	0.90
Inception	0.93	0.92	0.92	0.92
LSTM	0.94	0.90	0.92	0.95
Proposed Model	0.98	0.95	0.97	0.98

been made. The accuracy of our optimistic forecasts reaches an impressive 0.90. An F1-score of 0.90 is a good compromise between accuracy and recall. With a precision of 0.93, Inception has an exceptional degree of precision. A sensitivity of 0.92 indicates a high probability of a correct identification. The accuracy of 0.92 means that positive predictions may be made with confidence. An F1-score of 0.92 indicates that accuracy and recall are being used in tandem. When compared to other methods, LSTM's (Long Short-Term Memory) 0.94 accuracy stands out. When sensitivity is at 0.90, it means that the system is able to effectively recognize true positives. A positive predictive accuracy of 0.92 implies high precision. With an F1-score of 0.95, accuracy and recall are equally well-balanced. The proposed model has a higher accuracy than any other method we have tested (0.98). When used for positive identification, a sensitivity of 0.95 indicates a high degree of efficiency. With a precision of 0.97, we may be confident in our ability to make accurate forecasts. All indicators

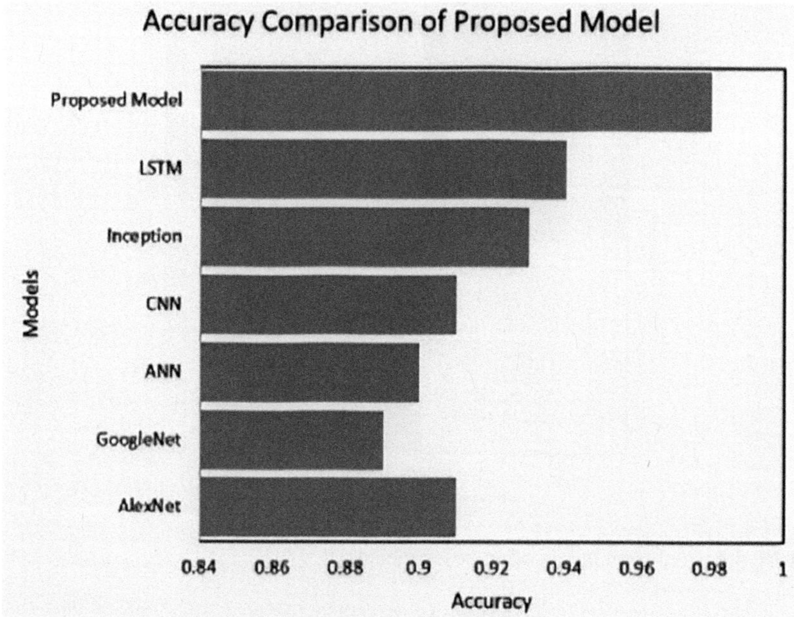

FIGURE 4.6 Model accuracy comparisons.

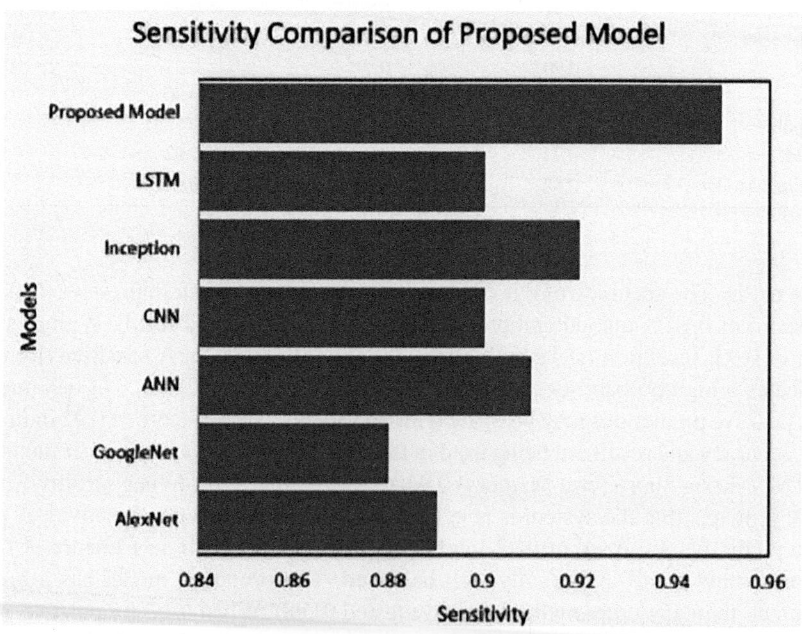

FIGURE 4.7 Analysis of model sensitivity.

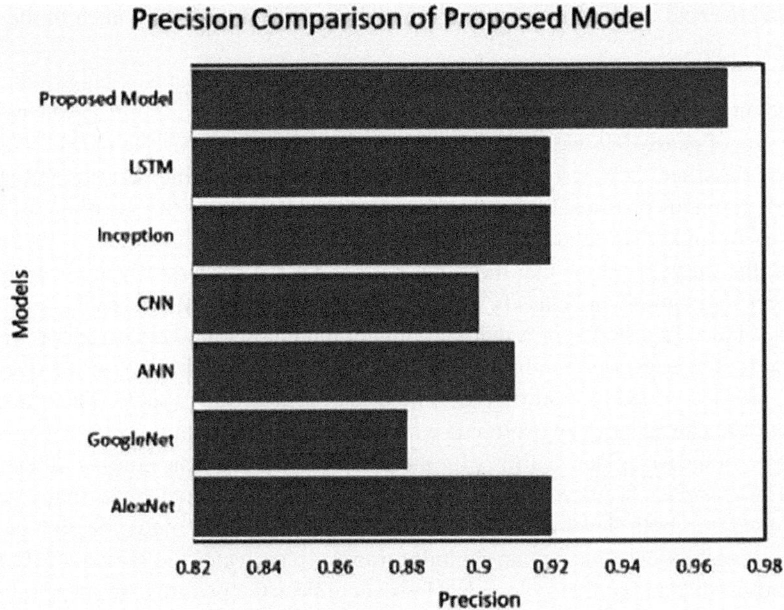

FIGURE 4.8 The precision of model comparisons.

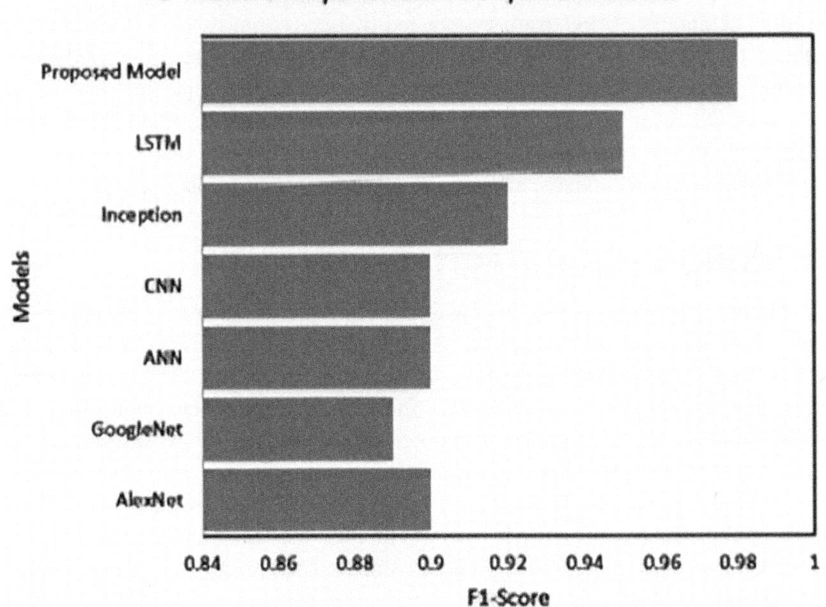

FIGURE 4.9 Model evaluation using the F1-score.

of effectiveness point to the proposed model's outstanding performance in the classification job.

When using a threshold of, the ROC curve for the model that was suggested using 5-fold and 10-fold cross-validation is shown in Figure 4.10. An impressive true positive rate of nearly 0.9 was attained, despite a low false positive rate of 0.1. The suggested classifier shows promise for application in differentiating between DR stages based on fundus pictures, with an AUC of 0.95 and 0.91, respectively, when 5-fold as well as 10-fold cross-validation is used.

In this study, we show that the suggested model can successfully analyze fundus pictures to diagnose and classify DR. The diagnostic accuracy, sensitivity, and specificity of the suggested approach are all higher than those of other current pretrained methods. The suggested method not only achieves excellent diagnostic accuracy but also excels in properly grading DR, which is of critical importance. There are two major obstacles that can be overcome with automated DR grading in clinical ophthalmology. In the first place, it allows for the possibility of real-time grading of telemedicine fundus photos. Access to specialist eye treatment is a problem for many people worldwide, in both developed and developing countries. Telemedicine applications that utilize fundus cameras can digitally transfer pictures of the retinas of diabetes patients to distant ophthalmologists. However, unless the pictures are interpreted by a specialist, the communication of a diagnosis is delayed. Theoretically, our suggested technology may deliver a diagnosis at the moment of image collection, providing patients and local healthcare providers with instantaneous insights. This has the ability to greatly reduce the need for time and effort. Second, examining physicians' manual DR grading in clinics may be inconsistent and inaccurate. Multiple studies provide a range of 0.62–0.87 for assessing inter-observer consistency in DR. In contrast, the DR diagnoses and grades produced by our system vastly outperform those produced by humans, who are prone to making mistakes. The suggested method overcomes these restrictions by facilitating precise diagnosis and quantitative measurement of DR severity, hence increasing people's access to treatment. Furthermore, it enables doctors to objectively compare the development of a disease and the efficacy of treatment across visits, allowing them to fine-tune medical actions.

4.12   CONCLUSION AND FUTURE WORK

By combining Deep Neural Networks with Genetic Algorithms and Firefly Algorithms, we introduce a unique and powerful learning principle called DGFM in this study. The first step is to normalize the raw dataset using the Standard Scalar technique. Then, a genetic algorithm is used to zero in on the most pertinent data points in the dataset. Dimensionality reduction is another area where the Firefly Algorithm helps out. For further categorization, the reduced dataset is loaded into a Deep Neural Network Model. On the freely accessible Kaggle EyePACS dataset, the DGFM model is shown to be effective. The model had the greatest classification accuracy of all the approaches we looked at, at 98.14%. These combined efforts demonstrate how DGFM may be used to great effect in normalization, feature extraction, dimensionality reduction, and classification applications. Without a large enough training dataset, a model won't be able to extract the characteristics it needs to correctly categorize fresh data.

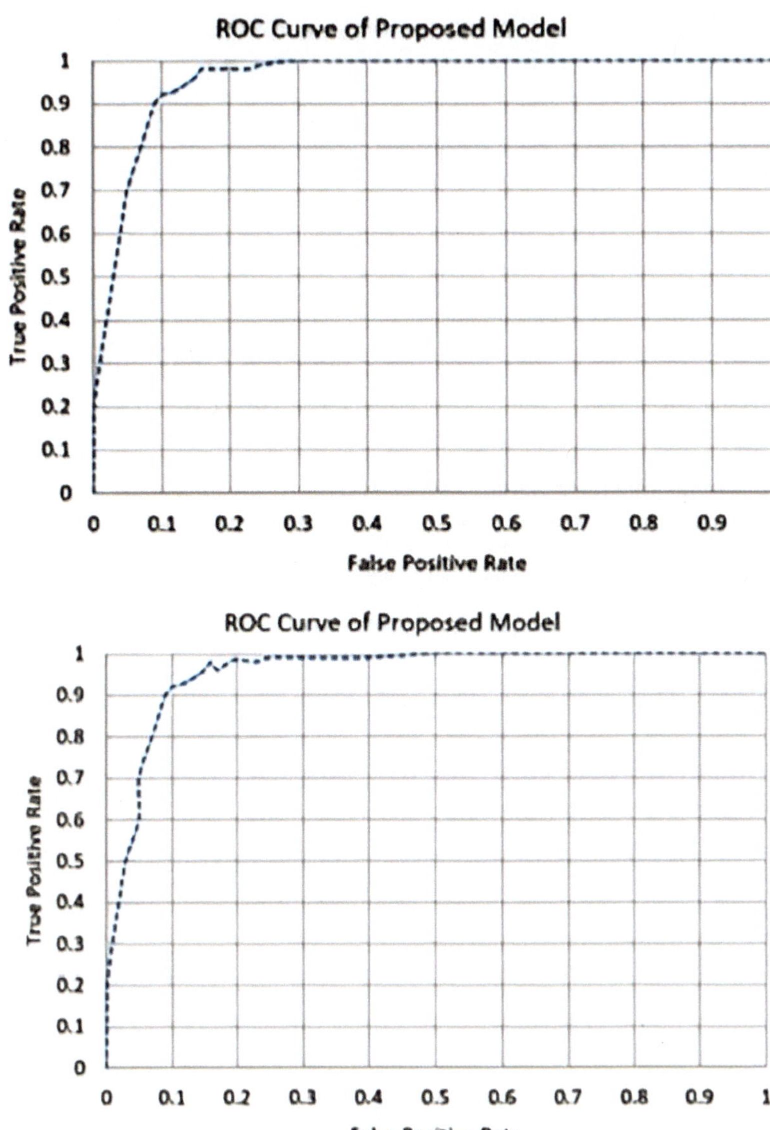

FIGURE 4.10 ROC plot for the model suggested if (a) 5-fold cross-validation (b) 10-fold cross-validation

Class-specific data augmentation, together with 5- and 10-fold cross-validation, was utilized to lessen the likelihood of overfitting and produce a more objective evaluation of the small dataset we had available. In the future, we want to train pictures from a variety of modalities using the suggested ensemble CNN model, which should significantly increase the accuracy of the proposed technique.

REFERENCES

[1] I. Giroti, J. K. A. Das, N. M. Harshith and G. Thahniyath, "Diabetic Retinopathy Detection & Classification using Efficient Net Model," 2023 International Conference on Artificial Intelligence and Applications (ICAIA) Alliance Technology Conference (ATCON-1), Bangalore, India, 2023, pp. 1–6, doi: 10.1109/ICAIA57370.2023.10169756.

[2] A. T. Nair, L. Anitha M. and M. N. Arun Kumar, "Disease Grading of Diabetic Retinopathy using Deep Learning Techniques," 2022 6th International Conference on Computing Methodologies and Communication (ICCMC), Erode, India, 2022, pp. 1019–1024, doi: 10.1109/ICCMC53470.2022.9754113.

[3] D. R. Raman, S. Nishanthi and P. Babysha, "Diagnosis of Diabetic Retinopathy by using EfficientNet-B7 CNN Architecture in Deep Learning," 2023 International Conference on Sustainable Computing and Smart Systems (ICSCSS), Coimbatore, India, 2023, pp. 430–435, doi: 10.1109/ICSCSS57650.2023.10169453.

[4] S. Valarmathi and R. Vijaybhanu, "A Survey on Diabetic Retinopathy Disease Detection and Classification Using Deep Learning Techniques," 2021 Seventh International Conference on Bio Signals, Images, and Instrumentation (ICBSII), Chennai, India, 2021, pp. 1–4, doi: 10.1109/ICBSII51839.2021.9445163.

[5] H. Jiang et al., "A Multi-Label Deep Learning Model with Interpretable Grad-CAM for Diabetic Retinopathy Classification," 2020 42nd Annual International Conference of the IEEE Engineering in Medicine & Biology Society (EMBC), Montreal, QC, Canada, 2020, pp. 1560–1563, doi: 10.1109/EMBC44109.2020.9175884.

[6] P. L. Jancy and B. Latha, "Deep Learning Techniques for Diabetic Retinopathy Diagnosis using Optical Coherence Tomography: A Review," 2022 International Conference on Advanced Computing Technologies and Applications (ICACTA), Coimbatore, India, 2022, pp. 1–4, doi: 10.1109/ICACTA54488.2022.9753418.

[7] S. Joshi, R. Kumar, P. K. Rai and S. Garg, "Diabetic Retinopathy Using Deep Learning," 2023 International Conference on Computational Intelligence and Sustainable Engineering Solutions (CISES), Greater Noida, India, 2023, pp. 145–149, doi: 10.1109/CISES58720.2023.10183562.

[8] P. Patra and T. Singh, "Diabetic Retinopathy Detection using an Improved ResNet50-InceptionV3 Structure," 2022 13th International Conference on Computing Communication and Networking Technologies (ICCCNT), Kharagpur, India, 2022, pp. 1–6, doi: 10.1109/ICCCNT54827.2022.9984253.

[9] A. Lands, A. J. Kottarathil, A. Biju, E. M. Jacob and S. Thomas, "Implementation of Deep Learning Based Algorithms for Diabetic Retinopathy Classification from Fundus Images," 2020 4th International Conference on Trends in Electronics and Informatics (ICOEI)(48184), Tirunelveli, India, 2020, pp. 1028–1032, doi: 10.1109/ICOEI48184.2020.9142878.

[10] Atul and S. Dhingra, "Classification of Diabetic Retinopathy Disease with Improved Transfer Learning Techniques using EfficientNets," 2022 10th International Conference on Reliability, Infocom Technologies and Optimization (Trends and Future Directions) (ICRITO), Noida, India, 2022, pp. 1–5, doi: 10.1109/ICRITO56286.2022.9965087.

[11] www.kaggle.com/datasets/eishkaran/diabetes-using-retinopathy-prediction Accessed on 12th June 2023

5 Liver Tumour Detection Using Machine Learning Techniques
A Systematic Review

Amrita Leima Singha and Khwairakpam Amitab

5.1 INTRODUCTION

An irregular expansion of tissue resulting from the rapid growth of cells is termed as tumour. These cells have no biological importance in the overall development of the human body. Tumours can be broadly classified into two categories: cancerous and non-cancerous. Liver cancer is common and life-threatening; it is essential to diagnose the disease accurately. There are different techniques for primary disease detection—clinically in the laboratory by imaging tests such as ultrasound, magnetic resonance imaging (MRI), and computed tomography (CT) scans (Almotairi et al., 2020). Generally, CT scan is preferred for the identification of liver tumours. It brings forth the 3D view of the abdomen, making it convenient to determine the exact location of tumour, its size, and the impact of the tumour on surrounding tissues (Gao et al., 2021). Contrast-enhanced CT (CECT) images are also often employed for diagnosing liver disease, but still, it is challenging because the difference in contrast between healthy and unhealthy parts of the organ is low. Furthermore, variations in contrast enhancement within the tumour area during CECT can occasionally be concealed by the contrast itself, potentially leading to uncertain assessments. This necessitates the development of a Computer-Aided Diagnosis (CAD) of liver diseases (Balagourouchetty et al., 2019). CAD employing texture information like grey level is also not accurate because the different abdomen disorders like tumours, cysts, or calculi are all delineated by grey level intensities. This might lead to confusion in identifying the correct disease (Sethi and Saini, 2016).

Machine learning (ML) is a subset of Artificial Intelligence (AI). ML models are intelligent and capable of learning from data. The model learns the patterns and relationships in the data during training and applies the knowledge gained on the testing data to predict the result. There are two types of ML: supervised and unsupervised. Supervised learning uses labelled data, which consists of labelled output and the corresponding input data. Common supervised learning techniques include linear regression, logistic regression, decision trees, k-nearest neighbour, support vector machine (SVM), random forest (RF), naive Bayes classification, and gradient

DOI: 10.1201/9781032635149-5

boosting. Unsupervised learning uses unlabelled data for training, which consists of only input data. It is used when the objective is to analyse the data with inferred information about it. Popular unsupervised learning techniques include k-means clustering and principal component analysis (PCA). Unlike conventional statistical methods based on hypothesis to derive the result, ML approaches do not use hypothesis-based methods for solving clinical problems. Hence, when applied to large datasets, ML models can analyse and find hidden patterns. This advantage makes ML-based methods more adequate and structured for diagnosing liver tumours. A subset of ML, deep learning (DL), is the state-of-the-art image detection, classification, and segmentation technique. DL is a neural network with multiple layers. The DL technique, such as convolutional neural networks (CNN), can learn the features, making it distinctively different from other AI techniques (Su et al., 2021).

The research articles considered in this systematic review were collected from the Web of Science (WoS) database (Clarivate, 2022). The query "TS = ((diagnosis OR detect* OR classif*) AND liver AND (tumour OR malignant) AND (CT OR computed tomography) AND (machine learning OR deep learning OR *net))" and Keywords: diagnosis, detect, classification, liver, tumour, malignant, CT, computed tomography, machine learning, deep learning were used to search the articles related to our topic in WoS database. The search result includes articles published till 30 March 2023. We applied PRISMA checklist 2020 (PRISMA, 2021) to select the relevant articles for the review. PRISMA aims to present a systematic and transparent analysis of the existing literature on the topic of research by following a predetermined set of criteria and methodology outlined in the PRISMA guidelines. The WoS search returned 50 articles. Only 33 articles were selected based on the PRISMA checklist, such as title, abstract, objectives, methods, results, relevance, clarity, completeness, methodology, originality, and contribution. Of the selected articles, 11 were review articles, and 22 were research articles.

Zhou et al. (2019) presented a review of AI applications in liver disease detection using medical imaging data. The authors highlighted AI's applications in medicines, including detecting and analysing focal liver lesions, facilitating treatment, and projecting treatment response. Nayantara et al. (2020) analysed different CAD systems for identifying benign and malignant lesions in CT images. Articles published from 1998 to 2000 were considered in their study, focusing on conventional and DL techniques for liver lesion detection. Wang et al. (2021) reviewed 125 research articles based on publication year, publication type, title and abstract, imaging modalities, and CAD approaches. It was observed that ML and DL techniques perform better than conventional techniques. Fahmy et al. (2022) reviewed the application of radiomics and AI to detect, segment, and manage Hepatocellular Carcinoma (HCC). The authors highlighted the capability of AI in the preoperative imaging of HCC. Feng et al. (2021) outlined the challenges encountered in the prior studies and future prospects for HCC diagnosis in medical images. Liu et al. (2021) reviewed AI techniques for detecting hepatitis, bringing forth its future scope and limitations. Xiang et al. (2021) evaluated the DL techniques for detecting liver disease based on imaging and the future prospects of DL. Survarachakan et al. (2022) also analysed DL models for liver, vessel, and lesion segmentation, classification of HCC, and metastatic cancer. It was observed that hybrid and ensembled techniques are more suitable for segmentation and combined methods for classification and detection. Azer (2019) evaluated the application of CNNs for detecting HCC and liver masses. It was observed that CNN showed better accuracy in the segmentation and classification of liver cancer. Rompianesi et al. (2022) reviewed AI-based techniques that include ML and DL for identifying colorectal cancer liver metastases (CRLM) patients. The authors observe that analysis of radiomics features based on ML and AI will be useful in predicting CRLM. Wei et al. (2020) discussed the importance of radiomics in liver disease treatment, like identifying and staging tumours, highlighting the limitations and future scope.

Few review papers are not systematic and have not mentioned how the research articles were selected in their study (Zhou et al., 2019; Nayantara et al., 2020; Wang et al., 2021; Fahmy et al., 2022; Feng et al., 2021; Liu et al., 2021; Xiang et al., 2021; Survarachakan et al., 2022; Azer, 2019; Rompianesi et al., 2022; Wei et al., 2020). Some review paper focuses on specific AI techniques (Survarachakan et al., 2022). Technologies are evolving rapidly, and better ML models are being introduced to detect liver tumours each passing day. The expeditious increase in the number of cancer cases and related deaths. Yu et al. (2021) necessitates an early solution for this. The recent advancement of ML in liver tumour detection has motivated us to review the existing literature on liver tumour detection using ML techniques. The review article includes recently published traditional, hybrid, ensemble, and deep learning techniques for liver tumour detection. This review will give an idea about the dataset, ML techniques, performance evaluation criteria, and other relevant information required in detecting liver tumour, which will help new researchers who wish to work in medical image analysis.

The rest of the chapter is organized as follows: Section 5.2 will explain the steps in liver tumour detection and summarize the work done by researchers. Section 5.3 discusses our observation of existing literature on liver tumour detection, and the chapter is concluded in Section 5.4 by presenting future work.

5.2 LIVER TUMOUR DETECTION

The detection of liver tumour using ML techniques involves several steps. The commonly used steps are as follows:

5.2.1 DATA COLLECTION

The first stage of liver tumour detection is medical imaging. Key imaging modalities include ultrasound, CT scans, MRI, and positron emission tomography (PET). The choice of imaging modality depends on factors such as the patient's clinical history, the type of tumour suspected, and the availability of imaging resources. Generally, CT imaging is the preferred modality. In CT images anatomy of the liver, tumour location, size, shape, and texture are visible. In addition, the images have high resolution, and movement due to respiratory gas does not affect the image quality. Researchers Zhou et al. (2019), Zhang et al. (2020), and Li et al. (2018) have used CT images. Li et al. (2018) conducted localization of tumours. There are few publicly available CT image datasets for liver tumour detection, which many researchers use for segmentation, classification, and detection. The Liver Tumour Segmentation (LiTS) benchmark dataset contains 201 CT images of the abdomen acquired from different patients, of which 194 CT scans consist of lesions and the rest are healthy liver (Bilic et al., 2023). Expert radiologists have carefully annotated by outlining the boundaries of the liver and any tumours within each CT scan. These annotations serve as ground truth data for training and evaluating ML algorithms. Another standard dataset many researchers employ is 3Dircadb. Yu et al. (2021), Devi and Seenivasagam (2020), Almotairi et al. (2020), and Li et al. (2018) have employed 3Dircadb in their work. 3Dircadb contains CT scans of 10 women and 10 men; 75% of the dataset is of patients with hepatic tumours. Researchers have also collected CT images from different hospitals and diagnostic centres (Balagourouchetty et al., 2019; Das et al., 2019; Yasaka et al., 2018; Zhang et al., 2021a; Hussain et al., 2022). Researchers use the dataset to train the ML models, benchmark their algorithms, and compare results. The dataset remains a valuable resource for researchers and medical professionals.

5.2.2 PRE-PROCESSING

After the dataset is acquired, pre-processing is the next significant step. The objective is to enhance the quality of the images by removing unwanted noise, contrast enhancement, sharpening, etc. Zhu et al. (2016) implemented Gaussian filtering and anisotropic diffusion for noise reduction and histogram equalization to normalize the intensity of the abdomen organs and contrast enhancement. Normalization is essential as the CT images are quite different from each other. Rela et al. (2023) have used histogram equalization for contrast enhancement and median filtering. Yu et al. (2021) applied Gaussian noise filtering, histogram equalization, and normalization. Zhang et al. (2021b) truncated the CT image in the range [-150, 250] Hounsfield unit (HU) scale, intending to eliminate irrelevant artefacts. Li et al. (2018) truncated the intensity values in the range [-200, 250] HU, Aslam et al. (2021) also applied [-100, 400] HU. Yu et al. (2021) used Gaussian filtering to reduce the noise, followed by histogram equalization to enhance the presentation of features, and normalization was also employed. Vorontsov et al. (2017) used principal component analysis whitening to pre-process images. Das et al. (2019) employed a guided filter for sharpening the edges of the liver. Hussain et al. (2022) converted the CT images to grayscale. The conversion reduces the computational cost and simplifies the algorithm. Training the supervised DL techniques requires a large dataset, and a sufficient dataset may not be available. Many researchers have used data augmentation to increase the dataset and data balancing (Aslam et al., 2021; Du et al., 2022; Li et al., 2018). Data augmentation is a technique to artificially increase the size and diversity of a dataset by applying various transformations and modifications to the existing data. The data augmentation can avoid overfitting and underfitting, increasing the overall prediction accuracy. Augmentation also makes the DL model more robust to noise, enlarging, rotation, and shift (Yasaka et al., 2018); Zhang et al. (2021a) have used data augmentation and normalization as pre-processing. The pre-processing technique depends on the specific goal and the characteristics of the input data.

5.2.3 Segmentation

Segmentation separates the liver or lesion from the abdomen CT; it decreases the complexity of the images and increases the classification accuracy. In the quantitative analysis of medical images, organ and substructure segmentation is the first step of the computerized detection process. Various techniques and algorithms have been developed for liver and lesion segmentation in CT images. Some popular liver and tumour segmentation techniques include thresholding, region growing, watershed, and DL techniques. Thresholding-based methods are simple yet effective techniques. It works by defining an intensity threshold value and classifying pixels in the image based on their intensity values. Jose et al. (2022) employed adaptive thresholding for liver segmentation. Region growing is a similarity-based segmentation technique. Adjacent pixels with similar intensities are grouped into regions or objects. Zhang et al. (2020) used 2D UNet for liver segmentation. Devi and Seenivasagam (2020) used region growing to segment liver from abdomen CT image. Balagourouchetty et al. (2019) segmented the liver lesions by region growing, region merging, and dynamic gradient thresholding. Sethi and Saini (2016) combined region growing with edge-based and thresholding techniques. Watershed segmentation works efficiently when the objects in the images are touching or overlapped. It simulates a flooding process from markers, creating boundaries where objects meet. Das et al. (2019) used the watershed segmentation technique to separate the liver from other organs, and the Gaussian mixture model segmented the cancerous lesion. Sethi and Saini (2016) used edge-based active contour models for segmenting the liver. Li et al. (2018) used H-DenseUNet for liver and tumour segmentation.

Supervised deep learning techniques have recently gained popularity in segmenting liver and lesions. Supervised techniques require a large amount of training data. The LiTS and 3Dircadb datasets are popular amongst researchers. Zhang et al. (2020) have used 2D U-net to extract the liver, and 3D FCN to segment liver tumour within the liver. Meddeb et al. (2022) have used a modified U-Net architecture to segment the spleen. Rela et al. (2023) segmented liver by adaptive thresholding and modified U-Net for segmenting tumours. Li et al. (2018) proposed a hybrid densely connected U-Net (H- DenseUNet). Yu et al. (2021) improved U-Net by introducing residual learning and multi-scale fusion (DResUNet) for liver tumour segmentation. Almotairi et al. (2020) adapted SegNet, a popular semantic segmentation architecture for the segmentation of road scenes in segmenting liver from CT images. Aslam et al. (2021) combined ResNet and U-net (ResUNet). Xue et al. (2021) applied V-Net to extract liver contours. Zhang et al. (2021b) proposed a DL-based interactive method (DeepRecS) for liver tumour segmentation.

Segmentation helps classifiers focus on discriminating between objects or regions of interest, improves feature extraction, and provides valuable contextual information. Most DL segmentation techniques have an accuracy of over 90% Almotairi et al. (2020), and U-Net is the most popular. Overfitting is one of the major concerns for segmentation algorithms. The ensemble strategy can alleviate overfitting problem (Zhu et al., 2016).

5.2.4 Feature Extraction and Selection

Feature extraction aims to capture relevant information from images. The choice of feature extraction technique depends on the specific task and data characteristics.

Radiomic refers to the extraction of a large number of features from medical images for use by ML classifiers. CT radiomic features can be used to differentiate tumours from other liver tissue. Feature selection reduces the dimension of the data by eliminating the less important features, which enhances the performance of ML algorithms designed for tumour detection. Hussain et al. (2022) have used histogram, texture, binary and rotational, scalability, and translational features. The correlation-based feature selection (CFS) technique was used, stating that CFS is better than principal component analysis. Sethi and Saini (2016) have extracted grey-level co-occurrence matrices (GLCM), discrete wavelet transform (DWT), and discrete curvelet transform (DCT) features from abdominal CT images. The optimum features were selected using a genetic algorithm (GA). Shaker et al. (2021) collected several features from CT images, and important features were selected using a statistical t-test for further evaluation. Rela et al. (2023) have extracted GLCM, GRLM, LTP, LBP, and shape features such as area, perimeter, and label-connected components. A new feature selection algorithm named GW-CTO was developed for use by neural network classifiers. Explicit feature extraction and selection are optional. DL techniques like CNN do not require feature extraction and selection because they can learn the important features during training. Du et al. (2022) compared the DL-based automatic feature learning model and SVM models that require radiomics feature selection, the authors found that the SMV classifier with radiomic features is more accurate.

5.2.5 Classification

Selected features are provided as input to the classifier for identifying the CT image of the patients as tumour or healthy. The classifiers are trained on the training data and validated on testing data. Researchers have used different ML-classifiers to detect liver tumours. Zhang et al. (2020) have detected the probabilistic distribution of the liver tumour using unsupervised fuzzy c-means clustering (FCM). Unsupervised FCM is useful when the labelled or ground truth training data is unavailable. Devi and Seenivasagam (2020) used support vector machines to classify liver tumours into three types: benign, malignant, and normal. Gao et al. (2021) used DL model integrated with Spatial Extractor-Temporal Encoder-Integration Classifier (STIC) for detecting hepatocellular carcinoma and intrahepatic cholangiocarcinoma. Balagourouchetty et al. (2019) used an ensemble FCNet classifier to classify liver lesions into six classes: normal, hepatocellular carcinoma, hemangioma, cyst, abscess, and liver metastasis. Ensemble FCNet is a deep neural network structured with three fully connected layers. Li et al. (2023) used Multi-Layer Perceptron (MLP) for examining the outer surface of the lung and liver to track tumour. MLP is a neural network composed of numerous interconnected layers. MLP consists of an input, hidden, and output layer. Each node of MLP uses an activation function to weigh inputs. Su et al. (2021) observed that AI can recognize and may even discover contemporary data on liver tumours, which radiologists may miss. AI has human-like problem-solving capabilities and can make decisions. Das et al. (2019) used a deep neural network classifier to classify liver cancer into hemangioma, hepatocellular carcinoma, and metastatic carcinoma (MET). The deep neural network has numerous hidden layers and can solve complex ML tasks. Yasaka et al. (2018) used CNN to differentiate hepatocellular carcinoma and non-HCC from liver lesions, hemangiomas, and cysts. Sethi and Saini (2016) used ANN to classify diseases of the abdomen. Zhu et al. (2016) used data and feature mixed ensemble-based extreme learning machine (DFEN-ELM) for one-class and two-class tumour detection. Extreme Learning Machines (ELM) is a single-hidden layer feed-forward neural network (Zhu et al., 2016). Hussain et al. (2022) employed random forest, J48, Logistic Model Tree (LMT), and Random Tree (RT) with numerous features for classification of multiclass liver tumours. RF and RT outperformed J48 and LMT. Random Forest is a machine learning technique that builds numerous decision trees during the training step and integrates their predictions to upgrade the overall accuracy and decrease overfitting. The random tree is a single decision tree where randomization techniques like feature selection or bootstrap sampling are employed to construct the tree. J48 is a decision tree technique used in classification tasks. LMT integrates decision trees and logistic regression techniques for classification tasks. Rela et al. (2023) used Hyperparameter-tuned Improved Deep Neural Network (HI-DNN) for liver tumour detection in CT images. HI-DNN hyperparameters are optimized for boosting performance, including learning rates, batch sizes, and layer configurations. Aslam et al. (2021) used ResUNet, which is a hybrid model constructed from UNet and ResNet architectures for liver tumour detection. ResUNet is an emerging deep learning technique created from U-Net and residual networks (ResNets). It is evident that deep learning techniques are gaining popularity and have achieved very high classification accuracy.

5.2.6 PERFORMANCE EVALUATION

Performance validation is conducted to check the feasibility of the classifier. Evaluating the ML model to claim superiority and suitability for clinical application is important. For evaluating liver and tumour segmentation techniques, dice similarity coefficient, volumetric overlap error, relative volume difference, and symmetric surface distance are commonly used by Zhang et al. (2020), Yu et al. (2021), and Vorontsov et al. (2017). To evaluate classification algorithms, accuracy Eq. (5.1), Tanimoto coefficient Eq. (5.2), and dice coefficient Eq. (5.3), area under the receiver operating characteristic curve (AUC), sensitivity Eq. (5.4), and specificity Eq. (5.5) are used (Li et al., 2023; Das et al., 2019; Devi and Seenivasagam, 2020). The accuracy Eq. (5.1) is widely accepted by many researchers.

$$Accuracy = \frac{TP + FN}{TP + TN + FP + FN} \tag{5.1}$$

$$Tanimoto\ coefficient = \frac{|TP|}{|TP| + |FP| + |FN|} \tag{5.2}$$

$$Dice\ coefficient = \frac{2 \times |TP|}{|TP| + |FP| + |FN|} \tag{5.3}$$

$$Sensitivity = \frac{TP}{TP + FN} \tag{5.4}$$

$$Specificity = \frac{TN}{TN + FP} \tag{5.5}$$

where TN, TP, FN, and FP are the true negative, true positive, false negative, and false positive, respectively. Zhang et al. (2020) designed 2DUNet + 3DFCN and achieved a dice global score of 96.7% for liver segmentation and 84.1% for tumour segmentation. Yu et al. (2021) designed DResUNet and achieved 96.5% for liver segmentation and 67.2% for tumour segmentation. Das et al. (2019) designed watershed Gaussian-based deep learning technique and achieved a classification accuracy of 99.38% and a Jaccard index of 98.18%. SVM classifier designed by Devi and Seenivasagam (2020) achieved 98.6% accuracy in categorizing liver lesions. Balagourouchetty et al. (2019) used Googlenet–LReLU transfer learning and could achieve 97.37% accuracy. Das et al. (2019) proposed deep CNN model with 99% accuracy. Li et al. (2018) designed DenseUNet for liver and tumour segmentation and achieved a dice global score of 96.5% for liver segmentation and 82.4% for tumour segmentation. It is evident from the results presented by researchers that the deep learning approaches are state-of-the-art in detecting and classifying liver tumours.

It is to be noted that the steps of liver tumour detection are different according to the machine learning technique employed. For example, CNN does not require feature extraction and selection, as the features are learned automatically.

5.3 DISCUSSION

Medical imaging has become an increasingly predominant approach in detecting liver tumours. Currently, the ML techniques used in liver tumour detection are highly advanced. This section will reflect on the dataset, preprocessing, segmentation, and classification techniques for liver tumour detection.

Modern ML models such as DL require a large dataset, and the unavailability of large datasets for training and validation of ML models is the major hurdle in achieving reliable results. Few datasets like LiTS Zhou et al. (2019); Li et al. (2018); 3Dircadb Li et al. (2018); Aslam et al. (2021) are publicly available. Several researchers have also used clinical datasets (Gao et al., 2021; Vorontsov et al., 2017). Developing a large dataset containing thousands of labelled CT images of healthy and cancerous patients in different age groups will help researchers develop more accurate and reliable ML-based CAD systems.

Most ML-based CAD systems for liver tumour detection apply pre-processing techniques like data augmentation and normalization. Medical images are affected by noise, which may distort the details in the images. Therefore, applying de-noising technique is considered an essential pre-processing technique. Researchers have also attempted to increase the resolution of the images by using super-resolution construction algorithms (Zhou et al., 2019; Zhang et al., 2020). This approach can significantly improve details in the image, thereby increasing accuracy.

Clinically, manual delineation or segmentation of liver and tumours visible in the CT images is preferred, but it is time-consuming and subjective to the experts. Researchers have proposed several automatic segmentation techniques. Researchers have used thresholding, region-based, watershed, and DL-based segmentation approaches. Supervised deep learning segmentation models have achieved remarkable segmentation accuracy in many other domains where large datasets are available. Few researchers have used supervised DL models to segment liver (Meddeb et al., 2022; Li et al., 2018; Almotairi et al., 2020), but achieving higher accuracy with limited data is challenging. Applying image enhancement techniques before segmentation of the liver and lesion in the liver can improve the result (Zhang et al., 2020; Devi and Seenivasagam, 2020; Das et al., 2019).

There are mainly two types of image features: texture features and radiology features. Medical experts visually analyse these features and diagnose the liver disease from the images. It is time-consuming and requires experienced, highly trained medical experts. CAD systems can automatically extract and select important features faster and inexpensively. However, it is challenging (Xue et al., 2021). Deep neural networks such as CNN can learn and extract the important features from the images (Nayantara et al., 2020) and are currently trending.

Researchers prefer traditional ML techniques over DL techniques for detecting liver tumours (Devi and Seenivasagam, 2020; Balagourouchetty et al., 2019). The reasons are scarcity of medical images required to train DL models—clinicians feel DL needs to be more illustrative—and lack of reasoning (Das et al., 2019). Despite all the challenges, ML and DL techniques have achieved accuracy above 90% (Devi and Seenivasagam, 2020); Balagourouchetty et al., 2019; Das et al., 2019). At present, manual diagnosis of liver tumours by doctors is still practice. But in the near future, with the availability of more datasets, DL-based CAD will be dominant.

5.4 CONCLUSION AND FUTURE WORK

This chapter reviews ML-based liver tumour detection techniques. The articles considered in this study were collected from the WoS database, and the relevant articles were systematically selected by following PRISMA guidelines. The steps involved in liver tumour detection are discussed, highlighting the state-of-the-art techniques. The CAD systems are capable of detecting tumours with high accuracy. However, there is still scope for developing more reliable and accurate CAD. Advanced DL models are promising, but more labelled datasets to train the models are needed. CAD systems capable of detecting tumours accurately at an early stage will enable timely intervention and potentially increase the chances of successful treatment and survival.

Based on our review, the following are a few future scopes that researchers can contribute to ML-based CAD for liver tumour detection.

(1) Data collection for training the ML model is challenging. Building a large dataset containing images labeled by medical experts will be the most important future scope.
(2) Fusion of features extracted from multiple imaging modalities will improve the reliability.

(3) Multi-stage classification techniques can be used for weak pathological features. It can classify complex diseases accurately.

(4) Classifying segmented liver lesions, rather than detecting tumours within segmented liver images, can yield higher accuracy but requires more computational resources.

The limitation of this article is using only the WoS database to search articles related to liver tumour detection. Future review papers can consider keywords not included in the search query and more academic research databases.

REFERENCES

Almotairi, S., Kareem, G., Aouf, M., Almutairi, B., and Salem, M. A.-M. (2020). Liver tumor segmentation in CT scans using modified segnet. *Sensors*, 20(5):1516.

Aslam, M. S., Younas, M., Sarwar, M. U., Shah, M. A., Khan, A., Uddin, M. I., Ahmad, S., Firdausi, M., and Zaindin, M. (2021). Liver-tumor detection using CNN resunet. *Computers, Materials & Continua*, 67:1899–1914.

Azer, S. A. (2019). Deep learning with convolutional neural networks for identification of liver masses and hepatocellular carcinoma: A systematic review. *World Journal of Gastrointestinal Oncology*, 11(12):1218.

Balagourouchetty, L., Pragatheeswaran, J. K., Pottakkat, B., and Ramkumar, G. (2019). Googlenet-based ensemble fcnet classifier for focal liver lesion diagnosis. *IEEE Journal of Biomedical and Health Informatics*, 24(6):1686–1694.

Bilic, P., Christ, P., Li, H. B., Vorontsov, E., Ben-Cohen, A., Kaissis, G., Szeskin, A., Jacobs, C., Mamani, G. E. H., Chartrand, G., et al. (2023). The liver tumor segmentation benchmark (lits). *Medical Image Analysis*, 84:102680.

Clarivate. (2022). *Web of Science*. www.webofscience.com/wos/woscc/basic-search.

Das, A., Acharya, U. R., Panda, S. S., and Sabut, S. (2019). Deep learning based liver cancer detection using watershed transform and gaussian mixture model techniques. *Cognitive Systems Research*, 54:165–175.

Devi, R. M. and Seenivasagam, V. (2020). Automatic segmentation and classification of liver tumor from CT image using feature difference and SVM based classifier-soft computing technique. *Soft Computing*, 24:18591–18598.

Du, L., Yuan, J., Gan, M., Li, Z., Wang, P., Hou, Z., and Wang, C. (2022). A comparative study between deep learning and radiomics models in grading liver tumors using hepatobiliary phase contrast-enhanced MR images. *BMC Medical Imaging*, 22(1):1–9.

Fahmy, D., Alksas, A., Elnakib, A., Mahmoud, A., Kandil, H., Khalil, A., Ghazal, M., van Bogaert, E., Contractor, S., and El-Baz, A. (2022). The role of radiomics and AI technologies in the segmentation, detection, and management of hepatocellular carcinoma. *Cancers*, 14(24):6123.

Feng, B., Ma, X.-H., Wang, S., Cai, W., Liu, X.-B., and Zhao, X.-M. (2021). Application of artificial intelligence in preoperative imaging of hepatocellular carcinoma: Current status and future perspectives. *World Journal of Gastroenterology*, 27(32):5341.

Gao, R., Zhao, S., Aishanjiang, K., Cai, H., Wei, T., Zhang, Y., Liu, Z., Zhou, J., Han, B., Wang, J., et al. (2021). Deep learning for differential diagnosis of malignant hepatic tumors based on multi-phase contrast-enhanced CT and clinical data. *Journal of Hematology & Oncology*, 14(1):1–7.

Hussain, M., Saher, N., and Qadri, S. (2022). Computer vision approach for liver tumor classification using CT dataset. *Applied Artificial Intelligence*, 36(1):2055395.

Jose, R., Chacko, S., Jayakumar, J., and Jarin, T. (2022). Liver tumor classification using optimal opposition-based grey wolf optimization. *International Journal of Pattern Recognition and Artificial Intelligence*, 36(16):2240005.

Li, G., Zhang, X., Song, X., Duan, L., Wang, G., Xiao, Q., Li, J., Liang, L., Bai, L., and Bai, S. (2023). Machine learning for predicting accuracy of lung and liver tumor motion tracking using radiomic features. *Quantitative Imaging in Medicine and Surgery*, 13(3):1605.

Li, X., Chen, H., Qi, X., Dou, Q., Fu, C.-W., and Heng, P.-A. (2018). H-denseunet: Hybrid densely connected unet for liver and tumor segmentation from CT volumes. *IEEE Transactions on Medical Imaging*, 37(12):2663–2674.

Liu, W., Liu, X., Peng, M., Chen, G.-Q., Liu, P.-H., Cui, X.-W., Jiang, F., and Diet- rich, C. F. (2021). Artificial intelligence for hepatitis evaluation. *World Journal of Gastroenterology*, 27(34):5715.

Meddeb, A., Kossen, T., Bressem, K. K., Molinski, N., Hamm, B., and Nagel, S. N. (2022). Two-stage deep learning model for automated segmentation and classification of splenomegaly. *Cancers*, 14(22):5476.

Nayantara, P. V., Kamath, S., Manjunath, K., and Rajagopal, K. (2020). Computer-aided diagnosis of liver lesions using CT images: A systematic review. *Computers in Biology and Medicine*, 127:104035.

PRISMA. (2021). *Prisma Checklist*. https://prisma-statement.org/PRISMAStatement/Checklist.

Rela, M., Suryakari, N. R., and Patil, R. R. (2023). A diagnosis system by u-net and deep neural network enabled with optimal feature selection for liver tumor detection using CT images. *Multimedia Tools and Applications*, 82(3):3185–3227.

Rompianesi, G., Pegoraro, F., Ceresa, C. D., Montalti, R., and Troisi, R. I. (2022). Artificial intelligence in the diagnosis and management of colorectal cancer liver metastases. *World Journal of Gastroenterology*, 28(1):108.

Sethi, G., and Saini, B. S. (2016). Computer aided diagnosis system for abdomen diseases in computed tomography images. *Biocybernetics and Biomedical Engineering*, 36(1):42–55.

Shaker, R., Wilke, C., Ober, C., and Lawrence, J. (2021). Machine learning model development for quantitative analysis of CT heterogeneity in canine hepatic masses may predict histologic malignancy. *Veterinary Radiology & Ultrasound*, 62(6):711–719.

Su, T.-H., Wu, C.-H., and Kao, J.-H. (2021). Artificial intelligence in precision medicine in hepatology. *Journal of Gastroenterology and Hepatology*, 36(3):569–580.

Survarachakan, S., Prasad, P. J. R., Naseem, R., de Frutos, J. P., Kumar, R. P., Langø, T., Cheikh, F. A., Elle, O. J., and Lindseth, F. (2022). Deep learning for image-based liver analysis—a comprehensive review focusing on malignant lesions. *Artificial Intelligence in Medicine*, 102331.

Vorontsov, E., Tang, A., Roy, D., Pal, C. J., and Kadoury, S. (2017). Metastatic liver tumour segmentation with a neural network-guided 3d deformable model. *Medical & Biological Engineering & Computing*, 55:127–139.

Wang, S., Liu, X., Zhao, J., Liu, Y., Liu, S., Liu, Y., and Zhao, J. (2021). Computer auxiliary diagnosis technique of detecting cholangiocarcinoma based on medical imaging: A review. *Computer Methods and Programs in Biomedicine*, 208:106265.

Wei, J., Jiang, H., Gu, D., Niu, M., Fu, F., Han, Y., Song, B., and Tian, J. (2020). Radiomics in liver diseases: Current progress and future opportunities. *Liver Inter- national*, 40(9):2050–2063.

Xiang, K., Jiang, B., and Shang, D. (2021). The overview of the deep learning integrated into the medical imaging of liver: A review. *Hepatology International*, 15:868–880.

Xue, Z., Li, P., Zhang, L., Lu, X., Zhu, G., Shen, P., Shah, S. A. A., and Bennamoun, M. (2021). Multi-modal co-learning for liver lesion segmentation on pet-ct images. *IEEE Transactions on Medical Imaging*, 40(12):3531–3542.

Yasaka, K., Akai, H., Abe, O., and Kiryu, S. (2018). Deep learning with convolutional neural network for differentiation of liver masses at dynamic contrast-enhanced CT: A preliminary study. *Radiology*, 286(3):887–896.

Yu, A., Liu, Z., Sheng, V. S., Song, Y., Liu, X., Ma, C., Wang, W., and Ma, C. (2021). Ct segmentation of liver and tumors fused multi-scale features. *Intelligent Automation & Soft Computing*, 30(2).

Zhang, Y., Jiang, B., Wu, J., Ji, D., Liu, Y., Chen, Y., Wu, E. X., and Tang, X. (2020). Deep learning initialized and gradient enhanced level-set based segmentation for liver tumor from CT images. *IEEE Access*, 8:76056–76068.

Zhang, Y., Li, H., Du, J., Qin, J., Wang, T., Chen, Y., Liu, B., Gao, W., Ma, G., and Lei, B. (2021a). 3d multi-attention guided multi-task learning network for automatic gastric tumor segmentation and lymph node classification. *IEEE Transactions on Medical Imaging*, 40(6):1618–1631.

Zhang, Y., Peng, C., Peng, L., Xu, Y., Lin, L., Tong, R., Peng, Z., Mao, X., Hu, H., Chen, Y.-W., et al. (2021b). Deeprecs: From recist diameters to precise liver tumor segmentation. *IEEE Journal of Biomedical and Health Informatics*, 26(2):614–625.

Zhou, L.-Q., Wang, J.-Y., Yu, S.-Y., Wu, G.-G., Wei, Q., Deng, Y.-B., Wu, X.-L., Cui, X.-W., and Dietrich, C. F. (2019). Artificial intelligence in medical imaging of the liver. *World journal of gastroenterology*, 25(6):672.

Zhu, W., Huang, W., Lin, Z., Yang, Y., Huang, S., and Zhou, J. (2016). Data and feature mixed ensemble based extreme learning machine for medical object detection and segmentation. *Multimedia Tools and Applications*, 75:2815–2837.

6 Deep Learning in Photoacoustic Tomographic Image Reconstruction

Bondita Paul and Rusha Patra

6.1 INTRODUCTION

Photoacoustic tomographic (PAT) imaging, also known as optoacoustic tomographic (OAT) imaging, is a non-invasive biomedical imaging technique that relies on the photoacoustic effect within tissue. It combines the benefits of both optical and ultrasound imaging modalities. Over the past years, researchers have extensively explored the applications of this methodology. Because PAI offers several advantages, including higher spatial resolution for the visualization of microbiological tissue, rich contrast, great penetration depth, higher functional and structural information, and better tolerance to variations in the speed of sound. Moreover, its implementation is cost-effective compared to other optical molecular imaging techniques like diffusion optical tomography. PAT finds application in imaging small animals and human tissues, including in-vitro and in-vivo imaging [1], microvascular tissue studies [2], monitoring oxy-hemoglobin saturation, cerebral functional imaging, tumor detection [3], breast cancer detection, skin cancer detection, inflammatory arthritis [4], and beyond. In 1880, Alexander Graham Bell discovered the Photoacoustic (PA) effect during his experiment involving the illumination of a small amount of sunlight into an optically absorbing material, resulting in the production of audible sound [5]. This discovery led to the development of PA imaging in 1990, first in non-biological media and later in biological tissues [5]. In PAT, the fundamental concept involves illuminating biological tissue with a time-varying laser source. This leads to the absorption of photons by tissue particles, giving rise to the generation of acoustic pressure waves. These resultant pressure signals are then captured by ultrasonic transducers situated at various positions along the sample's boundary. From these measured acoustic pressures, the initial pressure distribution within the medium is reconstructed, enabling visualization of the internal structure of the tissue. Moreover, other optical properties such as absorption and scattering coefficient can also be estimated from this data.

DOI: 10.1201/9781032635149-6

6.2 FUNDAMENTALS OF PHOTOACOUSTIC TOMOGRAPHY: PRINCIPLES AND RECONSTRUCTION

PAT is a hybrid method that capitalizes on the photoacoustic effect, a natural occurrence where absorbed electromagnetic energy transforms into acoustic waves through thermal and stress confinement conditions. PAT comprises two problems, namely, forward and inverse problems. The forward problem involves calculating the boundary pressure given a known source, while the inverse problem focuses on reconstructing the source based on the measured pressure values at the boundary. Moreover, photoacoustic reconstruction can be performed in the time domain or frequency domain. In the time domain, a nanosecond pulsed laser source is used, while in the frequency domain, an intensity-modulated light source irradiates the sample. The frequency domain (FD) implementation of optoacoustic tomography offers simplicity in the reconstruction process and can operate with cost-effective light sources compared to the time domain approach. PAT imaging allows for two types of reconstruction: cross-sectional or 2D reconstruction and volumetric or 3D reconstruction. The primary objective of a PAT system is to recover the initial pressure distribution from the measured PA signal data.

6.2.1 PRINCIPLE OF PAT

In PAT, a time-varying laser illuminates the sample, causing tissue particles to absorb photons and convert light energy into heat. This leads to thermal expansion, generating acoustic pressure waves. The ultrasonic transducer captures the pressure signals at the boundary. Figure 6.1 depicts the PAT model representation.

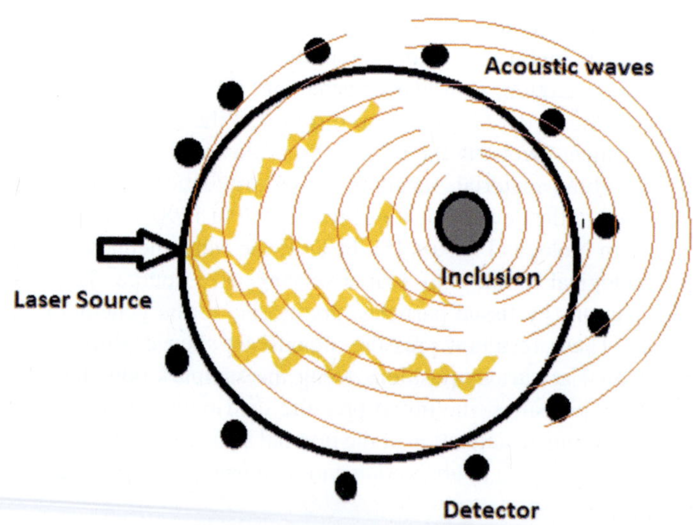

FIGURE 6.1 Representation of the PAT model.

In the depicted illustration, a circular medium is exposed to a laser source, causing scattering and absorption of light within the medium, particularly by an inclusion. The phenomenon of the photoacoustic effect gives rise to the generation of a sound wave at the inclusion, and this wave travels through the medium. Ultrasonic detectors, strategically positioned along the boundary, capture and measure these propagated sound waves. During the laser pulse illumination in PAT, the duration of the pulse should be much less. Based on these two common assumptions are typically made. The first assumption is thermal confinement, where it is assumed that the heat conductance does not significantly affect the neighboring regions of the tissue within the image region dimension. The second assumption is stress confinement, implying that the volume expansion is negligible. As a result of these assumptions, the initial pressure distribution ($p_0(r)$) can be directly proportional to the total optical absorbed energy ($H(r)$), which can be expressed as

$$p_0(r) = p(r, t = 0) = \Gamma \cdot H(r) \tag{6.1}$$

where $\Gamma = \dfrac{\beta c_{ac}^2}{C_p}$ is the dimensionless Gruneisen parameter, which is a proportional constant, is the thermal expansion coefficient, is the specific heat coefficient, and c_{ac} represents the sound velocity in the tissue medium. $r = (X, Y, Z)$ represents the positions in 3D space and t is the time. Again, $H(r)$ can be expressed by the multiplication of the absorption coefficient $\mu_a(r)$ and light fluence rate or photon density $\Phi(r, \mu_a, \mu_s, g)$ in the tissue medium.

$$H(r) = \mu_a(r) \cdot \Phi\ (r, \mu_a, \mu_s, g) \tag{6.2}$$

where μ_s is the scattering coefficient and g is the anisotropic factor.

6.2.2 Optical Properties of Tissue

Biological tissue exhibits various optical properties, including the absorption coefficient (μ_a), scattering coefficient (μ_s), and anisotropy factor (g). The absorption coefficient of tissue components is dependent on the wavelength of the incident light, typically ranging from 0.01 to 0.5 cm^{-1} [6]. Scattering occurs in tissue due to the differing refractive indices between tissue components and the surrounding medium. The scattering coefficient in tissue typically falls within the range of 20 to 200 cm^{-1} [6], particularly in the near-infrared (NIR) region. The anisotropy factor represents the average cosine of the scattering angle, and in tissue, it typically ranges from 0.8 to 0.98 [6]. In the NIR range (700–1100 nm), the optical absorption is considerably lower than the scattering coefficient (i.e., $\mu_s \gg \mu_a$), enabling NIR light to penetrate more deeply into tissue compared to visible light.

6.2.3 Time Domain PAT

In time-domain photoacoustic imaging, the complete pulse period is utilized for generating acoustic signals, whether induced optically or with RF/microwave. This approach employs pulsed light sources, particularly for optoacoustic imaging, with optical pulses typically lasting below 10 ns [7]. This allows for high-resolution imaging but requires complex setups and costly sources. As an example, generating ultra-short, high-energy light pulses often involves a tunable optical parametric oscillator laser that's powered by a Q-switched Nd: YAG laser. However, this setup can be quite costly. Significant advancements have occurred in time domain PAT over the past decade, with pulse laser sources being extensively employed [8–53]. The Helmholtz equation describes the propagation of the acoustic field in the time domain which is given by Eq. (6.3).

$$\left(\nabla^2 - \frac{1}{c_{ac}^2}\frac{\partial^2}{\partial t^2}\right)P(r,t) = -\frac{\beta}{C_p}\frac{\partial H(r,t)}{\partial t} \tag{6.3}$$

where P is the pressure measured at the detector at time t. $H(r,t)$ is the product of the spatial and temporal components can be written as [9]

$$H(r,t) = H_r(r)H_t(t) \tag{6.4}$$

Since the duration of the laser pulse is very short, the temporal components can be expressed by the delta function, that is, $H_t(t) = \delta(t)$. Using Green's function, the solution to the forward problem (Eq. (6.3)) is given by

$$P(r_d,t) = \frac{\beta}{4\pi C_p}\frac{\partial}{\partial t}\left[\int \frac{dr}{|r-r_d|}H(r)\delta\left(t - \frac{|r-r_d|}{c_{ac}}\right)\right] \tag{6.5}$$

where $|r-r_d|$ represents the distance between the position of the image voxel (r) and the detector position (r_d).

6.2.4 Frequency Domain PAT

In contrast to the pulsed excitation utilized in time-domain photoacoustic imaging, continuous wave (CW) sources are predominantly employed in frequency-domain (FD) photoacoustic (FDPA) imaging. FDPA employs modulated light intensity to generate the PA signals. While time-domain systems often require costly and bulky sources like OPO-Lasers or RF/microwave amplifiers, frequency-domain setups make use of more cost-efficient sources such as diode lasers or narrowband LEDs. This choice of source also ensures lower laser fluence in the frequency domain, contributing to safer operation conditions for patients. The development of frequency-domain optoacoustic imaging has been documented in previous works [2, 54–56]. In the frequency domain, the propagation equation of the photoacoustic wave field is given by taking Fourier transform of Eq. (6.3).

$$\left(\nabla^2 + k^2\right)P(r,\omega) = -\frac{j\omega\beta}{C_p}H(r,\omega) \tag{6.6}$$

where ω is the angular frequency modulation, k is the wave number ($k = \omega/c_{ac}$). Here optical absorbed energy density can be written as

$$H(r,\omega) = \Gamma \mu_a(r) \cdot \Phi(r,\omega) \tag{6.7}$$

Similar to the time domain, the forward solution in the frequency domain is given by

$$P(r_d,\omega) = \frac{j\omega\beta}{4\pi C_p} \int \frac{dr}{|r - r_d|} H(r,\omega) \exp(jk|r - r_d|) \tag{6.8}$$

There are numerous algorithms have been developed in the past years to solve the inverse problem in the PAT system. The image reconstruction methods are explained in the next section.

6.2.5 Image Reconstruction

The main goal of the PAT system is to recover the initial pressure and the optical parameters. The reconstruction of PA images is a challenging task due to the ill-posed nature of the inverse problem. To address this issue, various reconstruction algorithms have been developed, including filtered back projection (FBP), delay-and-sum, fast Fourier transformation (FFT), time reversal (TR), model-based inversion techniques, and deep learning-based methods, in recent years.

In the time domain approach, the back projection algorithm [8–19] is widely utilized in PAT image reconstruction due to its simplicity. This algorithm relies on a closed-form analytical inversion formula that applies to both 2D and 3D images [8], akin to the Radon transformation. It is adaptable to various geometries, making it advantageous. Another benefit is its implementation feasibility in both Fourier domain and spatial-temporal domain. However, the conventional back projection algorithm has its limitations. It does not provide exact results and tends to introduce artifacts into the reconstructed image. Minor or negative values of optical absorption can lead to variations in the recovered image. In the FBP algorithm, the initial pressure is derived using Eq. (6.1), followed by the application of a filter function. The modified back projection algorithm is expressed as follows:

$$H_r(r) = -\frac{1}{2\pi c^2 \Gamma} \int_{t-R/c} \frac{1}{t} \left[\frac{\partial P(r,t)}{\partial t} - \frac{P(r,t)}{t} \right] dA' \tag{6.9}$$

FFT technique has been extensively employed in various studies [8, 10, 24–31] for PA imaging. Fourier reconstruction algorithms have demonstrated superior performance compared to conventional Back Projection algorithms while offering enhanced speed. However, it's important to note that the FFT method utilized in photoacoustic imaging involves interpolation within the Fourier space domain, which can introduce artifacts into the reconstructed images. The TR method has been employed in various works [10, 24, 32–37, 55]. In this technique, the pressure profile is re-emitted on the surface in reverse chronological order, originating from zero initial conditions at $t = T$, and then traced backward in time to obtain the initial pressure distribution at $t = 0$. The iterative image reconstruction technique has been introduced and developed in a series of works [2, 38–43, 56]. This method is commonly utilized for the reconstruction of both 2D and 3D images. While providing quicker and superior quality imaging compared to FBP algorithms, it's worth noting that this technique comes at a higher computational cost. This approach plays a crucial role in artifact removal and noise reduction, proving especially advantageous in scenarios involving incomplete data. The iterative algorithm [38–43] initiates with an initially assumed image dataset and continually refines the data by iteratively updating it based on the disparities between the actual and computed image datasets. Least square and conjugate gradient are some examples of iterative inversion algorithms. Model-based iterative method [8, 44–49, 55] is the most popular method to solve the inverse problem in the PAT system. Here, numerous regularization techniques are used to remove noise and artifacts. This algorithm is employed to construct the model matrix, aiding in the reconstruction of the initial pressure image. In time domain model-based optoacoustic tomographic (OAT) image reconstruction, a high-dimensional sparse matrix is formulated, leading to increased memory requirements and computational complexity, which pose challenges for real-world imaging applications. To address this issue, various regularization schemes (total variation, Tikhonov, L_1 norm, and so on) are employed to enhance the recovery of the sparse matrix while also reducing the number of required detectors. In [44], a modified weighted interpolated matrix model inversion method (IMMI) was introduced, outperforming the interpolated model matrix inversion for different transducer angles. The linear connection between the acquired pressure signals, or projections, and the corresponding relation between them are given in Eqs. (6.5) and (6.8), this relationship can be expressed in a discrete form using a matrix representation:

$$Ax = P \tag{6.10}$$

Here P is the PA signal, A is the model matrix of the medium, and x denotes the initial pressure distribution. Since A is an ill-posed matrix, a direct solution to this equation is not possible. Therefore, to solve this, some optimization techniques were employed. In [55] using the green function, the authors developed the expression for the model matrix for a 3D circular phantom as

$$W(\omega) = -jAe^{j\Phi_a} \begin{pmatrix} w_{11} & \cdot & \cdot & w_{1v} \\ \cdot & & & \cdot \\ \cdot & & & \cdot \\ w_{n1} & \cdot & \cdot & w_{nv} \end{pmatrix}, \text{ where } w_{nv} = \frac{\omega e^{\left(j\left(\frac{\omega}{c_{ac}} \right) |r(v) - r_d(n)| \right)}}{|r(v) - r_d(n)|} \tag{6.11}$$

Here $r(v)$ and $r_d(n)$ represent the image voxel positions and the detector's locations on the boundary of the geometry, respectively, A is a constant and Φ_a is a phase constant. The forward model of the phantom is given by

$$\tilde{p} = \bar{W}X \text{, where } \bar{W} = \begin{pmatrix} W(\omega_1) \\ \vdots \\ W(\omega_F) \end{pmatrix} \text{ and } \tilde{p} = \begin{pmatrix} p(\omega_1) \\ \vdots \\ p(\omega_F) \end{pmatrix} \quad (6.12)$$

Ultimately, the solution to Eq. (6.12) can be obtained through the utilization of Tikhonov regularization, expressed as follows [55].

$$X_0 = \arg\min\left(\left\|\mathrm{Re}(\bar{W})X - \mathrm{Re}(\tilde{p})\right\|_2^2 + \left\|\mathrm{Im}(\bar{W})X - \mathrm{Im}(\tilde{p})\right\|_2^2 + \lambda\|X\|_2^2\right), \text{ sub. to } X \geq 0 \quad (6.13)$$

In this context, *Re* and *Im* correspond to the actual and imaginary segments of $\bar{W}$ and $\tilde{p}$. The regularization parameter (λ) was chosen at the point where the L-curve exhibits an inflection [57]. Addressing the optimization problem outlined in Eq. (6.13) was achieved via the least squares method (LSQR), involving a total of 100 iterations. The final solution of X represents the reconstructed initial pressure distribution of the PAT image. In PAT K-wave toolbox in MATLAB is very helpful for simulation. Over the past few years, within the field of PA image reconstruction, deep learning techniques leveraging convolutional neural networks (CNNs) have gained substantial recognition [50–53, 63–65, 71–78, 82]. The deep learning architectures are described in the next section.

6.3 DEEP NEURAL NETWORKS: ARCHITECTURE, TRAINING, OPTIMIZATION

Deep learning is a subset of machine learning that harnesses the power of artificial neural networks to decipher intricate patterns and relationships within data. Unlike traditional programming, deep learning doesn't require explicit coding for every aspect. This approach has gained immense popularity due to enhanced processing capabilities and the abundance of extensive datasets. Its foundation lies in artificial neural networks also known as deep neural networks (DNNs), mimicking the structure and function of biological neurons in the human brain, enabling them to learn from vast volumes of data. At its core, deep learning employs neural networks to address complex problems. These networks consist of interconnected layers of nodes, resembling the brain's structure, and process data through transformations. At the core of deep learning lies the utilization of deep neural networks, consisting of numerous layers. These networks unveil intricate data representations by discovering layered patterns and features in the data. Unlike conventional approaches, deep learning algorithms possess the ability to autonomously learn and refine information without the need for manual crafting of features. Deep learning's success spans a multitude of fields, encompassing visual identification, linguistic comprehension, speech comprehension, and recommendation systems. Notable architectural examples include Convolutional Neural Networks (CNNs), Recurrent Neural Networks (RNNs), and Deep Belief Networks (DBNs). The training of deep neural networks requires substantial data and computational resources. However, the advent of cloud computing and specialized hardware, like GPUs, has eased the process of training deep networks. Deep learning encompasses a variety of techniques in machine learning, spanning supervised, unsupervised, and reinforcement learning domains. It harnesses neural networks to enhance predictive accuracy, uncover patterns, and refine decision-making processes.

In supervised learning, neural networks predict or classify data using labeled datasets, taking both input features and target variables. Learning occurs through adjusting predictions based on the error between predicted and actual targets, known as backpropagation. CNN and RNN are deployed for tasks like image recognition, sentiment analysis, and language translation. Unsupervised learning involves neural networks identifying patterns or grouping data without labels. No target variables are used; instead, the network autonomously uncovers hidden relationships in datasets. Autoencoders and generative models perform tasks like clustering, reducing dimensions, and spotting anomalies. In reinforcement learning, agents learn to make decisions to optimize rewards within an environment. Agents interact with the environment, take actions, and observe rewards. Incorporating techniques such as Deep Q networks and Deep Deterministic Policy Gradient (DDPG), deep reinforcement learning elevates capabilities in areas like robotics and interactive gaming.

DNN consists of both single-layer and multi-layer. In a single-layer network, inputs are directly linked to outputs through a modified linear function, often termed a perceptron. Multi-layer neural networks extend this concept, organizing neurons in layers, including input, hidden, and output layers. This architecture is known as a feed-forward network. A standard Neural Network consists of three types of layers:

1. Input Layer: This initial layer receives the input data, with the number of neurons matching the total features (e.g., pixels in an image).
2. Hidden Layer: The input from the Input Layer flows into the hidden layers. Multiple hidden layers can exist, each potentially with a different number of neurons, typically exceeding the feature count. Neurons in each layer process input through weights and biases, followed by activation functions for nonlinearity.
3. Output Layer: The output of the Hidden Layer is processed through a logistic function (like sigmoid or SoftMax), transforming it into probability scores for each class.

The data is input into the model and generates outputs through a process known as feedforward. The error is then computed using functions like cross-entropy or square loss, indicating the network's performance. To minimize this error, backpropagation is employed, involving the calculation of derivatives within the model. This iterative process aims to enhance the model's accuracy.

Deep Learning has strengths like high accuracy and scalability, but it also has notable drawbacks. It demands substantial data and computational resources for training and optimization, making it resource-intensive. Additionally, it relies heavily on extensive labeled data, which can be costly and time-consuming to obtain. Hence, while Deep Learning offers advantages, its computational demands, data requirements, and interpretability issues must be carefully considered when applying it to specific tasks. DNNs hold immense promise in the realms of medical imaging technology, clinical data analysis, healthcare diagnosis, and related healthcare challenges. They are being actively explored and implemented, not only in pre-clinical but also in clinical settings.

6.3.1 ARCHITECTURE

Deep learning researchers have developed a range of layer types and architectures to accommodate various use cases and data formats, such as images or sequential data. Prominent DL architectures encompass stacked autoencoders, deep Boltzmann machines, RNNs, Feedforward neural networks (FFNs), CNN, Transformer neural networks, etc. Among these, the CNN model garners the most widespread usage in computer vision and image processing, constituting a subject of extensive exploration within the field [51].

Convolutional Neural Networks (CNN): A CNN is a multilayer neural network inspired by the visual cortex of animals. In this architecture, early layers detect basic features like edges, while subsequent layers combine these features to identify more complex attributes in the input. A typical CNN configuration encompasses successive layers of convolution, pooling, activation, fully connected, normalization layer, and dropout. The convolution layers include trainable filters (or kernels) with small dimensions in width and height, matching the depth of the input volume (usually 3 for image input). For downsampling the spatial dimension of data, pooling layers are applied. Pooling involves sliding a 2D filter across each feature map channel, summarizing features within its covered region. It can also reduce the computation complexity and make the network more robust to variations in positions and size of features. Two types of pooling are max pooling and average pooling. Activation functions introduce non-linearity in the outputs of certain layers (e.g., convolutional and fully connected layers). Widely adopted activation functions comprise sigmoid, SoftMax, tanh, rectified linear unit (ReLU), and its variants such as Leaky ReLU. Notably, ReLU gains prominence due to its robust non-linearity and facile gradient computation. The classification layer, often a fully connected layer, facilitates the linkage of feature maps and outputs. It processes the input from the preceding layer and performs the ultimate classification or regression task. Integration of normalization layers between convolutional layers and activation functions expedites training and mitigates vulnerability to network initialization challenges. These layers effectuate transformations that maintain mean activation proximal to zero and activate standard deviation proximal to one. Batch normalization emerges as the norm for such normalization, enjoying widespread adoption. The composition of the training dataset critically impacts the model's effectiveness, with loss functions serving as performance evaluators. The applications of CNN are image classification, image segmentation, object detection, audio processing, video analysis, and so on.

Many CNN architectures have been designed in the past few years for image reconstruction and denoising. Most of the researchers use pre-trained models of deep neural networks (DNNs) because they are much faster and easier than training a network that is designed from scratch. Some examples of pre-trained CNN are LeNet, Alexnet, Googlenet, Resnet, VGGnet, Inception, U-Net, and many more. Pretrained networks are already trained on a huge number of images. The architecture can also be designed from scratch. Among them, the U-Net [58] stands as the predominant CNN architecture for employing deep learning in sparse tomographic image reconstruction using post-processing techniques. It possesses attributes highly suitable for artifact elimination, including its multilevel decomposition and multichannel filtering [59]. Additionally, it has shown competitive performance to iterative methods in mitigating sparse PAT image artifacts in both synthetic and experimental datasets. The U-Net architecture has been depicted in Figure 6.2.

For network training, the U-Net [59] architecture has demonstrated success in medical image segmentation and reconstruction, particularly with limited data. The network comprises an encoder and a dimensionally symmetric decoder, both consisting of consecutive convolutional layers. The encoder adheres to a conventional convolutional network structure, iteratively applying a pair of 3×3 convolutions (without padding). Subsequently, a ReLU activation is employed, and downsampling is carried out through 2×2 max pooling. Here, each convolutional layer's output undergoes halving image size through the max pooling layer. For example, if an image with dimension $32 \times 32 \times 3$ (width × height × depth) is fed into the model, then for the convolution layer with 64 filters the image dimension will be $32 \times 32 \times 64$, and for max pooling with stride 2 the dimension becomes $16 \times 16 \times 64$. Feature channels are doubled at each downsampling step. This compression in the encoder is reversed symmetrically via upsampling layers in the decoder, restoring the original image dimensions. In the decoder, the upsampling is followed by a 2×2 convolution to reduce feature channels, merging with trimmed feature maps originating from the encoder pathway, and two 3×3 convolutions with ReLU. Skip connections concatenate equal-resolution layers, compensating for spatial resolution loss. This preserves fine details and relevant information from previous encoder layers, enhancing generalization and aiding in accurate reconstruction. In the final layer, a 1×1 convolution is utilized to transform a 64-part feature vector into the intended number of classes. Overall, the network includes 23 convolutional layers.

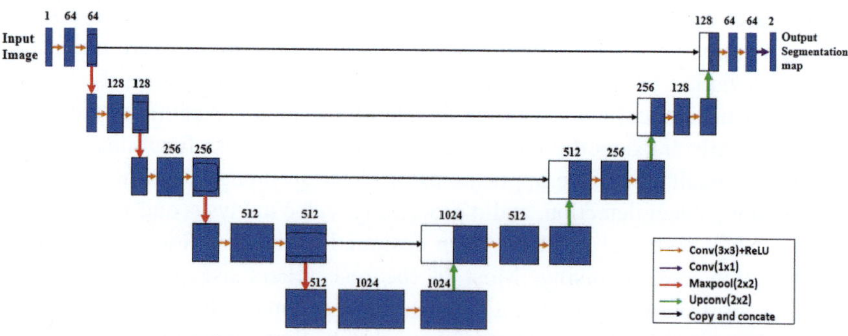

FIGURE 6.2 U-Net CNN architecture. Multi-channel feature maps, depicted in blue boxes with channel numbers atop, are accompanied by replicated feature maps illustrated in white boxes. Arrows symbolize the various operations undertaken.

6.3.2 TRAINING

Training a DNN involves finding the optimal weights for its neurons to make accurate predictions. Initially, random weights are assigned, and the network processes the training data. A loss function assesses the prediction error compared to the actual outcome. Backpropagation, a crucial neural network training method, can be quite sensitive to small changes in settings like initialization. This instability is more pronounced in deep networks. Using gradient descent, the weights are adjusted through backpropagation, a method to efficiently calculate gradients. This process iterates, updating weights until a satisfactory set is achieved. The success of a deep learning model depends on its training data. The construction of the dataset remains a pivotal concern in DL. A central role is played by the Loss Function (LF); it assesses how well the network learns the task during training. There are various LFs such as Mean Square Error (MSE), Mean Absolute Error (MAE) or L_1 loss, Huber loss, or Smooth MAE. These LFs are called regression loss. The classification LF are cross-entropy loss or negative log-likelihood, hinge loss. Selecting a suitable LF can be a challenging task, as it's not always clear which one to opt for or even what exactly a loss function is and how it impacts the training of a neural network. For images, the MSE is commonly used as the LF. The MSE is also known as square loss or L_2 loss. If the actual and predicted values are represented as Y_i and $\overline{Y}_i$, then MSE can be expressed as

$$MSE = \frac{1}{N}\sum_{i}^{N}(Y_i - \overline{Y}_i)^2 \tag{6.14}$$

Other metrics like structural similarity index (SSIM) and peak signal-to-noise ratio (PSNR), which measure the quality of the image, have also been incorporated into the LF. Some essential terms are used in the training process described as follows:

- Epoch: This represents how many times the algorithm processes the entire training dataset.
- Sample: An individual row of data extracted from the dataset.
- Batch: This denotes the number of samples grouped together for the purpose of adjusting the model parameters collectively.
- Learning Rate: It guides the extent to which the model's weights should be adjusted.
- Loss Function: This function measures the difference between predicted and actual values, quantifying the model's accuracy.
- Weights/Bias: These are adjustable elements in the model that influence the interaction between neurons.

6.3.3 OPTIMIZATION

Optimizer algorithms are crucial methods for enhancing the performance of deep learning models. These algorithms, also known as optimizers, significantly impact the accuracy and speed of model training. In essence, an optimizer is a tool that adjusts attributes like weights and learning rates of a neural network during training, aiming to minimize the LF and enhance accuracy. Since deep learning models consist of numerous parameters, selecting suitable weights is a complex task, prompting the need for appropriate optimization algorithms. The choice of optimizer can influence the model's outcome, and while trying all possibilities might seem tempting, it's time-consuming, especially with large datasets. Various optimizers are Gradient Descent, Stochastic Gradient Descent, and others like RMSProp, Adagrad, AdaDelta, Momentum, and Adam [60]. Gradient descent stands as a highly favored technique for optimization, especially in the realm of neural networks. It's a widespread method employed to fine-tune neural network parameters. Gradient descent operates as follows:

- Commencing with initial coefficients, it evaluates their associated cost and endeavors to locate a reduced cost.
- It adjusts the coefficients in the direction of lower weight values.
- This cycle continues iteratively until a local minimum is attained, signifying a point where further progress is inhibited.

Gradient descent is effective in many cases but has drawbacks. It becomes costly to compute gradients with large data sizes. While suitable for convex functions, it lacks guidance for traversing gradients in nonconvex functions. Therefore, to mitigate these challenges stochastic gradient descent (SGD) method was developed. It offers a solution by randomly selecting data batches, leading to faster convergence. SGD with momentum accelerates convergence by adding a fraction of the previous update to the current one. Mini-batch gradient descent, a variant of SGD, uses subsets of data for faster computation. AdaGrad adjusts learning rates individually for each iteration, making it effective for sparse datasets. RMS Prop enhances AdaGrad's robustness and efficiency, keeping the learning rate adaptive. AdaDelta improves upon AdaGrad and RMS Prop by addressing their limitations, offering stable learning rates, and preventing stagnation. Adam optimizer, short for Adaptive Moment Estimation, combines features of AdaGrad and RMSProp, dynamically adjusting learning rates based on past gradients and their variances, leading to faster convergence and improved performance. The Adam optimizer is commonly favored in PAT image reconstruction due to its advantageous characteristics.

6.4 DEEP CNN FOR PAT RECONSTRUCTION: ARCHITECTURES, TRAINING, DATA AUGMENTATION, PERFORMANCE EVALUATION

Deep convolutional neural networks (CNNs) have achieved significant success in computer vision, prompting the rise of supervised learning-based reconstruction in medical imaging [61]. This method exploits the network's ability to learn optimal features through weight and filter adjustments, effectively handling challenges from ill-posed inverse problems. A prevalent machine learning (ML) approach works within the image domain, using distorted images processed by traditional reconstruction under ill-posed conditions for training [52, 62–65]. However, ML applied to reconstructed images often struggles to recover subtle signals due to data loss during image reconstruction. Using adaptable neural networks, deep learning excels across domains, even outperforming comparable algorithms. While it has been applied broadly, its recent use in image reconstruction is evident [52, 59, 64, 66–70]. In this process, a CNN learns to relate measured data to the desired reconstructed image. Tuned with training images, the CNN's adjustable weights enable accurate image reconstruction. Deep learning reconstruction involves one network evaluation, adapting itself to specific tasks and phantom classes. When conventional algorithms are applied to sparse data challenges in PAT, they produce subpar images filled with pronounced under-sampling artifacts. In certain scenarios, these imperfections can be lessened through iterative image reconstruction techniques that incorporate prior knowledge like smoothness, total variation (TV), or sparsity limitations. However, these methods are often time-intensive because of the repetitive solving of both forward and adjoint problems. Additionally, iterative methods have drawbacks including heavy reliance on model assumptions that may not hold in practical scenarios. To address these concerns, the researchers developed direct and efficient reconstruction approaches rooted in deep learning. In contrast to iterative methods, a CNN was employed, pre-trained on a dataset, for image reconstruction. The actual reconstruction only requires a single assessment of the trained network, providing the desired outcome. The DNN architectures, designed for PAT image reconstruction, are discussed in the next section.

6.4.1 ARCHITECTURES

There are numerous CNN architectures were designed for PAT image reconstruction. In [50, 51, 64, 71–78], the authors introduced different modified U-Net CNN architecture for PAT image reconstruction. The U-Net is a fully convolutional network structured as an encoder-decoder with skip connections. The encoder comprises four blocks, each passing the signal through two convolution layers followed by ReLU activation. Max pooling reduces image size and increases filter count in each block, enhancing feature extraction. The decoder mirrors this structure, replacing downsampling with upsampling. Skip connections concatenate encoder outputs with decoder upsampled images, preserving higher frequencies lost in downsampling and aiding gradient flow. Fully dense (FD) U-Net was employed in [71, 72]. In the FD U-Net architecture, the input image X goes through a multi-level breakdown in the contracting path of the FD U-Net [71]. This process entails diminishing the spatial dimensions of the feature maps using a max-pooling operation. This facilitates the network in capturing both small-scale and large-scale features, which are pivotal for addressing artifacts at various levels. During the expanding phase, the acquired feature maps are magnified via a deconvolution operator and amalgamated to produce an image (Y) as output that matches the dimensions of the input image (X). In this context, deconvolution is akin to reversing the convolution process. In the FD U-Net architecture, each spatial tier (s) uses a dense block with a growth rate (ks). The growth rate adjusts at each level to keep a consistent number of convolutional layers across dense blocks, ensuring computational efficiency. The enlarged feature maps merge with similar-sized maps from the contracting path, using a 1×1 convolution to reduce them to the intended size. In a dense block, each layer connects to all previous layers, promoting feature reuse and diversification. Dense connectivity allows for deeper networks, addressing issues like the vanishing gradient problem. The dense block applies residual learning, transforming input images efficiently and restoring desired artifact-free images. This architecture's effectiveness lies in its ability to efficiently capture and combine multi-scale features, enabling enhanced artifact removal while efficiently training deeper networks through dense connectivity and residual learning. The FD U-Net consists of a substantial 82 convolution and deconvolution layers, in contrast to the U-Net's more modest 23 layers. A novel technique, named Pixel-wise Deep Learning (Pixel-DL), was devised specifically for addressing sparse and restricted-view PAT image reconstruction [72]. Pixel-DL utilizes a physics-guided pixel-wise interpolation strategy to extract relevant information from sensor data, directly feeding it into an FD U-Net CNN to facilitate image reconstruction. This approach eliminates the requirement for an initial inversion and enhances image quality by leveraging more sensor data. Pixel-DL's performance, evaluated using SSIM and PSNR metrics, surpassed conventional PAT reconstruction methods and other direct learned methods in simulated experiments involving diverse vasculature phantoms for training and testing.

Another modified version of U-Net known as Residual U-Net was implemented in [64, 73, 74]. For residual U-Net an additive skip connection (residual connection) adds the back-projected output of the U-Net, leveraging simpler residual images for effective training. In [64] a deep learning method for PAT using sparse data involves applying a linear reconstruction algorithm (FBP) to sparse data, followed by a residual U-Net with tuned weights based on training data. Two percent Gaussian noise was added to the PA signal. CNN evaluation is non-iterative and comparable in effort to standard FBP for PAT. The results indicated deep learning's feasibility and promise for PAT image reconstruction. In [73] a non-iterative deep learning reconstruction method called DALnet was developed to handle challenges like non-ideal impulse response function (IRF), spatial under-sampling, and limited view. DALnet combines universal back-projection (UBP) with dynamic aperture length (DAL) correction for limited view and IRF issues and a convolutional neural network (CNN) for spatial under-sampling. This network architecture design is the same as residual U-Net. DALnet achieves real-time high-resolution PA projection imaging, surpassing TV minimization in speed and error metrics in comparison to FBP and iterative methods.

Another neural network framework called ConvU-Net [75] and DU-Net [76] were introduced for PA imaging reconstruction directly from the raw PA data captured by multifrequency ultrasound sensors. An end-to-end network is trained to compare performance when transducers encompass the region of interest, capturing varying frequency spectrum information. In comparison to the U-net architecture, notable modifications have been made to the skip connections in the first stage of DU-Net. Specifically, these connections have been adapted to link a convolutional layer with a kernel size of (20×3) and a stride of (20×1). Additionally, an initial convolutional layer is introduced to process the input image before feeding it into the subsequent layers. The convolutional layers in both the contracting and expanding paths employ a kernel size of 3 and a stride of 1. The input to this network comprises 120 channels of multi-frequency sensor data. Through the U-net process, time-domain information is transformed into the spatial domain, resulting in a 128×128-pixel output image. To introduce nonlinearity, the leaky rectified linear unit (ReLU) activation function is utilized. As for the optimization algorithm, Adam has been chosen for this study. Numerical simulations reveal the superior performance of the proposed framework over conventional reconstruction methods. This approach outperforms the U-net on test datasets, evaluated by various indexes. Y-Net [50, 77] and S-Net [51] were also developed based on U-Net for PAT image reconstruction. Authors in [50] introduced Y-Net, a novel CNN architecture with two intersecting encoder paths. Y-Net uses two distinct input types: representing texture structure from conventional algorithms and encompassing high-dimensional features extracted from raw signals. The network is trained using k-Wave PA simulation data and evaluated on a test set. Experimental results show the feasibility and robustness of the proposed method compared to other models and conventional approaches. Y-Net's performance may benefit from an improved beamforming algorithm to address artifacts. A deep learning framework (S-Net) for image reconstruction in limited-view PAT using sparse data was developed in [51]. The proposed approach involves an initial FBP algorithm application followed by artifact removal using a CNN. U-Net and S-Net architectures for the CNN were explored here. Both networks enhance image quality, with U-Net outperforming and being comparable to iterative TV minimization. These reconstruction networks enable real-time application, unlike slower iterative methods.

6.4.2 TRAINING

Most of the CNN architectures are trained using the Keras software, Pytorch, a user-friendly API in Python, for training and evaluating the U-net model. Keras operates on top of TensorFlow, an open-source machine intelligence library. This combination facilitated the streamlined implementation of the customized U-net. Adam and a stochastic gradient with momentum algorithm optimizer are utilized for network training. In [52] the U-Net network was trained using pairs of datasets (x_i, y_i), where x_i represents artefactual images and y_i represents artifact-free images. The network was trained with various types of data, including simulated data with different absorber sizes and experimentally acquired data. The network's goal was to minimize pre-defined loss functions (L_1-norm and L_2-norm) by adjusting its parameters in each iteration. Adam optimization algorithm was used for training. The training process took around 50 seconds per epoch (60 numbers of epochs). For testing, different sub-sampled data with varying numbers of projections, ranging from 8 to 256 projections were used. The testing and image recovery process was very fast, taking about 0.1 seconds per image. This rapid image reconstruction significantly outperformed conventional iterative methods that use signals from all 512 available projections.

6.4.3 DATA AUGMENTATION

Data augmentation is a technique in deep learning that enhances the quality of training data for artificial neural networks. It works by expanding the training dataset through the addition of variations to existing data samples. This can be achieved manually by introducing alterations like noise addition, resizing, or rotation to the data. Alternatively, algorithms can automatically generate new data samples. Data augmentation is crucial in deep learning as it addresses the need for extensive data, particularly when collecting a vast number of images isn't feasible. This process aids in dataset enlargement and diversity introduction. Common augmentation operations include rotation, shearing, zooming, cropping, flipping, and brightness adjustment. In frameworks like Keras, data augmentation can be performed using tools like the Image Data Generator class, which offers parameters for controlling augmentation operations such as rotation, brightness, shear, and zoom. Here data augmentation has been explained for PAT image reconstruction.

In [72] training data were expanded using data augmentation techniques. For instance, in the case of synthetic vasculature phantoms (340×340 pixels), images were scaled (0.5 to 2 scaling factor), rotated (0–359 degrees), and translated to generate variations. A total of 500 training images were constructed from these phantoms. Multiple iterations of this process were combined to create training images. The mouse brain vasculature dataset involved applying a vessel Ness filter and generating new images from filtered volumes. Similar augmentation processes were applied to the "High-Resolution Fundus Image Database" and the "ELCAP Public Lung Image Database." Here the images were divided into 500 training and 50 testing. During the simulation phase, a MATLAB toolbox known as k-Wave [79] was employed to replicate the process of acquiring photoacoustic data. Each image intended for training and testing underwent normalization and was considered a photoacoustic source situated on a grid.

In [50] the dataset for training is generated using the MATLAB toolbox k-Wave. In the simulation setup depicted a linear array transducer is positioned at the top of the region of interest (ROI). The region of interest (ROI) spans 38.4×38.4 mm and is probed using a linear array containing 128 elements to capture Photoacoustic (PA) signals from the specimen. Raw data is gathered from the sensor, serving as the foundation for generating beamformed images and reference data for both training and testing needs. All images are normalized to dimensions of 128×128 pixels, with a sound velocity of 1500 m/s being established. The center frequency of the transducer is 7 MHz with an 80% fractional bandwidth. An input size of 2560×128 is designated for PA signals, achieving an SNR of 60 dB. The dataset is further enriched with artificial segmented vessels obtained from the public fundus oculi DRIVE [48] dataset. For data preparation, the entire blood vessel structure within the fundus oculi is divided into four equal segments. Then, random rotations (90°, 180°, 270°) are introduced, and two segmented blood vessels are overlaid. This augmented dataset is subsequently incorporated into the k-Wave simulation toolbox, where it serves as the initial pressure distribution. The final dataset consists of 4700 training sets and 400 test sets. These sets are produced using the specialized k-Wave toolbox in MATLAB, designed specifically for simulating Photoacoustic scenarios. This comprehensive dataset serves as the foundation for training and evaluating the developed approach.

6.4.4 Performance Evaluation

The performance of the CNN architecture for PAT image reconstruction is evaluated using various indexes called PSNR, SSIM, SNR, and relative L_2 error. The SSIM quantifies the quality of an estimated image, with a higher value indicating better quality. It is defined as follows:

$$SSIM = \frac{\left(2\mu_x\mu_y + c_1\right)\left(2\sigma_{xy} + c_2\right)}{\left(\mu_x^2 + \mu_y^2 + c_1\right)\left(\sigma_x^2 + \sigma_y^2 + c_2\right)} \tag{6.15}$$

where μ_x and μ_y are the average values; σ_x^2 and σ_y^2 are variances; and σ_{xy} is the covariance of x and y windows. The PSNR is calculated in decibels (dB).

$$PSNR = 10\log_{10}\frac{peakvalue^2}{MSE} \tag{6.16}$$

Here, MSE is mean square error. The Signal-to-Noise Ratio (SNR) is expressed as the logarithmic ratio between the peak signal intensity and the standard deviation of background intensities, focusing solely on signal and noise levels.

$$SNR = 10\log_{10}\left(\frac{peak(X)}{\sigma_b}\right)^2 \tag{6.17}$$

where X denotes the reconstructed image and σ_b is the standard deviation of the background. The Relative L_2 reconstruction error is computed by measuring the difference between the reconstructed initial pressure (X_{CNN}) and the actual initial pressure (X_{ACT}), and then expressing it as

$$Error = \frac{\left\|X_{CNN} - X_{ACT}\right\|_2}{\left\|X_{ACT}\right\|_2} \tag{6.18}$$

The evaluation of image reconstruction from simulated data involved assessing image quality using these parameters, which gauge both global and local aspects. The quantitative values derived from these indexes were crucial for ensuring the robust training and testing of the proposed CNN architectures, accommodating variations across diverse datasets.

6.5 GENERATIVE ADVERSARIAL NETWORKS AND RECURRENT NEURAL NETWORKS FOR PAT IMAGING

Generative Adversarial Networks (GANs) and Recurrent Neural Networks (RNNs) are foundational architectures on which other deep learning structures are constructed.

6.5.1 GENERATIVE ADVERSARIAL NETWORKS

GANs constitute a compelling category of neural networks employed in unsupervised learning. It is a pivotal concept in deep learning, introduced by Ian J. Goodfellow in 2014. GANs encompass a dual neural network setup engaged in mutual competition, which are named as generator and discriminator. This setup adeptly dissects, comprehends, and emulates the intricate nuances present within a dataset. GANs fundamentally operate as a creative mechanism for generating new data closely resembling a given data distribution. For example, it enables the creation of novel images applicable in diverse deep learning domains, such as facial recognition and autonomous driving. In GANs, the Generator makes fake samples (like images or audio) and aims to trick the Discriminator. The Discriminator's job is to tell real from fake. Both are like computer brains, and they compete during training. This happens many times, making both the Generator and Discriminator improve with each round. In [80], authors introduced a new approach to reconstructing photo-acoustic (PA) images using a combination of traditional reconstruction and deep learning. A novel model called Ki-GAN was proposed to focus on rebuilding initial vessel PA pressure. This model performs well with different types of data, including full-sampled, sparse-sampled, and in vivo experimental data. To enhance deep learning-based imaging by infusing more knowledge Ki-GAN was developed. Here an Auto-Encoder (AE) was designed as the foundation of Ki-GAN, which consists of two parts: one that adapts AE to PA signals using a specialized kernel (PSSIK), and another that enforces constraints between PA signals and images using an Image Feature Supervision. Additionally, a Knowledge Embedding Branch (KEB) was introduced to provide texture information to the raw PA signals. This branch converts certified knowledge from a conventional method (DAS) into textural information. Here adversarial learning was also utilized to further improve the correlation between PA signals and vessel reconstruction. This generator network produces the reconstructed image and is trained using adversarial loss along with other constraints. This total loss considers different factors like adversarial loss, pixel loss, auxiliary loss, and textural loss. These components work together to improve the quality of reconstructed PA images.

In [81], a novel deep-learning model called WGAN-GP, which operates within the framework of the GAN was proposed, to address limited-view and limited-bandwidth artifacts in photoacoustic computed tomography (PACT) images. WGAN-GP is trained and evaluated using simulated disk data and TPM vascular images, demonstrating improved image quality metrics. Notably, WGAN-GP outperforms the U-Net model both qualitatively and quantitatively in experimental phantom and in vivo animal data. This capability to mitigate artifacts has significant potential for enhancing PACT image quality without requiring modifications to the imaging system or sacrificing imaging speed. This advancement holds promise for various PACT applications, including mapping tumor vasculature during thermal ablation and detecting blood clots during Sonothrombolysis. However, there are limitations to this method. Here forward model considers only ultrasound generation, neglecting optical excitation variations that occur in practice. Additionally, deep learning networks trained on specific targets are limited in recognizing only those resembling the training data, a common challenge. Despite its success, WGAN-GP's training time is longer than U-Net's. The model's performance on vessel data was improved by increasing the training data size and incorporating additional PA data sources. However, confirming the accuracy of the reconstructed structures in real-life images is still difficult. One way to address this challenge is by using special microbubbles that work with PACT to improve ultrasound imaging at the same time, helping the authors to validate this DL model.

6.5.2 Recurrent Neural Networks (RNNs)

RNNs are like memory-based versions of feedforward and CNN neural networks. They use past information to affect current input and output. Unlike usual networks, RNNs remember past inputs in sequences. But they can't predict using future events in one direction. RNNs are used for sequential or time-related tasks like language translation, speech recognition, and image descriptions. Within the realm of RNNs, various architectures exist (such as the widely used LSTM). The fundamental distinction is the presence of internal feedback in the network, emanating from hidden layers, the output layer, or a combination of both. In [82] the authors employed the Recurrent Inference Machines (RIM) architecture for accelerated PAT reconstruction, minimizing iterative time. RIMs, which fall under the category of recurrent neural networks (RNNs), were introduced as versatile solutions for addressing inverse problems [83]. It can infer the adjoint model and constrain the solution space through iterative re-evaluation. The authors achieved high-resolution reconstruction of photoacoustic images by incorporating approximated models within the likelihood gradient and training an iterative algorithm through the RIM architecture. This architecture consists of three convolution layers and two gated recurrent units (GRU) cells. This method improved speed and required fewer parameters. Here the network's generalization capabilities were also explored. Linear array sensors were used in the experiments.

6.6 HYBRID MODELS IN PAT IMAGE RECONSTRUCTION— COMBINING TRADITIONAL AND DEEP LEARNING METHODS

Hybrid Convolutional Neural Network (CNN) models [71, 73–78] have recently become crucial in PAT image reconstruction. These approaches have been used to achieve faster and enhanced image reconstruction. It can also provide accurate and efficient results for PAT image reconstruction. The traditional methods such as FBP, delay and sum, TR, and model-based iterative methods give better performance in the field of reconstruction and formation of the PAT images. However, these methods failed to remove the artifacts or noise from the reconstructed images. Therefore, to mitigate this problem deep learning networks have been used as a post-processing method. The combination of the traditional methods and deep learning network can remove the artifacts and enhance the quality of the reconstructed image. Deep CNN trains a large number of datasets and captures the complex pattern. The basic hybrid reconstruction framework is described as, first, the acoustic pressure that undergoes an initial reconstruction using the traditional method, resulting in an image X with artifacts. Subsequently, a CNN is utilized to correct the artifacts resulting from under-sampling within image X. The outcome is an image Y that is nearly free from such artifacts. This procedure can be cast as a supervised learning mission, where the primary goal is to obtain a restoration function capable of converting the input image X into the desired output image Y [64]. According to the literature survey in [50] a combination of CNN, specifically Y-Net, was used to address the limitations of deep learning methods in PA image reconstruction. This technique involves two steps: direct processing and post-processing. It takes raw PA data and an initial rough solution as input and learns a way to reconstruct without iterations. This bridges the gap between deep learning steps. Traditional methods like TR and delay and sum were compared with this approach. The drawback of deep learning is that it sometimes uses low-quality images in post-processing. Also, iterative schemes are time-consuming and limited by resources. In another approach [51], the author combined the FBP algorithm and CNN to enhance image quality and remove artifacts. The images were reconstructed using the FBP method. Due to the noise and artifacts the quality of the reconstructed images was degraded. Therefore, U-Net CNN architecture was used here as a post-processing technique to remove the artifacts from the reconstructed images and enhance the quality of the image. The network was trained using a large number of datasets. They tested different network structures and found that U-Net performed well, providing real-time results. A combination of TR and residual U-Net was proposed in [84]. In [71], a deep learning approach called FD U-Net was employed as a post-processing method for 2D PAT image reconstruction using a planar scanner with sparse data. The choice of TR for this study stemmed from its adaptability to various sensor setups, solid initial reconstruction, and computational efficiency compared to iterative techniques. The FD U-Net integrated dense connectivity into the U-Net CNN structure, enhancing efficiency and architecture. Diverse datasets and SSIM/PSNR-based experimental results underscored the method's potential.

6.7   CONCLUSION

In this chapter, deep learning has emerged as a powerful tool in the field of PAT image reconstruction. DL can solve the challenges associated with sparse and limited-view data of PAT. Leveraging the capabilities of CNNs, researchers have developed various innovative architectures, building upon the foundation of the popular U-Net model. These architectures address critical issues in PAT, such as artifact elimination, noise reduction, and image enhancement, leading to significant advancements in image quality and reconstruction speed.

The U-Net architecture, with its encoder-decoder structure and skip connections, serves as a fundamental building block for these advancements. Researchers have introduced modifications like residual connections, dynamic aperture length correction, and multi-frequency sensor integration to enhance the performance of U-Net-based models. These innovations have demonstrated impressive results in mitigating challenges like non-ideal impulse response functions, spatial under-sampling, limited view, and reflection artifacts. The training and data augmentations of CNN are discussed here. The performance of the networks is evaluated using four indexes. GANs and RNNs are performed well for image reconstruction. The different hybrid models combining both traditional and CNN architectures for PAT image reconstruction are explained as well. Overall, the integration of deep learning techniques, particularly modified U-Net architectures, into PAT image reconstruction has brought forth a paradigm shift in the field. The advancements showcased in various studies underscore the potential of deep learning to improve image quality, enhance artifact elimination, and accelerate reconstruction processes. As deep learning continues to evolve and new architectural innovations emerge, the future of PAT image reconstruction holds exciting possibilities for even more efficient, accurate, and practical imaging solutions in both research and clinical settings.

REFERENCES

[1] P. K. Upputuri, and M. Pramanik, "Recent advances toward preclinical and clinical translation of photoacoustic tomography: A review," Journal of Biomedical Optics, vol. 22, no. 4, p. 041006, 2017, doi: 10.1117/1.JBO.22.4.041006, PMID: 27893078.

[2] K. Qinglin, G. Rui, L. Jietao, and S. Xiaopeng, "Investigation on reconstruction for frequency domain photoacoustic imaging via TVAL3 regularization algorithm," IEEE Photonics Journal, vol. 10, pp. 1–1, 2018, doi:10.1109/JPHOT.2018.2869815.

[3] J. R. Rajian, G. Girishn, and X. Wang, "Photoacoustic tomography to identify inflammatory arthritis," Journal of Biomedical Optics, vol. 17, no. 9, 2012, doi: 10.1117/1. JBO.17.9.096013. PMID: 23085914; PMCID: PMC3442106.

[4] F. Kamyar, and N. Saffari, "A numerical model for the study of photoacoustic imaging of brain tumours," 2015, arXiv:1512.06792v1.

[5] P. K. Upputuri, and M. Pramanik, "Photoacoustic imaging in the second near-infrared window: A review," Journal of Biomedical Optics, vol. 24, no. 4, pp. 1–20, 2019, doi: 10.1117/1.JBO.24.4.040901.

[6] D. A. Boas, C. Pritris, and N. Ramanujam, Handbook of Biomedical Optics, CRC Press, Boca Raton, Florida, 2011.

[7] M. Mehrmohammadi, S. J. Yoon, D. Yeager, and S. Y. Emelianov, "Photoacoustic Imaging for Cancer Detection and Staging," Current Molecular Imaging, vol. 2, no. 1, pp. 89–105, 2013, doi:10.2174/2211555211302010010. PMID: 24032095; PMCID: PMC3769095.

[8] A. Petschke, and P. J. La Rivière, "Comparison of photoacoustic image reconstruction algorithms using the channelized Hotelling observer," Journal of Biomedical Optics, vol. 18, no. 2, p. 026009, 2013, doi: 10.1117/1.JBO.18.2.026009.

[9] H. Huang, G. Bustamante, R. Peterson, and J. Y. Ye, "An adaptive filtered back-projection for photoacoustic image reconstruction," Medical Physics, vol. 42, no. 5, pp. 2169–2178, 2015, doi:10.1118/1.4915532.

[10] S. Zheng, H. Duoduo, and Y. Yuan, "2-D image reconstruction of photoacoustic endoscopic imaging based on time-reversal," Computers in biology and medicine, vol. 76, pp. 60–68, ISSN 0010–4825, 2016, doi: 10.1016/j.compbiomed.2016.06.028.

[11] H. Duoduo, S. Zheng, and Y. Yuan, "Reconstruction of intravascular photoacoustic images based on filtered back projection algorithm," Chinese Journal of Biomedical Engineering, vol. 35, pp. 10–19, 2016, doi: 10.3969/j.issn.0258-8021.2016.01.002.

[12] C. Cai, X. Wang, K. Si, J. Qian, J. Luo, and C. Ma, "Feature coupling photoacoustic computed tomography for joint reconstruction of initial pressure and sound speed in vivo," Biomedical Optics Express, vol. 10, no. 7, pp. 3447–3462, 2019, doi: 10.1364/ BOE.10.003447. PMID: 31467789; PMCID: PMC6706027.

[13] V. M. Moock, E. A. Gutiérrez-Reyes, and C. García-Segundo, "Image reconstruction with the Heaviside equation in photoacoustic tomography accounting for dispersive acoustic media," Journal of Biomedical Optics, vol. 23, no. 7, p. 076010, 2018, doi: 10.1117/1.JBO.23.7.076010.

[14] Y. Wang, J. Li, T. Lu, L. Zhang, Z. Zhou, H. Zhao, and F. Gao, "Combined diffuse optical tomography and photoacoustic tomography for enhanced functional imaging of small animals: A methodological study on phantoms," Applied Optics, vol. 56, pp. 303–311, 2017, doi: 10.1364/AO.56.000303. PMID: 28085867

[15] L. Zeng, G. Liu, B. Shao, Z. Ren, and Z. Huang, "Image reconstruction of high-quality photoacoustic tomography using wavelet-analysis-based algor^{it}hm," 2nd International

Conference on Bioinformatics and Biomedical Engineering, Shanghai, pp. 2565–2570, 2008, doi: 10.1109/ICBBE.2008.975.

[16] X. L. Dean-Ben, R. Ma, D. Razansky, and V. Ntziachristos, "Statistical approach for optoacoustic image reconstruction in the presence of strong acoustic heterogeneities," IEEE Transactions on Medical Imaging, vol. 30, no. 2, pp. 401–8, 2010, doi: 10.1109/TMI.2010.2081683.

[17] J. Provost, and F. Lesage, "The application of compressed sensing for photo-acoustic tomography," IEEE Transactions on Medical Imaging, vol. 28, no. 4, pp. 585–94, 2009, doi: 10.1109/TMI.2008.2007825.

[18] M. A. Mastanduno, and S. Gambhir, "Quantitative photoacoustic image reconstruction improves accuracy in deep tissue structures," Biomedical Optics Express, vol. 7, no. 10, pp. 3811–3825, 2016, doi: 10.1364/BOE.7.003811.

[19] X. Liu, and D. Peng, "Regularized iterative weighted filtered back-projection for few-view data photoacoustic imaging", Computational and Mathematical Methods in Medicine, vol. 2016, pp. 1–8, p. 9732142, 2016, doi: 10.1155/2016/9732142.

[20] P. K. Upputuri, and M. Pramanik, "Pulsed laser diode based optoacoustic imaging of biological tissues," Biomedical Physics and Engineering Express, vol. 1, p. 045010, 2015, doi: 10. 1088/2057–1976/1/4/045010.

[21] P. K. Upputuri, and M. Pramanik, "Performance characterization of low-cost, high-speed, portable pulsed laser diode photoacoustic tomography (PLD-PAT) system," Biomedical Optics Express, vol. 6, no. 4, p. 4118, 2015, doi: 10.1364/BOE.6.004118.

[22] P. K. Upputuri, and M. Pramanik, "Dynamic in vivo imaging of small animal brain using pulsed laser diode-based photoacoustic tomography system," Journal of Biomedical Optics, vol. 22, pp. 90501–90504, 2017, doi: 10.1117/1.JBO.22.9.090501.

[23] B. T. Cox, S. Kara, S. R. Arridge, and P. C. Beard, "K-space propagation models for acoustically heterogeneous media: Application to biomedical photoacoustic," Journal of Acoustical Society of America, vol. 121, no. 6, pp. 3453–64, 2007, doi: 10.1121/1.2717409.

[24] M. Haltmeier, O. Scherzer, and G. Zangerl, "A Reconstruction algorithm for photoacoustic imaging based on the nonuniform FFT," IEEE Transactions on Medical Imaging, vol. 28, no. 11, 2009, doi: 10.1109/TMI.2009.2022623.

[25] P. Mohajerani, S. Kellnberger, and V. Ntziachristos, "Fast Fourier backprojection for frequency-domain optoacoustic tomography," Optics Letters, vol. 39, no. 18, pp. 5455–5458, 2014, doi: 10.1364/OL.39.005455. PMID: 26466296.

[26] R. Schulze, G. Zangerl, M. Holotta, D. Meyer, F. Handle, R. Nuster, G. Paltauf, and O. Scherzer, "On the use of frequency-domain reconstruction algorithms for photoacoustic imaging," Journal of Biomedical Optics, vol. 16, no. 8, p. 086002, 2011, doi: 10.1117/1.3605696.

[27] T. Berer, A. Hochreiner, H. Roitner, and P. Burgholzer, "Reconstruction algorithms for remote photoacoustic imaging," IEEE International Ultrasonics Symposium (IUS), pp. 1–4, 2012, doi: 10.1109/ULTSYM.2012.0579.

[28] B. E. Treeby, J. Jaros, and B. T. Cox, "Advanced photoacoustic image reconstruction using the k-Wave toolbox," Proceedings SPIE 9708, Photons Plus Ultrasound: Imaging and Sensing, vol. 97082P, 2016, doi: 10.1117/12.2209254.

[29] R. W. Schoonover and M. A. Anastasio, "Image reconstruction in photoacoustic tomography involving layered acoustic media," Journal of Optical Society of America A, vol. 28, no. 6, pp. 1114–1120, 2011, doi: 10.1364/JOSAA.28.001114. PMID: 21643397; PMCID: PMC3273907.

[30] K. Kondo, T. Namita, M. Yamakawa, and T. Shiina, "Three-dimensional photoacoustic reconstruction for sparse array using compressed sensing based on k-space algorithm," IEEE International Ultrasonics Symposium (IUS), Tours, France, 2016, pp. 1–3, 2016, doi: 10.1109/ULTSYM.2016.7728883.

[31] E. Batbayar, J. Y. Lee, W. Ham, E. Tumenjargal, C. Song, and S. Roh, "Implementation of medical image reconstruction algorithm for photoacoustic imaging using k-wave toolkit," IEEE 17th International Conference on Bioinformatics and Bioengineering (BIBE), Washington, DC, USA, 2017, pp. 508–513, 2016, doi:10.1109/BIBE.2017.000-3.

[32] S. Schoeder, M. Kronbichler, and W. A. Wall, "Photoacoustic image reconstruction: Material detection and acoustical heterogeneities," Inverse Problems, vol. 33, no. 5, p. 055010, 2017, doi: 10.1088/1361-6420/aa635b.

[33] R. J. Zemp, "Quantitative photoacoustic tomography with multiple optical sources," Applied Optics, vol. 49, pp. 3566–3572, 2010, doi: 10.1364/AO.49.003566.

[34] B. Cong, K. Kondo, M. Yamakawa, T. Shiina, "Photoacoustic image reconstruction quality enhancement based on optimum focusing by calculating mean acoustic sound-speed," IEEE International Ultrasonics Symposium, IUS, pp. 1368–1371, 2014, doi: 10.1109/ULTSYM.2014.0338.

[35] P. Warbal and S. Ratank, "A comparative study of some photoacoustic image reconstruction algorithm for inhomogeneous phantom," WESPAC, New Delhi, India 2018.

[36] C. Huang, "Image reconstruction in photoacoustic computed tomography with acoustically heterogeneous media," All Theses and Dissertations (ETDs), p. 1308, 2014.

[37] B. E. Treeby, J. Laufer, E. Zhang, F. Norris, M. Lythgoe, P. Beard, and B. Cox, "Acoustic attenuation compensation in photoacoustic tomography: Application to high-resolution 3D imaging of vascular networks in mice," Journal of Biomedical Optics, vol. 18, no. 3, p. 7899, 2011, doi: 10.1117/12.874530.

[38] A. Javaherian, and S. Holman, "A multi-grid iterative method for photoacoustic tomography," IEEE Transactions on Medical Imaging, vol. 36, no. 3, pp. 696–706, 2017, doi: 10.1109/TMI.2016.2625272.

[39] K. Wang, R. Su, and A. A. Oraevsky, "Investigation of iterative image reconstruction in three-dimensional optoacoustic tomography," Physics in Medicine and Biology, vol. 57, no. 17, pp. 5399–5423, 2012, doi: 10.1088/0031-9155/57/17/5399.

[40] C. Huang, K. Wang, L. Nie, and L. V. Wang, "Full-wave iterative image reconstruction in photoacoustic tomography with acoustically inhomogeneous media," IEEE Transactions on Medical Imaging, vol. 32, no. 6, pp. 1097–1110, 2013, doi: 10.1109/TMI.2013.2254496.

[41] B. Banerjee, S. Bagchi, R. M. Vasu, and D. Roy, "Quantitative photoacoustic tomography from boundary pressure measurements: Noniterative recovery of optical absorption coefficient from the reconstructed absorbed energy map," Journal of Optical Society of America A, vol. 25, no. 9, pp. 2347–2356, 2008, doi: 10.1364/josaa.25.002347. PMID: 18758563.

[42] P. Omidi, M. Zafar, M. Mozaffarzadeh, A. Hariri, X. Haung, M. Orooji, and M. Nasiriavanaki, "A novel dictionary-based image reconstruction for photoacoustic computed tomography," Applied Sciences, vol. 8, no. 9, p. 1570, 2018, doi: 10.3390/app8091570.

[43] T. Jetzfellner, D. Razansky, A. Rosenthal, R. Schulz, K. H. Englmeier, and V. Ntziachristos, "Performance of iterative optoacoustic tomography with experimental data," Applied Physics Letters, vol. 95, no. 1, pp. 013703–013703, 2009, doi: 10.1063/1.3167280.

[44] X. L. Dean-Ben, R. Ma, A. Rosenthal, V. Ntziachristos, and D. Razansky, "Weighted model-based optoacoustic reconstruction in acoustic scattering media," Physics in Medicine and Biology, vol. 58, no. 16, pp. 5555–5566, 2013, doi: 10.1088/0031-9155/58/16/5555.

[45] K. J. Francis, P. Mishra, P. Rajalakshmi, S. S. Channappayya, and A. Richhariya, "A simple and accurate matrix for model-based photoacoustic imaging," 2016 IEEE 18th International Conference on e-Health Networking, Applications, and Services (Healthcom), Munich, Germany, pp. 1–5, 2016, doi: 10.1109/HealthCom.2016.7749481.

[46] L. Ding, X. L. Deán-Ben, and D. Razansky, "Real-time model-based inversion in cross-sectional optoacoustic tomography," IEEE Transactions on Medical Imaging, vol. 35, no. 8, pp. 1883–1891, 2016, doi: 10.1109/TMI.2016.2536779.

[47] M. Mozaffarzadeh, A. Mahloojifar, M. Nasiriavanaki, and M. Orooji, "Model-based photoacoustic image reconstruction using compressed sensing and smoothed L0 norm," Proc. SPIE 10494, Photons Plus Ultrasound: Imaging and Sensing 2018, 104943Z, 2018, doi: 10.1117/12.2291535.

[48] S. Biton, N. Arbel, G. Drozdov, G. Gilboa, and A. Rosenthal, "Optoacoustic model-based inversion using anisotropic adaptive total-variation regularization," Photoacoustics, vol. 16, p. 100142, ISSN 2213–5979, 2019, doi: 10.1016/j.pacs.2019.100142.

[49] M. Bhatt, S. Gutta, and P. Yalavarthy, "Exponential filtering of singular values improves photoacoustic image reconstruction," Journal of the Optical Society of America A, Optics, Image Science, and Vision, vol. 33, no. 9, pp. 1785–1792, 2016, doi: 10.1364/JOSAA.33.001785.

[50] H. Lan, D. Jiang, C. Yang, and F. Gao, "Y-Net: Hybrid deep learning image reconstruction for photoacoustic tomography in vivo," Photoacoustics, vol. 20, p. 100197, ISSN 2213–5979, 2020, doi: 10.1016/j.pacs.2020.100197.

[51] S. Antholzer, M. Haltmeier, R. Nuster, and J. Schwab, "Photoacoustic image reconstruction via deep learning," Proceedings of SPIE 10494, Photons Plus Ultrasound: Imaging and Sensing, 104944U, 2018, doi: 10.1117/12.2290676.

[52] N. Davoudi, X.L. Deán-Ben, and D. Razansky, "Deep learning optoacoustic tomography with sparse data," Nature Machine Intelligence, vol. 1, no. 10, pp. 453–460, 2019, doi: 10.1038/s42256-019-0095-3.

[53] A. Hauptmann, B. Cox, F. Lucka, N. Huynh, B. Marta, P. Beard, and S. Arridge, "Approximate k-space models and deep learning for fast photoacoustic reconstruction," Machine Learning for Medical Image Reconstruction (MLMIR), Lecture Notes in Computer Science, vol. 11074, Springer, Cham. 2018, doi: 10.1007/978-3-030-00129-2_12.

[54] N. Baddour, "Theory and analysis of frequency-domain photoacoustic tomography," Journal of the Acoustical Society of America A, vol. 123, no. 5, pp. 2577–90, 2008, doi: 10.1121/1.2897132.

[55] P. Mohajerani, S. Kellnberger, and V. Ntziachristos, "Frequency domain optoacoustic tomography using amplitude and phase," Photoacoustics, vol. 2, no. 3, pp. 114–118, 2014, doi: 10.1016/j.pacs.2014.06.002.

[56] H. -M. Schwab, M. F. Beckmann, and G. Schmitz, "Iterative photoacoustic reconstruction in heterogeneous media using the Kaczmarz method," IEEE International Ultrasonics Symposium, Chicago, IL, USA, pp. 33–36, 2014, doi: 10.1109/ULTSYM.2014.0009.

[57] P. C. Hansen, and D. P. O'Leary, "The use of the l-curve in the regularization of discrete Ill-posed problems," SIAM Journal on Scientific Computing, vol. 14, no. 6, pp. 1487–1503, 1993, doi: 10.1137/0914086.

[58] O. Ronneberger, P. Fischer, and T. Brox, "U-net: Convolutional networks for biomedical image segmentation," Medical Image Computing and Computer-Assisted Intervention—MICCAI 2015, Lecture Notes in Computer Science, vol. 9351, Springer, Cham, pp. 234–241, 2015, doi: 10.1007/978-3-319-24574-4_28.

[59] K. H. Jin, M. T. McCann, E. Froustey, and M. Unser, "Deep Convolutional Neural Network for Inverse Problems in Imaging," IEEE Transactions on Image Processing, vol. 26, no. 9, pp. 4509–4522, 2017, doi: 10.1109/TIP.2017.2713099.

[60] D. P. Kingma, and J. Ba, "Adam: A method for stochastic optimization," arXiv:1412.6980, 2014.

[61] J. G. Lee, S. Jun, Y. W. Cho, H. Lee, G. B. Kim, J. B. Seo, and N. Kim, "Deep learning in medical imaging: General overview," Korean Journal of Radiology, vol. 18, no. 4, pp. 570–584, 2017, doi: 10.3348/kjr.2017.18.4.570. PMID: 28670152; PMCID: PMC5447633.

[62] M. T. McCann, K. H. Jin, and M. Unser, "Convolutional neural networks for inverse problems in imaging: A review," IEEE Signal Processing Magazine, vol. 34, no. 6, pp. 85–95, 2017, doi: 10.1109/MSP.2017.2739299.

[63] C. Cai, K. Deng, C. Ma, and J. Luo, "End-to-end deep neural network for optical inversion in quantitative photoacoustic imaging," Optics Letters, vol. 43, no. 12, pp. 2752–2755, 2018, doi: 10.1364/OL.43.002752.

[64] S. Antholzer, M. Haltmeier, and J. Schwab, "Deep learning for photoacoustic tomography from sparse data," Inverse Problems in Science and Engineering, vol. 27, no. 7, pp. 987–1005, 2019, doi: 10.1080/17415977.2018.1518444. PMID: 31057659

[65] N. Awasthi, K. R. Prabhakar, S. K. Kalva, M. Pramanik, R. V. Babu, and P. K. Yalavarthy, "PA-fuse: Deep supervised approach for the fusion of photoacoustic images with distinct reconstruction characteristics," Biomedical Optics Express, vol. 10, no. 5, pp. 2227–2243, 2019, doi: 10.1364/BOE.10.002227. PMID: 31149371; PMCID: PMC6524595.

[66] H. Chen, Y. Zhang, W. Zhang, P. Liao, K. Li, J. Zhou, and G. Wang, "Low-dose CT via convolutional neural network," Biomedical Optics Express, vol. 8, no. 2, pp. 679–694, 2017, doi: 10.1364/BOE.8.000679. PMID: 28270976; PMCID: PMC5330597

[67] B. Kelly, T. P. Matthews, and M. A. Anastasio, "Deep learning-guided image reconstruction from incomplete data," arXiv:1709.00584, 2017.

[68] Y. Han, J. J. Yoo, and J. C. Ye, "Deep residual learning for compressed sensing CT reconstruction via persistent homology analysis," arXiv: abs/1611.06391, 2016.

[69] G. Wang, "A perspective on deep imaging," IEEE Access, vol. 4, pp. 8914–8924, 2016, doi: 10.1109/ACCESS.2016.2624938.

[70] H. Zhang, L. Li, K. Qiao, L. Wang, B. Yan, and G. Hu, "Image prediction for limited-angle tomography via deep learning with convolutional neural network," arXiv:1607.08707, 2016.

[71] S. Guan, A. A. Khan, S. Sikdar, and P. V. Chitnis, "Fully dense U-Net for 2-D sparse photoacoustic tomography artifact removal," IEEE Journal of Biomedical and Health Informatics, vol. 24, no. 2, pp. 568–576, 2020, doi: 10.1109/JBHI.2019.2912935.

[72] S. Guan, A. A. Khan, S. Sikdar, and P. V. Chitnis, "Limited-view and sparse photoacoustic tomography for neuroimaging with deep learning," Scientific Reports, vol. 10, no. 8510, 2020, doi.org/10.1038/s41598-020-65235-2.

[73] J. Schwab, S. Antholzer, R. Nuster, and M. Haltmeier, "Real-time photoacoustic projection imaging using deep learning," arXiv:1801.06693, 2018.

[74] H. Shahid, A. Khalid, X. Liu, M. Irfan, and D. Ta, "A deep learning approach for the photoacoustic tomography recovery from undersampled measurements," Frontiers in Neuroscience, vol. 15, no. 18, 2021, doi.org/10.3389/fnins.2021.598693.

[75] H. Lan, C. Yang, D. Jiang, and F. Gao, "Deep learning approach to reconstruct the photoacoustic image using multi-frequency data," IEEE International Ultrasonics Symposium (IUS), Glasgow, UK, pp. 487–489, 2019, doi: 10.1109/ULTSYM.2019.8926287.

[76] H. Lan, C. Yang, D. Jiang, and F. Gao, "Reconstruct the photoacoustic image based on deep learning with multi-frequency ring-shape transducer array," in 41st Annual International Conference of the IEEE Engineering in Medicine and Biology Society (EMBC), Berlin, Germany, pp. 7115–7118, 2019, doi: 10.1109/EMBC.2019.8856590.

[77] H. Lan, K. Zhou, C. Yang, J. Liu, S. Gao, and F. Gao, "Hybrid neural network for photoacoustic imaging reconstruction" in 41st Annual International Conference of the IEEE Engineering in Medicine and Biology Society (EMBC), IEEE, Berlin, Germany, pp. 6367–6370, 2019, doi: 10.1109/EMBC.2019.8857019.

[78] T. Tong, W. Huang, K. Wang, Z. He, L. Yin, X. Yang, S. Zhang, and J. Tian, "Domain transform network for photoacoustic tomography from limited-view and sparsely sampled data," Photoacoustics, vol. 19, p. 100190, 2020, doi: 10.1016/j.pacs.2020.100190. PMID: 32617261; PMCID: PMC7322684.

[79] B. E. Treeby, and B. T. Cox, "k-Wave: MATLAB toolbox for the simulation and reconstruction of photoacoustic wave fields," Journal of Biomedical Optics, vol. 15, no. 2, pp. 021314–12, 2010, doi: 10.1117/1.3360308.

[80] H. Lan, C. Yang, J. Cheng, J. Liu, S. Gao, F. Gao, and K. Zhou, "Ki-GAN: Knowledge infusion generative adversarial network for photoacoustic image reconstruction

in Vivo," in Medical Image Computing and Computer Assisted Intervention—MIC-CAI 2019, Lecture Notes in Computer Science, vol. 11764. Springer, Cham, 2019, doi: 10.1007/978-3-030-32239-7_31.

[81] T. Vu, M. Li, H. Humayun, Y. Zhou, and J. Yao, "A generative adversarial network for artifact removal in photoacoustic computed tomography with a linear-array transducer," Experimental Biology and Medicine (Maywood, N.J.), vol. 245, no. 7, pp. 597–605, 2020, doi: 10.1177/1535370220914285.

[82] C. Yang, H. Lan, and F. Gao, "Accelerated photoacoustic tomography reconstruction via recurrent inference machines," in 41st Annual International Conference of the IEEE Engineering in Medicine and Biology Society (EMBC), Berlin, Germany, pp. 6371–6374, 2019, doi: 10.1109/EMBC.2019.8856290.

[83] P. Putzky, and M. Welling, "Recurrent inference machines for solving inverse problems," 2017, doi: 10.48550/arXiv.1706.04008.

[84] P. Farnia, M. Mohammadi, E. Najafzadeh, M. Alimohamadi, B. Makkiabadi and A. Ahmadian, "High-quality photoacoustic image reconstruction based on deep convolutional neural network: Towards intra-operative photoacoustic imaging," Biomedical Physics and Engineering Express, vol. 6, no. 4, IOP Publishing Ltd., 2020, doi: 10.1088/2057-1976/ab9a10.

7 Design and Development of Computer-Aided Diagnosis to Detect Lung Cancer Disease by Using Intelligent Deep Learning Principle

Jayaraj R., Sivakamasundari N., Satyajeet Sahoo, Niranjana S., and Ramkumar G.

7.1 INTRODUCTION

Lung cancer refers to the uncontrolled proliferation of cells in the lungs of a human being. As the main cause of death over the past few decades, lung cancer ranks among the world's worst diseases. In terms of annual deaths, it surpasses even those caused by breast, prostate, and colon cancers. The number of people diagnosed with and lost to lung cancer has risen dramatically. Non-small cell lung carcinoma (NSCLC) accounts for 85–88% of lung cancer cases, while small cell lung carcinoma (SCLC) accounts for 12–15%. Due to its invasiveness and heterogeneity, lung cancer needs early identification and treatment in order to improve the overall five-year survival rate [1]. Cigarette smoking is associated with a higher risk of developing lung cancer.

Approximately 81% of the 127,070 deaths from lung cancer in 2023 will be attributable to smoking cigarettes, with passive smoking accounting for an additional 3560 deaths. Lung nodules can be either benign or cancerous, the latter being far less common. Benign nodules in the lungs don't go somewhere else in the body and tend to stay put. Nodules in the lungs are often noncancerous. Factors such as diet, stress, heredity, local injury, and radiation exposure have been proposed as possible causes of benign tumors [2]. However, malignant lung nodules can rapidly metastasize throughout the body via the lymphatic or circulatory systems. If a malignant lung tumor is caught early enough, surgery and chemotherapy can be effective treatments.

DOI: 10.1201/9781032635149-7

Early identification with CT and MRI, two routine medical tests, has been shown to significantly increase patient survival rates. Sequential Flood Feature Selection Algorithms (SFFSA) and Genetic Algorithms (GA) are two examples of feature extraction techniques that were traditionally employed by previous intelligence systems to assist in creating ideal features [3]. Many effective medical image processing tools can attribute their success to their incorporation of deep learning algorithms, which are utilized in CAD systems to automatically extract picture attributes.

Small-cell lung cancer and non-small-cell lung cancer are the two most common forms of lung cancer. Among the causes of lung cancer are tobacco use (in smokers and nonsmokers alike), environmental tobacco smoke, hazardous air particles, sexual orientation, genetics, age, etc. Among the leading causes of lung cancer is a lifetime of tobacco use. Lung cancer can be diagnosed based on the presence of a number of symptoms, such as yellow fingers, anxiety, chronic disease, weariness, allergies, wheezing and roaring, coughing up blood, even little quantities, hoarseness, shortness of breath, bone pain, headache, trouble swallowing, and chest discomfort. Lung cancer is seen on X-ray, Figure 7.1.

With its high-contrast pictures and three-dimensional data, computed tomography (CT) scans are among the most effective diagnostic tools for people with lung cancer and chronic kidney disease. Manual review of medical photographs is costly, time-consuming, and prone to error because of a worldwide dearth of nephrologists and radiologists. Radiologists rely heavily on CT scans to detect lung and renal problems. However, the procedure is greatly impacted by the need for a second opinion because of the scarcity of healthcare specialists [4]. This suggests that the early diagnosis of lung illnesses and renal disorders including kidney stones, cysts, and tumors is crucial in minimizing kidney failure and lung cancer.

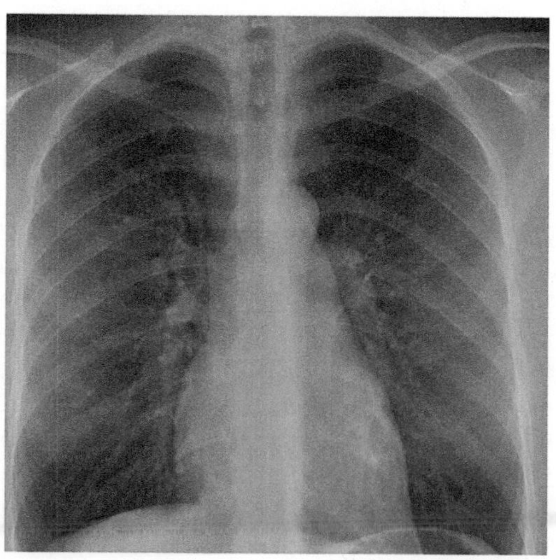

FIGURE 7.1 Lung cancer sample image.

Lung cancer identification and categorization using CAD systems has been the subject of much research. The performance of CAD systems in detecting lung nodules and cancer in medical imaging is superior to that of professional radiologists. The four main components of a CAD-based lung cancer detection system are image processing, ROI extraction, feature selection, and categorization. As the CAD system uses image processing to gather trustworthy features, the precision and responsiveness of the system greatly benefit from feature selection and categorization. The difficulty is in determining whether a nodule is benign or cancerous. Numerous researchers have used deep learning methods to improve radiologists' diagnostic precision. Studies have shown that CAD systems powered by deep learning may greatly enhance the speed and precision with which medical professionals can identify and treat common malignancies like lung and breast. By employing novel network architectures, CAD systems powered by deep learning can automatically extract complex information from raw pictures. Nevertheless, there are drawbacks to CAD systems that rely on deep learning, such as limited sensitivity, high FP, and lengthy processing times. Consequently, there is an immediate requirement for a quick, low-cost, and highly sensitive CAD system based on deep learning for predicting lung cancer.

Investigations into lung imaging methods based on deep learning have focused mostly on the identification, segmentation, and classification of benign and malignant pulmonary nodules. If we want better results from our deep learning models, we need to come up with new network architectures and loss functions, and that's where most of the research effort goes. Review articles on deep learning methods have been published by a number of academic organizations recently [5]. Many novel deep learning approaches and applications appear each year, though, due to the field's fast evolution. In this work, we present a novel methodology for exploiting chest X-ray pictures to diagnose lung disorders such as pneumonia and Covid-19. The foundation of our method is the use of the INNOT (Improved Neural Network and Optimization Technique). Due to the risk of picture deterioration in X-ray imaging, we employ a two-stage technique consisting of median filtering and histogram equalization to improve image quality.

To choose the best characteristics to feed into an Artificial Neural Network (ANN) for classification, we use the fuzzy particle swarm optimization (FPSO) method. In this stage, we choose the most important and differentiating attributes to feed into the ANN. By combining these, we have a robust and very successful system for accurate illness prediction, one that is well-suited to the difficulties of chest X-ray pictures.

7.2 RELATED WORKS

In our day and age, lung cancer is the second-most common cancer stereotype after breast cancer. Similarly to other malignancies, the survival rate for this one is low. The early detection of lung cancer by screening is possible. Early detection and treatment of an illness improves the likelihood of a successful outcome. The most popular and efficient method of screening for lung cancer is computed tomography (CT). Visual interpretation of CT scan pictures, however, is challenging, time-consuming, and might result in incorrect malignancy interpretation. Therefore, the identification of lung disorders requires the use of computer-assisted approaches. There are a number of methods described in the books. Using CT scan image processing, the authors of [6] provide a unique method for detecting and classifying lung cancer. Several preprocessing methods are used for smoothing and improving the images. Researchers then use thresholding and edge detection to isolate the lung tumor inside the area of interest (ROI). Furthermore, a support vector machine (SVM) classifier is used to categorize the retrieved ROI based on its many geometrical properties into benign and malignant categories. We discovered that our suggested technique is very accurate in detecting lung cancer nodules and estimating the severity level.

Common people's lives can be severely disrupted by lung infections. Conditions affecting the lungs, such as TB, pneumonia, lung cancer, and chronic obstructive pulmonary disease, require prompt medical attention. Due to its widespread availability and low cost, chest X-rays are often used as a diagnostic tool for a variety of lung disorders. Radiologists and pulmonologists face a formidable challenge when tasked with categorizing illnesses from chest X-rays. When it comes to diagnosing illnesses, computer-aided diagnosis (CAD) systems are helpful since they allow clinicians to do quantitative analysis on chest X-rays. The diagnosis accuracy of such systems may be maximized if they were better able to draw judgments about disease types from X-ray images. The shortage of qualified radiologists only makes everything more precarious. It is unrealistic to expect technicians and care providers to be trained for the influx of demand in such a short amount of time. Researchers employ cutting-edge technology to find a solution. Early identification of lung issues using the accessible chest X-ray picture may be a good fit for machine learning-based algorithms, which might yield consistent findings. This means that high-quality algorithms applied to chest X-ray pictures may one day allow us to put a numerical value on the extent of lung disease. In [7], the author describes in depth the publicly available chest X-ray image databases that may be used to diagnose a wide range of lung disorders.

Lung diseases are a broad term that encompasses a wide range of lung-related conditions, such as pneumonia, TB, lung cancer, and many more. Three million people every year lose their lives to COPD (chronic obstructive lung disease), making it the third-biggest cause of mortality on the planet. A prompt response to disease prevention requires early identification. Imaging techniques such as computed tomography (CT) and chest X-rays can diagnose these conditions. This is because there is a lot of overlap across lung illnesses and even within a single condition, making it difficult to diagnose accurately. up his study of lung disorders, author [8] zeroed up on the fact that there is little variance across classes but a lot of diversity within classes. Normal, lung cancer, pneumonia, and TB are four classes that are classified using the suggested method's combination of pre-processing, data augmentation, and deep learning. By augmenting data with DCGAN, we can better portray underrepresented groups. Using a publicly accessible dataset, we conduct a thorough evaluation of the suggested methodology and find that it outperforms the state-of-the-art methods by a significant margin.

The effects of lung cancer are devastating. Lung cancer identification based on medical records has been used before, but it has shown poor results. Classifying people with and without lung cancer using AI algorithms is more accurate and time-efficient. Lung cancer diagnosis determined by medical records is time-consuming and expensive. After diagnosis, lung cancer has a relatively low survival rate. Lung cancer may be diagnosed quickly and effectively using AI-based diagnostic technologies. Nevertheless, there are a number of caveats to the existing body of research. For instance, some strategies have a very long computing time but great accuracy, while others have a shorter computation time but lower accuracy. In order to identify lung cancer at an early stage and with high accuracy, researchers [9] propose a diagnosis method based on deep convolutional neural networks. We used a deep convolutional neural network trained on data obtained from the public Kaggle library to diagnose lung cancer with high precision. We have also utilized certain max, min, standard deviation, and variance threshold preprocessing and feature selection methods.

All areas of medicine have advanced in recent years, but cancer diagnosis in particular has come a long way. Nonetheless, it remains the leading cause of mortality worldwide. Twenty percent of all cancer cases are exclusively attributable to colon and lung cancers. Both prognosis and treatment success rate improve with earlier-stage cancer detection. In this respect, diagnostic phases are particularly important places for artificial intelligence-based aid toolboxes to shine. Author [10] used three small-footprint deep learning networks to categorize photos of colon and lung cancer in three different settings. In the context of the transfer learning concept, we used pre-trained models such as AlexNet, SqueezeNet, and ShuflleNet. In the first case, CNNs were employed to detect lung and colon cancers. Each model's outcomes for classification were given independently as SoftMax classification results. In the second instance, the SVM classifier was trained using just the image attributes returned by the pre-trained model. In the last instance, a principal component analysis (PCA) was run on the retrieved features of the networks to aid in refining the investigation. The reliability of classification was further enhanced by feeding the revised feature sets produced by the feature selection technique into SVM. The third scenario provided the clearest visuals of colon and lung cancer. The ShuffleNet was shown to have a classification accuracy of 99.93% for the colon cancer dataset and 97.92% for the lung cancer dataset.

7.3 METHODOLOGY

In order to foresee lung disorders, this study presents a novel framework called Improved Neural Network and Optimization Technique (INNOT). We devised a two-step improvement strategy incorporating median filtering and histogram equalization to solve the difficulties posed by picture quality decrease during X-ray imaging. Choosing the right features is a crucial part of the preprocessing that comes before using an ANN for categorization. The FPSO method is used for this aim. The suggested model's architecture is depicted in Figure 7.2.

7.4 IMAGE PREPROCESSING

In order to employ X-ray pictures of lung cancer in machine learning or deep learning models, they must first undergo extensive preprocessing. Data quality, noise levels, and the suitability of the pictures for analysis may all be improved with careful preparation. Collect a database of X-rays of the lungs that includes both lung cancer cases and healthy lungs. Add a label (positive or negative) to each photograph to

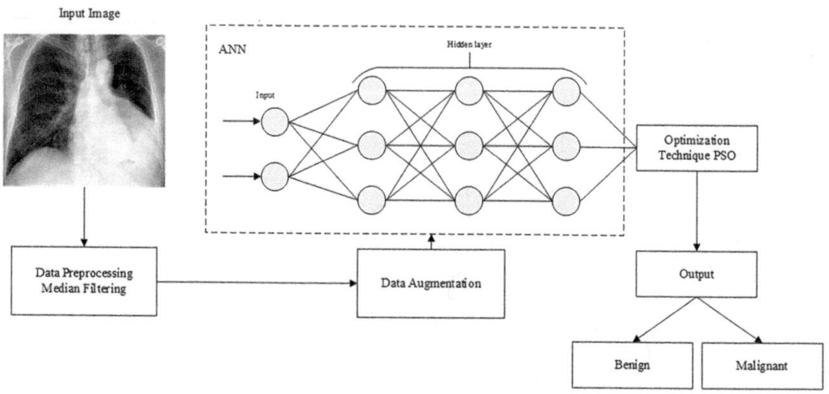

FIGURE 7.2 Architecture of proposed model.

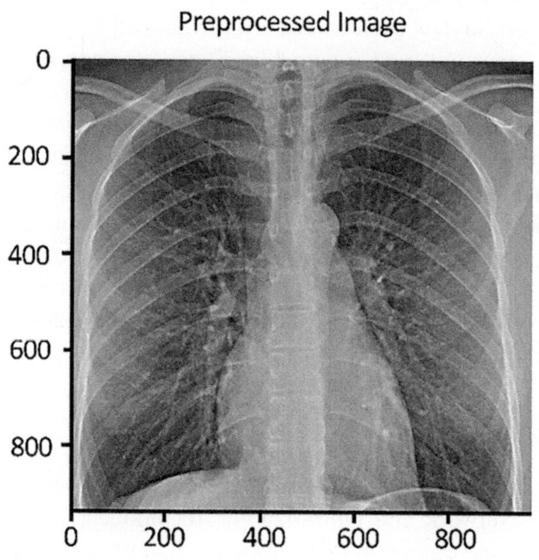

FIGURE 7.3 Preprocessed image.

indicate whether or not lung cancer is visible. Discard any photos that have already been used. Take care of any problems with the data's quality, such as blurry pictures or incorrectly oriented photographs. Median filtering is a standard preprocessing method utilized to lessen the impact of noise and boost image quality. It works especially well when dealing with salt-and-pepper noise, which causes random bright and dark spots to appear in an otherwise normal image. Image before any processing is shown in Figure 7.3. Median filtering is effective because it replaces every pixel's numerical value with the median value of its adjacent pixel values, which is less susceptible to extreme values and more capable of maintaining the image's edges and finer features.

7.5 IMAGE AUGMENTATION

X-ray image enhancement for lung cancer detection is a useful method for expanding and improving your training dataset. To make your model more robust and accurate, you may apply several adjustments to the source photos. Simulate image flaws by adding noise, such as Gaussian noise. Image augmentation often involves the addition of noise, and Gaussian noise is a frequent form of noise to use. It generates noise similar to that which may be seen in real-world imaging by simulating random fluctuations in pixel values. In Gaussian (normal) noise, the variance is roughly normally distributed about some central value. You may make your machine learning or deep learning models more robust by training them on noisy data by including Gaussian noise in the picture augmentation process. Particularly in medical imaging applications, such as lung cancer diagnosis, it is crucial to regulate the amount of noise supplied to guarantee that the pictures remain diagnostically correct. Figure 7.4 displays the unaltered and enhanced versions of the photograph.

7.6 FEATURE EXTRACTION

In order to make sense of the raw pixel data in medical pictures like X-ray lung scans, feature extraction is a vital stage in the analysis process. Machine learning and deep learning models take these depictions, or features, as inputs to accomplish tasks like lung disease diagnosis, anomaly detection, and classification. In order to extract relevant features from a picture, histogram-based feature extraction analyzes the distribution of pixel intensities in the histogram. Image contrast, brightness, and general texture may all be gleaned via this technique. Histogram equalization is used to increase contrast in a picture by resampling pixel intensities throughout the whole range.

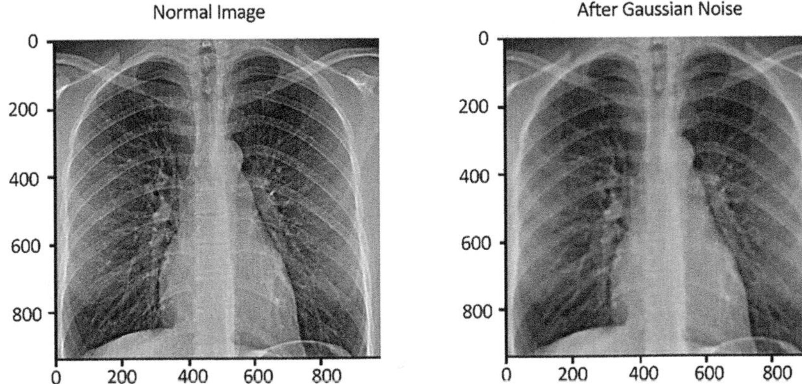

FIGURE 7.4 Normal image and after adding Gaussian noise.

7.7 ARTIFICIAL NEURAL NETWORK

Biological neural networks in the human brain serve as inspiration for Artificial Neural Networks (ANNs), which are computer models. ANNs are crucial to the fields of machine learning and deep learning because of their ability to infer hidden meaning from datasets. They find widespread use in identifying patterns and prediction tasks including image and speech recognition, NLP, and a host of others. Artificial Neural Networks (ANNs) are a common and successful method in the analysis of medical images for detecting lung cancer in X-ray pictures. Artificial neural networks (ANNs) are a sort of ML models that take their cues from the brain's neural architecture. They are well-suited for jobs such as picture categorization and medical diagnosis because of their prowess in learning complicated patterns and correlations within data.

An ANN is a computer program that mimics the functions of a network of real neurons to perform tasks such as data analysis. An ANN consists of the following primary parts:

1. Neurons (Nodes)
   - Neurons are computing elements that simulate the function of real neurons.
   - Neurons receive data, process it, and then release some kind of signal.
   - Every neuron in an ANN is given a weight that indicates how much its input is valued overall.
2. Layers
   - The neurons in an ANN are arranged in layers. Layers can be categorized as either input, concealed, or output.
   - Raw data or features are received by the input layer, whereas the final forecast or result is generated by the output layer.
   - To the extent that they exist, hidden layers serve as intermediary layers that develop sophisticated representations of the incoming data.
3. Connections (Synapses)
   - Connections between neurons act like synapses in organic brain networks by allowing information to flow between neurons.
   - The significance or weight of a link in the overall flow of data is represented by its size.
4. Activation Function
   - With the help of an activation function, neurons may perform calculations in a non-linear fashion, allowing the network to accurately represent complicated connections.
   - Sigmoid, tanh, and ReLU (Rectified Linear Unit) are typical activation functions.
5. Feedforward Propagation
   - Feedforward propagation refers to the method by which an input is sent through the many layers of a network in order to generate a desired output.
   - Each layer's neurons are fed data from the layer below them and outputs are generated based on the weighted sum of those inputs as well as an activation function.

6. Training and Learning
   - Training is the process through which ANNs acquire knowledge from their inputs. The network learns by comparing its predictions with its actual results and then adjusting its weights accordingly.
   - Optimization methods, such as gradient descent, are commonly used to make this modification by minimizing a loss function that characterizes the model's prediction error.
7. Backpropagation
   - By recalculating the loss function's gradients with regard to the network's weights, we get backpropagation. Throughout training, the weights are adjusted based on these gradients.
   - The term "backpropagation" refers to the process of sending an error signal from the output layer to the hidden layers below.
8. Deep Neural Networks (DNNs)
   - Deep neural networks (DNNs) are artificial neural networks (ANNs) having more than one hidden layer.
   - In order to learn complex and hierarchical features from data, deep learning makes use of DNNs' expressive capabilities.

Because of their impressive capacity to self-teach using available data, artificial neural networks have been widely used. An ANN's architecture, size, and configuration are all determined by the nature of the issue at hand and the data being used. Collect a database of X-rays that includes both lung cancer patients and controls. Enhance the model's generalization by preprocessing the pictures using scaling, normalization, and enhancement. Using the training data, teach the neural network how to perform. The network is trained to identify characteristics and trends that separate instances with and without lung cancer. Whenever the model has been trained and improved, it should be tested on a separate testing dataset to determine how well it performs in the real world.

7.8 FPSO TECHNIQUE

To improve its efficiency in finding solutions to optimization issues, the FPSO method takes cues from fuzzy logic. Particle swarm optimization (PSO) is a well-known method for finding optimum or near-optimal solutions; it was developed after observing the cooperative nature of birds and fish.

The FPSO method is a hybrid of the PSO algorithm with fuzzy logic, a mathematical foundation for handling fuzziness and imprecision. Fuzzy logic's ability to describe linguistic variables and rules makes it well-suited for tackling optimization issues with ambiguous or incomplete constraints. By taking into account the particle's position and velocity as well as the uncertainty associated with the problem's restrictions and objectives, fuzzy logic is applied to adjust the update rules of the PSO algorithm in the context of FPSO. The goal of FPSO's use of fuzzy logic is to make the optimization process more resilient and flexible, particularly when faced with complicated and unpredictable optimization landscapes.

These are the building blocks of the FPSO algorithm:

1. Initialization: The particles' placements and velocities should first be generated at random within the solution space.
2. Fuzzy Inference: Fuzzy logic relies on previously established linguistic norms to assign a degree of significance to each particle's membership in various subsets of the solution space.
3. Fitness Evaluation: Apply a classification algorithm to the collected data to determine how fit each particle is. This is a perfect application for fuzzy logic, which can account for the uncertainty and imprecision of the features' contributions.
4. Update Particle Velocity and Position: Modify the PSO update rules to account for fuzzy inference, and then apply them to the particle velocities and locations.
5. Update Personal and Global Best: Maintain the most recent best local and best global locations for every particle.
6. Termination Criteria: Inquire about the presence of stopping conditions, such as the attainment of a desired solution or the completion of a predetermined number of repetitions.

Extracting useful information from medical pictures, including CT scans, is a common part of making a lung cancer diagnosis. When just the most useful features are employed in the method of categorization, computation time is reduced and diagnostic model accuracy is improved by feature selection. In cases when the optimization issue contains unclear or incorrect data, FPSO's use of fuzzy logic enables a more adaptable and nuanced exploration of the solution space. However, it should be noted that the effectiveness of FPSO depends on the appropriateness of the language norms and the degree to which the fuzzy logic notions are implemented.

Parameter tuning, issue characteristics, and the quality of the fuzzy logic rules given are all contributors to FPSO's success, as they are with any optimization method. It is advisable to try different values for the parameters and see what works best for a certain situation. By applying FPSO, we can better understand which factors contribute most to the diagnostic accuracy of our lung cancer models for categorization. Due to the nature of medical image analysis, fuzzy logic allows for the insertion of ambiguous or vague information regarding the importance of characteristics.

7.9   HYBRID ANN-PSO

In ANN-PSO, the weights and biases of an ANN are optimized with the help of PSO. The PSO technique uses particles to represent various ANN weight and bias configurations. During PSO training, the efficiency with which an ANN completes a given job serves as the "fitness function" to be measured.

Algorithm Steps:

• Begin by setting the initial values for the ANN weights and biases represented by the particles in the population.

- Determine every particle's fitness level depending on how well it did on the training data used by the ANN.
- Make adjustments to the particle's speed and location in light of its current and previous locations as well as those of its neighbors.
- Repeatedly iterate over generations to give particles more time to investigate several options and eventually settle on the best one.
- The best particle (solution) discovered over the iterations is the optimal ANN setup.

When optimizing ANN parameters with PSO, you may increase convergence and generalizability and prevent getting trapped in local minima during training. The success of ANN-PSO, however, is conditional on a number of variables, including the nature of the issue, the structure of the ANN selected, the PSO variables, and the quality of the training data. In order to put ANN-PSO into action, it is necessary to either combine existing PSO and ANN libraries or to write both sets of code from scratch. The ANN may be implemented using a library like TensorFlow or Keras or PyTorch, whereas the optimization can utilize a library like PSO or a bespoke implementation. Make sure the PSO settings and ANN design are finely tuned for the best outcomes.

7.10 RESULTS AND DISCUSSION

7.10.1 IMPLEMENTATION DETAIL

The suggested model was run using Google Colab Pro Plus, with the parameters described next. The software stack includes versions 3.8.10 of Python, 2.9.0 of Keras, and 2.9.2 of TensorFlow. The graphics processing unit (GPU) "NVIDIA A100-SXM" has 11.6 CUDA cores and 8GB of RAM.

7.10.2 EXPERIMENTAL SETUP

The 2,242,243 input photos were split into two sets, one for training and one for testing. In order to find the most effective model, a series of experiments were run using a total of six different networks: MobileNet, AlexNet, Inception, EfficientNet, CNN, and the suggested network. The upper layers of these networks have to be modified to accommodate the new data. A 1024-layer, 512-layer, and 256-layer network with the ReLU activation function and a 4-layer network with the softmax activation function were substituted for all other networks except the proposed model.

Experiments comparing the proposed model to MobileNet, AlexNet, Inception, EfficientNet, and CNN were also done for multi-class classification. The accuracy, precision, recall, and F1-score were utilized to compare the suggested approach to other pre-trained networks. The term "accuracy" is used to characterize the degree to which Eq. (7.1) positively predicted value is similar to observed values. Precision (Pr) measures how often a good outcome is properly predicted. The solution may be found in Eq. (7.2). The proportion of correct predictions is proportional to the recall (Re), which is calculated using Eq. (7.3). Using Eq. (7.4), we can see that F1-Score is the harmonic mean of Re and Pr with a weighting factor applied.

$$Accuracy = \frac{TPos + TNeg}{TPos + TNeg + FPos + FNeg} \tag{7.1}$$

where TPos represents True Positive, TNeg denotes True Negative, FPos denotes False Positive, and FNeg represents False Negative.

$$Precision = \frac{TPos}{TPoS + FPos} \tag{7.2}$$

$$Recall = \frac{TPos}{TPos + FNeg} \tag{7.3}$$

$$F1 - Score = \frac{2 \times Precision \times Recall}{Precison + Recall} \tag{7.4}$$

7.11 EXPERIMENTAL RESULT

Different models, including MobileNet, AlexNet, Inception, EfficientNet, CNN, and the suggested modified Xception model, are compared in Table 7.1 for their Train Accuracy, Validation Accuracy, and Test Accuracy. Accuracy levels for MobileNet ranged from 80.81 to 82.41 to 84.16% during training, validation, and testing, correspondingly. Alternatively, the suggested model achieved the highest possible Train, Validation, and Test Accuracy of 98.42%, 97.92%, and 97.19%.

Figures 7.5 and 7.6 show the accuracy and loss curves for the aforementioned four models, respectively. In terms of accuracy and loss curves, MobileNet performed the worst, at around 80%. Results from training and validating the suggested model indicated an accuracy of less than 98% and a loss of roughly 1%. The suggested model, on the other hand, got a 99% Train Accuracy and a 1% Validation Accuracy loss. Another reason why deep learning model epochs aren't always the same is that when validation loss didn't go down after 10 training cycles, an early termination callback was triggered.

TABLE 7.1

Accuracy for Different Models

Model	Train Accuracy	Validation Accuracy	Test Accuracy
MobileNet	0.80	0.82	0.84
AlexNet	0.90	0.90	0.92
Inception	0.92	0.91	0.92
EfficientNet	0.95	0.93	0.93
CNN	0.93	0.93	0.93
Proposed	0.98	0.97	0.97

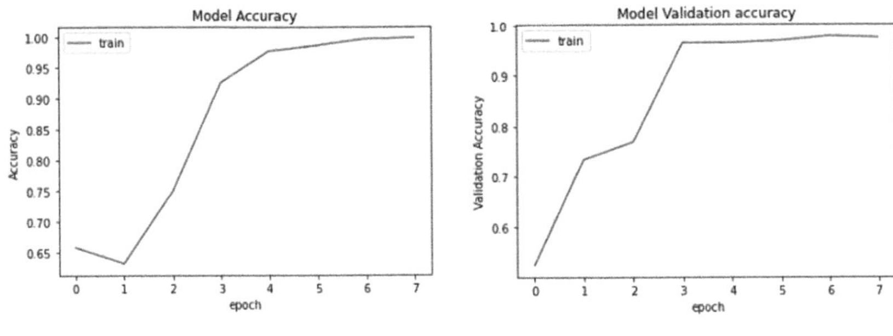

FIGURE 7.5 Validation of the proposed model and its accuracy graph.

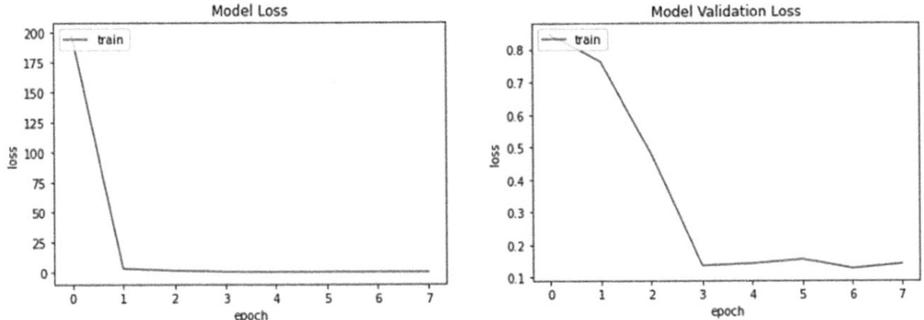

FIGURE 7.6 Graph showing the proposed model's loss and the loss during validation.

TABLE 7.2
Performance Evaluation of Various Models

Model	Precision	Recall	F1-Score
MobileNet	0.82	0.84	0.85
AlexNet	0.92	0.92	0.93
Inception	0.94	0.93	0.93
EfficientNet	0.97	0.95	0.94
CNN	0.95	0.95	0.94
Proposed	0.98	0.97	0.98

Table 7.2 and Figures 7.7, 7.8, and 7.9 detail the Precision, Recall, and F1-Score measures along with other model performance indicators. Classification model performance is often measured using these indicators, especially in high-stakes domains like medical diagnosis and picture recognition. The accuracy of a model is measured by how many times it correctly predicts as positive compared to how many occasions it incorrectly predicts as positive. The Precision values for these models go from 0.82 for MobileNet to 0.98 for the Suggested model. False positive predictions

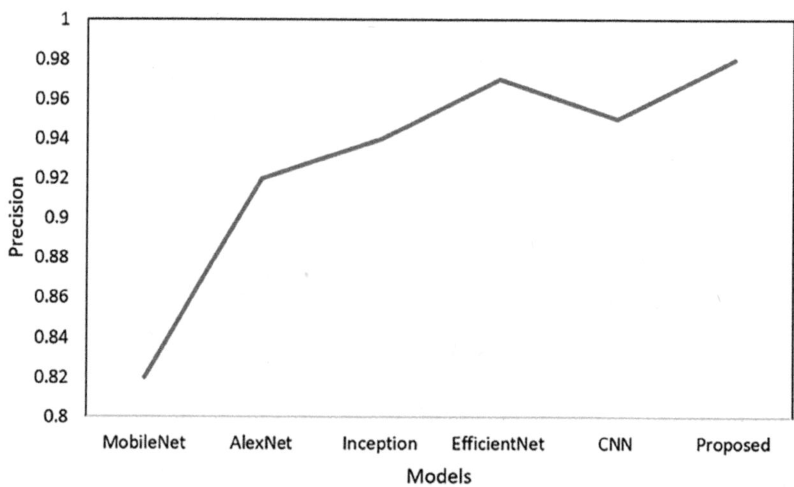

FIGURE 7.7 Accurate evaluation of the new model.

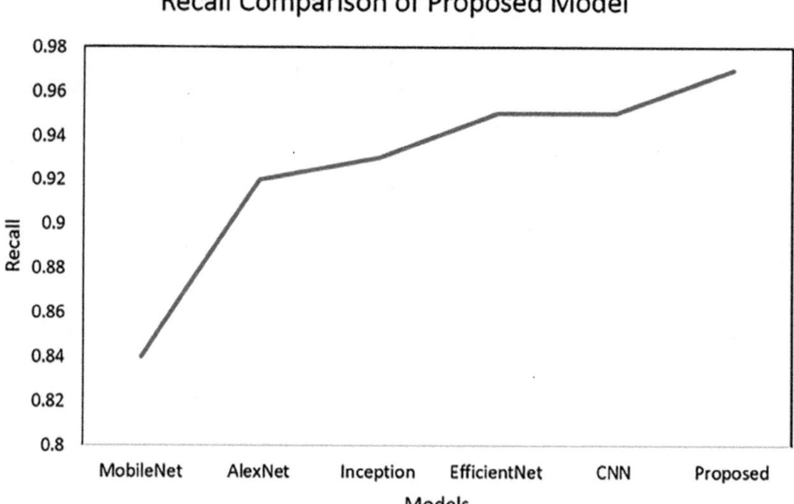

FIGURE 7.8 Model proposal recall and comparison.

are less likely to occur when the Precision score is high. The term "recall" refers to the rate at which positive occurrences are accurately anticipated relative to the total number of actual positive cases. The range of values for Recall in this table begins at 0.84 for MobileNet and ends at 0.97 for Suggested. If the model has a high Recall, it successfully captures positive examples. The F1-Score provides a well-rounded

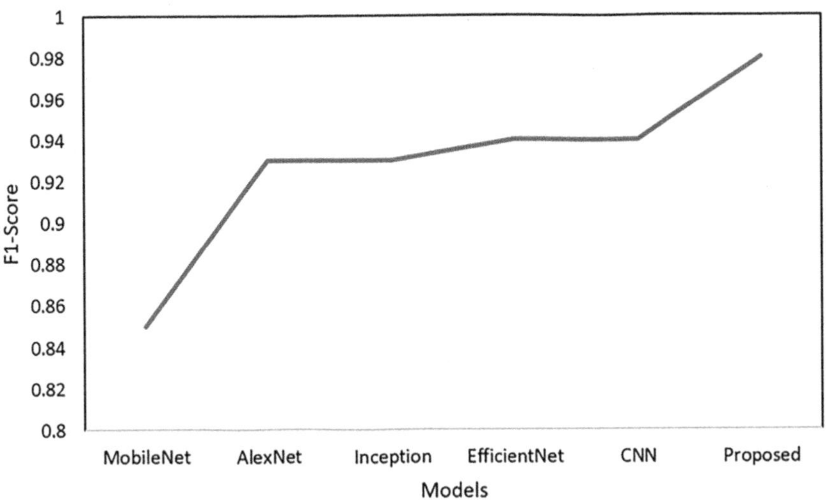

FIGURE 7.9 Model comparison using F1-Score.

measure of a model's efficacy by averaging its Precision and Recall scores. Table 7.2 displays F1-Score values between 0.85 (for MobileNet) and 0.98 (for Proposed). While there is some variation regarding effectiveness among the models across the measures, the "Proposed" model regularly outperforms the other two. It appears that the "Proposed" model has the best balance of Precision and Recall and is the most accurate and precise in recognizing affirmative situations. Table 7.2 provides a streamlined comparison of various models' prediction abilities, facilitating choice of their fitness for certain uses or activities.

Figure 7.10 is a visual depiction of the confusion matrices, which show the general effectiveness of the models. The test dataset includes 1063 samples altogether, with 480 samples coming from the lung cancer picture and 583 samples coming from the healthy image. Diseased individuals are indicated by the label "1," whereas healthy individuals are indicated by the label "0." Using the updated model, 579 normal samples and 478 cancerous lung tissue samples can be appropriately recognized from the matrix. Ninety-eight percent of test data samples were correctly identified by the model.

The computation durations, in seconds, for various models are shown in Table 7.3 and Figure 7.11. In real-time applications or other circumstances where time is of the essence, computation time is a crucial component in evaluating the efficacy and viability of models. MobileNet needs 1106 seconds for calculations. The predicted accuracy of this model, as well as any potential trade-offs with computing speed, should be considered while assessing its effectiveness. AlexNet has been shown to do computations in 968 seconds less time. Even though the model is less resource-intensive to run than MobileNet, its accuracy and other performance indicators should still be taken into account. The time needed to calculate Inception is 1070 seconds.

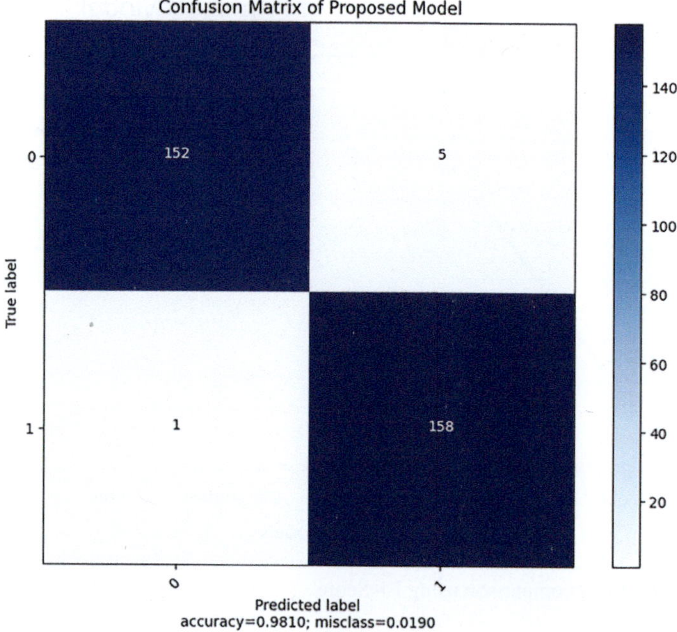

FIGURE 7.10 Confusion matrix of proposed model.

TABLE 7.3

Computational Time of Multiple Models

Model	Computation Time (sec)
MobileNet	1106
AlexNet	968
Inception	1070
EfficientNet	1073
CNN	971
Proposed	776

Its accuracy and other parameters should be studied alongside this time since it finds a balance between computing speed and effectiveness. EfficientNet's computation time is 1073 seconds, which is quite close to Inception's. The tradeoffs between computing efficiency and performance are analogous. CNN It takes 971 milliseconds to calculate. Performance measurements should be interpreted in light of the fact that it delivers only moderate computing speed. Proposed stands out with a shorter 776-second computation time, making it a clear frontrunner. This is evidence of its very accurate processing and prediction abilities. This chart does a great job of highlighting the differing computing efficiencies of these models, which sheds light on their potential applications in the real world. It's a great resource for determining

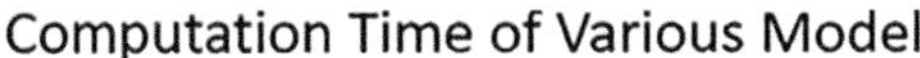

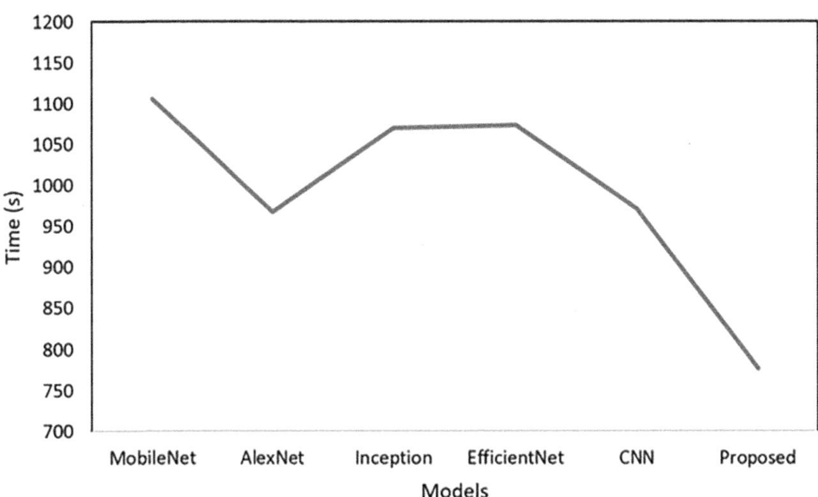

FIGURE 7.11 Computation time of various models.

which models offer the best trade-off between computational effort and accuracy in predictions.

7.12 CONCLUSION AND FUTURE SCOPE

Malignant tumors or abnormal growths within the lungs can be detected for lung cancer through diagnostic imaging and other medical procedures. The ability to diagnose lung cancer early and accurately is crucial for prompt treatment and better patient outcomes. In this research, we present a novel methodology for analyzing chest X-rays to detect lung disorders including pneumonia and Covid-19. The INNOT (Improved Neural Network and Optimization Technique) is the foundation of our method. To combat the gradual deterioration of picture quality during X-ray imaging, we use a two-stage improvement approach consisting of median filtering and histogram equalization. We use the fuzzy particle swarm optimization (FPSO) method to pick the best features before feeding them into an Artificial Neural Network (ANN) for classification. The proposed model is evaluated in light of existing, cutting-edge methods. The effectiveness and sturdiness of our concept have been demonstrated experimentally. The results demonstrate that, in comparison to other modern approaches, the suggested INNOT-based approach achieves the maximum efficiency and the lowest inaccuracy. Our approach's high accuracy (98.42%), sensitivity (97.77%), and specificity (97.63%) in predicting disease is evidence of its outstanding effectiveness. More advanced algorithms, such as Squeeze and Excitation, Transformer Block, and Dense Block, may be integrated into future studies to boost the effectiveness of the proposed method. This development has the potential to improve the accuracy and efficiency of diagnosing lung cancer. Though each of Squeeze and Excitation, Dense Block, and Vision Transformer may be used independently, they all work better together to maximize efficiency and insight. The study's overarching goal is to contribute to more precise and efficient diagnostic approaches by expanding the current state of the art in lung cancer detection through the investigation of these cutting-edge algorithmic innovations and their combinations.

REFERENCES

[1] S. Saini, A. Maithani, D. Dhiman and A. Bisht, "Analysis of Different Machine Learning Algorithms Used for Identification of Lung Cancer Disease," in 2021 9th International Conference on Reliability, Infocom Technologies and Optimization (Trends and Future Directions) (ICRITO), Noida, India, 2021, pp. 1–5, doi: 10.1109/ICRITO51393.2021.9596308.

[2] D. Hişam and E. Hişam, "Deep Learning Models for Classifying Cancer and COVID-19 Lung Diseases," in 2021 Innovations in Intelligent Systems and Applications Conference (ASYU), Elazig, Turkey, 2021, pp. 1–4, doi: 10.1109/ASYU52992.2021.9598993.

[3] N. Nawreen, U. Hany and T. Islam, "Lung Cancer Detection and Classification using CT Scan Image Processing," in 2021 International Conference on Automation, Control and Mechatronics for Industry 4.0 (ACMI), Rajshahi, Bangladesh, 2021, pp. 1–6, doi: 10.1109/ACMI53878.2021.9528297.

[4] V. G. Sreena, N. Ponraj and P. L. Deepa, "Study on Public Chest X-ray Data Sets for Lung Disease Classification," in 2021 3rd International Conference on Signal Processing and Communication (ICPSC), Coimbatore, India, 2021, pp. 54–58, doi: 10.1109/ICSPC51351.2021.9451726.

[5] S. K. H. Bukhari and L. Fahad, "Lung Disease Detection using Deep Learning," in 2022 17th International Conference on Emerging Technologies (ICET), Swabi, Pakistan, 2022, pp. 154–159, doi: 10.1109/ICET56601.2022.10004651.

[6] B. Zhou, X. Yang, X. Zhang, W. J. Curran and T. Liu, "Ultrasound Elastography for Lung Disease Assessment," IEEE Transactions on Ultrasonics, Ferroelectrics, and Frequency Control, vol. 67, no. 11, pp. 2249–2257, 2020, doi: 10.1109/TUFFC.2020.3026536.

[7] G. Zaman Khan et al., "An Efficient Deep Learning Model based Diagnosis System for Lung Cancer Disease," in 2023 4th International Conference on Computing, Mathematics and Engineering Technologies (iCoMET), Sukkur, Pakistan, 2023, pp. 1–6, doi: 10.1109/iCoMET57998.2023.10099357.

[8] S. Mukherjee and S. U. Bohra, "Lung Cancer Disease Diagnosis Using Machine Learning Approach," in 2020 3rd International Conference on Intelligent Sustainable Systems (ICISS), Thoothukudi, India, 2020, pp. 207–211, doi: 10.1109/ICISS49785.2020.9315909.

[9] S. Al-Ofary and H. O. Ilhan, "Classification of PCA Based Reduced Deep Features by SVM for Diagnosing Lung and Colon Cancer," in 2023 5th International Congress on Human-Computer Interaction, Optimization and Robotic Applications (HORA), Istanbul, Turkiye, 2023, pp. 1–5, doi: 10.1109/HORA58378.2023.10156720.

[10] D. Gupta and S. Dawn, "Detection and Staging of Lung Cancer from CT Scan Images by Deep Learning," 2023 International Conference on Disruptive Technologies (ICDT), Greater Noida, India, 2023, pp. 274–278, doi: 10.1109/ICDT57929.2023.10151194.

8 Novel Methodology to Predict and Classify Liver Diseases Based on Hybrid Deep Learning Strategy

Sathesh Abraham Leo E., Rajalakshmi R.,
Kavitha T., Prathima C., and Anitha G.

8.1 INTRODUCTION

The liver is the biggest internal organ. It is in charge of all metabolic processes in the body, from converting food into useful chemicals to storing those compounds until they are needed by the cells. The liver, an organ unique to vertebrates, is positioned on the right side of the abdomen, just below the rib cage. It helps with things like digestion, metabolism, getting rid of waste, building immunity, and storing nutrients. Among its primary functions are the elimination of waste products, the prevention of disease, and the maintenance of normal hormone levels and bile production [1]. A variety of problems and liver disorders might arise if the liver fails to properly carry out these tasks.

The term "liver disease" is used to describe conditions caused by dysfunction of the liver. A damaged or inflamed liver may have devastating effects on one's health because of the numerous important bodily processes it supports. Liver disease can be difficult to identify since its early signs are often overlooked. Due to the liver's ability to continue functioning while being partially destroyed, many liver disorders go undetected until it is too late to treat them. Potentially saving lives, an early diagnosis is essential. While the earliest signs of these illnesses are invisible to even the most seasoned doctor, they are detectable. By catching health problems early, patients' lifespans can be greatly extended. Liver tumors form when aberrant cells proliferate in the organ [2]. Cancerous tumors of the liver are rare but do occur. Liver cancer ranks third in terms of cancer mortality rates worldwide. The survival rate and likelihood of a complete recovery from liver cancer are both significantly increased by prompt diagnosis and treatment. It used to be that doctors' clinical expertise was the only guide in making a diagnosis of liver disease. Depending only on a doctor's

DOI: 10.1201/9781032635149-8

experience to spot the first lesions of liver disease can be a time-consuming and frustrating process, as well as a potentially subjective one.

Liver disease, seen in Figure 8.1, is a growing public health crisis throughout the world, since it impairs the liver's ability to metabolize protein, hormones, and minerals. Liver biopsies are the "gold standard" for diagnosing disease and fibrosis in the liver. Cirrhosis from excessive alcohol use as well as fatty liver disease from being overweight are the leading causes of liver cancer and other liver-related illnesses. The presence of the hepatitis B and C viruses is also a major influence. The incidence of liver cancer increased by almost 3% yearly. However, the technique of obtaining a liver biopsy is intrusive and requires surgical operations on patients, which are both costly and time-consuming [3]. Together with technical developments, several scientific studies are currently conducted to uncover and improve non-invasive procedures. Nevertheless, it is important to keep in mind that the diagnoses of non-invasive techniques have not yet been acknowledged worldwide and that the adoption rate varies greatly between nations. However, such treatments serve as screenings, allowing doctors to narrow down the pool of people who will need a biopsy. Quicker than conventional biopsies, these diagnostic techniques allow for quicker therapy implementation after their results. These medical issues have, therefore, received a lot of focus in recent years in terms of how to improve future liver tests and how to create individualized treatment programs. The goal is to create a non-invasive diagnostic approach that can replace histopathological analyses and biopsies.

The causes and outcomes of various liver illnesses are used to classify them into distinct groups. Infection, injury, medication or toxin exposure, procedure, or genetic abnormalities (such as hemochromatosis) can all play a role in causing this condition. Hepatitis, cirrhosis, and stones are all possible outcomes of the aforementioned

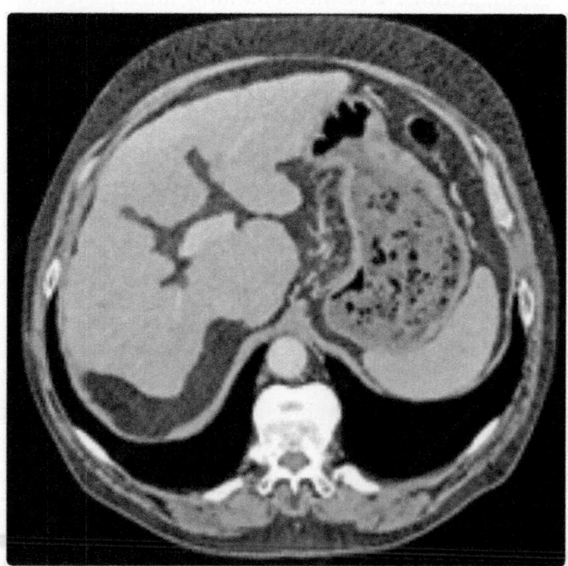

FIGURE 8.1 Liver disease.

conditions, and they can obstruct the liver, induce fatty infiltration of the liver, and even lead to liver cancer in extremely rare circumstances. As with the accumulation and concentration of hazardous components like iron or copper, genetic defects can impede critical liver activities and cause buildup of these substances.

Lipid buildup in the liver is a hallmark of non-alcoholic fatty liver disease (NAFLD), one of the most common forms of liver disease. Non-alcoholic steatohepatitis is characterized by inflammation and damage to the liver cells. One of the worst liver illnesses is cirrhosis [4]. As a result of this condition, good tissue is replaced by scar tissue. Hence, the liver suffers irreversible harm and becomes dysfunctional. Acute hepatitis, when the liver gets inflamed quickly, and chronic hepatitis, which occurs when the liver gets irritated and damaged slowly over an extended amount of time, are the two most common types of hepatitis. Hepatitis A, B, C, D, and E are the official designations for these viruses in the order in which they were identified.

HAV is the virus responsible for hepatitis A. The usual vectors of transmission include tainted food and drink. Sexual intercourse and, less frequently, blood transfusions are potentially potential vectors for transmission. The symptoms of hepatitis B are quite similar. Nevertheless, in this scenario, transmission occurs through contact with any contaminated body fluid. Acute and chronic manifestations exist. The latter, if unchecked, can progress to cancer of the liver or lead to hepatic failure. The progression of hepatitis C is quite like that of the first two. However, it is spread by direct contact with a carrier's blood. It may take up to 10 years after infection for the first signs to show. Like hepatitis B, hepatitis C can manifest in both acute and chronic forms. Obesity and diabetes pose a new and potentially catastrophic hazard to the liver, which has traditionally been connected with drinking and hepatitis. The chance of dying from advanced fatty liver disease is roughly seven times higher than the risk from any other cause. Fatty liver disease is a quiet "killer," and by the time the signs of liver impairment manifest, the situation is dire.

There is a correlation between heavy drinking and liver damage. Finally, the benefits of exercise, a good diet, and weight maintenance on liver health are well documented [5]. Histopathological examinations have long been the gold standard for generating a definitive diagnosis and medical report for patients. Efficiency in data collecting, processing, and visualization has emerged because of developments in ICT, particularly artificial intelligence (AI) and machine learning (ML). When doctors take into account the results of AI and ML models in addition to the data gleaned via clinical approaches, they may make more informed judgments about diagnosing disease.

Machine learning's subfield known as "deep learning" consists mainly of a multilayered neural network. By teaching computers to recognize data types like text, pictures, and sounds with only a small amount of training data, deep learning attempts to give computers the same analytical learning skills as humans by understanding the intrinsic structures as well as representational details of sample data. The scope of deep learning's impact is expanding daily. For tasks including image identification, speech recognition, and picture production, several deep learning approaches like the convolutional neural network (CNN), long short-term memory (LSTM), and transformer have been on par with or even beyond human performance. In this study, we describe a novel deep learning architecture for analyzing CT scan data from clinical settings to categorize nonalcoholic fatty liver disease. In order to automatically detect liver disorders in CT scan pictures, our method combines Long Short-Term Memory (LSTM) with a powerful CNN. Feature selection in the field of medical data classification is analogous to selecting a subset of variables or picking a collection of characteristics to describe a given dataset. A selection of relevant features that aid in correct categorization will be identified in this phase. To do so, we use the Ant Lion Optimization (ALO) method.

8.2 RELATED WORKS

The human liver plays a crucial role in the body. Early detection or diagnosis of the condition is crucial. This is a major step toward early illness prevention requiring little to no treatment. Liver function tests and their outcomes are examples of conventional procedures. Liver illness is notoriously difficult to diagnose early on. This is because the onset of symptoms coincides with the advanced stages of the disease. This machine learning approach aids in early illness identification by singling out factors that contribute to the development of deadly liver damage. Due to the apparent sensitivity of the indications, it is challenging for doctors and scientists to predict the disease in its early stages. When it's already too late, people will realize the consequences. The project aims to enhance the lives of those affected by the disease via the application of machine learning methods. Liver illness is notoriously hard to detect, and its symptoms often don't manifest until it's too late. To differentiate between those with liver illness and those without, Author [6] employs a categorization strategy, further subdividing those with liver disease by staging and subtype. Precautions are also included in case you have any symptoms. As a result, ML methods have been used to diagnose liver disease in people.

Chronic liver disease is extremely common, and NAFLD is the main cause of liver-related morbidity and death globally. It is believed that anywhere from 25% of the overall population to 90% of obese as well as diabetic individuals are affected by the condition. Many individuals are hard to detect and treat because they have no obvious symptoms. Nevertheless, the current gold-standard method for diagnosis, the liver biopsy, has limitations that have led to an international need for the development of a non-invasive method of diagnosis and technique that can identify the illness with excellent precision at its earliest irreversible stage, is economical, simple to use, as well as offering a reproducible evaluation. The team we worked with has decades of experience in metrology, so we knew we could use it to design a power impedance-based diagnostic process for NAFLD earlier than usual, which would be ideal for this purpose. The most significant advances made in research tools are highlighted in this piece of writing.

The prevalence of liver illness has increased dramatically in recent years. Liver disease is on the rise due to a number of factors. These include, but are not limited to, increased alcohol intake, exposure to toxic fumes, eating contaminated food, and using drugs like opiates and cocaine. Liver disease is a leading cause of many other life-threatening conditions, including cancer of the liver. Semi-supervised machine learning algorithms have been described in [8] study to improve liver disease categorization. Techniques for classification for predicting liver illness are being developed, and researchers are looking at using datasets of liver patients as training data. The suggested research uses a model based on a combination of SVM and K-Means algorithms to analyze the whole extent of liver disease in individuals. Liver illness that has persisted for at least six months is considered chronic. As a result, the population under consideration will be segregated into those with and without liver illness. The total amount of people who have been afflicted by liver disease is calculated using SVM classifiers, and the extent of that damage is calculated using the hybrid k means clustering approach. High prediction accuracy is therefore shown in the results of the suggested hybrid K-Means clustering model.

Medical image processing is one area where convolutional neural networks (CNNs) have proven to be exceptionally effective. Object categorization, picture reconstruction, and tissue characterization are only some of the uses of CNNs in ultrasound (US) imaging. Contrary to popular belief, CNNs are not impervious to adversarial assaults; even little changes to the input data can have a major impact on the effectiveness of the model and lead to inaccurate results. In order to counter ultrasonic (US) imaging, the author [9] creates a new type of adversarial assault. The United States uses radio frequency waves to recreate pictures. Through the use of zeroth order optimization, we are able to pinpoint the tiniest changes to the image reconstruction variables that lead to incorrect results, including those that are associated with attenuation correction and amplitude compression. We use a deep learning model built for fatty liver disease detection to demonstrate our method and show that the suggested adversarial attack had a 48% success rate.

Liver illness, second only to heart disease, is a major killer of Americans. As it is usually too late to treat liver disease when it is diagnosed. The amount of persons with liver disease is rising due to several reasons, including increased alcohol consumption, exposure to toxic gases, consumption of impure water, and others. In the early stages of liver disease, such health characteristics may be used to make predictions using machine learning models for forecasting. Author [10] uses the Indian Liver Patient Dataset (ILPD), which is based on Indian patients, and the Random Forest (RF) procedure, which predicts illness using multiple preprocessing approaches, to construct the machine learning model. Through univariate and bivariate analysis, we examine the data for skewness, outliers, and imbalance; next, we employ appropriate algorithms to eliminate the outliers and a variety of oversampling and undersampling methods to restore statistical parity. Utilizing grid search as well as feature selection, hyperparameter tweaking further hones the model. The completed model has a perfect score on every measure we tested it with, and it's also 100% accurate.

8.3 METHODOLOGY

8.3.1 DATA ACQUISITION

Collecting a dataset of liver plain CT scans was the primary objective of the MLTI architecture. Figure 8.2 displays the two types of benign and malignant liver tumor CT scans present in the dataset. CT scans from one hundred patients were chosen for analysis. We used 512 × 512 pixel CT images of liver tumors from 10 different patients. So that we may get reliable outcomes, we have included 1000 24-bit JPEGs in the sample.

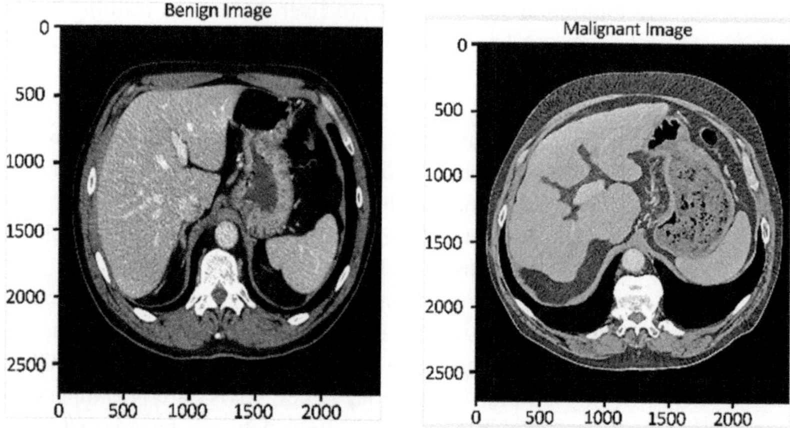

FIGURE 8.2 Benign and malignant image.

8.3.2 DATA PREPROCESSING

Preparing as well as cleaning unprocessed information for use in analysis or modeling is known as "data preprocessing," and it is an essential part of the data science pipeline. All data-driven methods, including machine learning models, rely on having clean, well-structured input data in order to perform optimally. The purpose of data preprocessing is to prepare the raw data for analysis by cleaning it up, standardizing it, and removing any outliers like missing numbers or discrepancies. Locate and address any dataset gaps. Rows with missing values can be removed or imputed using methods like mean, median, or interpolation, according to the number and kind of missing data. The unaltered picture is displayed in Figure 8.3.

8.3.3 FEATURE EXTRACTION

In data preparation and machine learning, feature extraction is a step taken to glean useful information from raw data. With feature extraction, you may reduce the number of dimensions your data occupies while still keeping the information you need for analysis and modeling. Selecting the most important features from a large pool of candidates is the goal of feature selection methods. The most informative details for this study or model are contained in this subset. Methods like the chi-square test and recursive feature removal are often used in the realm of feature selection.

8.3.4 CLASSIFICATION MODEL—LSTM

To overcome the challenge of vanishing gradients and accurately record persistent dependencies in sequential data, researchers developed a recurrent neural network (RNN) structure known as LSTM. Machine learning for the detection of speech, statistical analysis of time series, recognition of handwriting, and many more all use

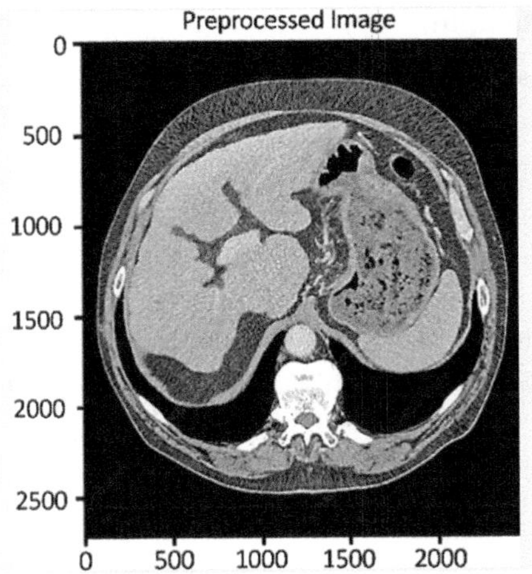

FIGURE 8.3 Preprocessed image.

sequential information, and LSTMs have grown into an essential building component in these areas. Next, we describe the main parts and the roles they play:

1. Memory Cell

The memory cell, seen here as a horizontal line crossing the top of the LSTM units, is the brain of the recurrent neural network. An LSTM system is useful for simulating lengthy sequences because of its memory cell's ability to remember data through long intervals of time.

2. Gates

The input and output of an LSTM is regulated by three distinct kinds of gates:

a. Forget Gate

Tossing out some or all of the data stored in a memory cell from the prior time step is controlled by this gate. Every storage cell's output is an amount that ranges from 0 to 1, based on the current input as well as the hidden state (output) from the previous time step. Forget this knowledge altogether if the value is zero, and remember it well if it's one.

b. Input Gate

It is the responsibility of the input gate to determine what fresh data will be written into the memory device. It takes the current input as well as the hidden state from the earlier time step and produces a potential vector of fresh values that could potentially be committed to the storage cell.

c. Output Gate

Whether portions of the memory cell have been employed to calculate the current time step's output is determined by the output gate. It takes into account the present input and the prior concealed state and then outputs a filtered version of the information inside the memory cell.

3. Hidden State (Output)

At every single step, the result of the LSTM unit represents the hidden state, frequently abbreviated as "h." The result is the memory cell's content after being altered by the output gate.

In-depth explanation of how LSTM is computed:

1. You will be given the current input in addition to the prior secret state.
2. Determine what data from the memory cell can be forgotten by computing the forget gate.
3. To update the data stored in the memory cell, you must first determine its input gate as well as the candidate vector.
4. Using the candidate vector determined by the forget as well as input gates, upgrade the memory cell with the combined contents of the old memory cell as well as the vector.
5. The result (hidden state) for the present time step can be filtered from the contents of the memory cell, hence it's important to determine the output gate.
6. Send the result (the concealed state) on to the next time step, as well as continue doing so until all inputs have been exhausted.

Since LSTMs may be layered to construct deeper structures, they can simulate intricate relationships in sequential information. These more complex LSTM networks are widely employed in state-of-the-art natural language processing applications including machine translation as well as sentiment analysis. Long short-term memories (LSTMs) have been helpful in the resolution of many practical issues, particularly those requiring sequential information, and they remain a hotspot for study in the area of deep learning.

8.3.5 Convolutional Neural Network

To handle and analyze visual data like photos and videos, one sort of deep learning model called a CNN was developed. With its groundbreaking performance in computer vision tasks, CNNs have quickly become the standard architecture for a wide range of image-related software. The visual functioning in the human visual cortex served as inspiration for these systems, and their outstanding capacity to effortlessly acquire hierarchical patterns from raw input has been established.

1. Convolutional Layers

CNNs rely heavily on their convolutional layers as their foundation. When applied to an input picture, a convolutional layer's collection of learnable filters (also known as kernels) generates feature maps that are indicative of the image's underlying patterns and characteristics. By using element-wise multiplication and summing as they glide through the whole input picture, these filters are able to efficiently capture local patterns.

2. Activation Function

An activation coefficient is applied incrementally to the feature maps following the convolution procedure. Rectified Linear Unit (ReLU) is a popular activation function in CNNs since it converts negative values to zero while leaving positive values unaffected. By introducing non-linearity to the system, ReLU facilitates its ability to learn more intricate patterns.

3. Pooling Layers

Through the use of pooling layers, the spatial extents of the feature maps may be shrunk without losing any of the crucial details. Maximum pooling as well as average pooling are two common methods of aggregation through pooling. The feature maps can be downsampled by using max pooling, which chooses the maximum value inside a certain window, or by using average pooling, which determines the average value throughout the window.

4. Fully Connected Layers

Finally, the feature maps are streamlined into a one-dimensional vector after passing through numerous pooling and convolutional layers. Next, we link this vector to a dense layer or many dense layers, which are also called fully linked layers. The fully connected layers master the task of final categorization or regression by learning abstract visualizations and inter-feature interactions.

5. Dropout (Optional)

Dropout can be used among layers that are completely linked to reduce the likelihood of overfitting and increase generalization. Every training iteration, dropout inactivates a small percentage of neurons at random, making the system more resilient by forcing it to use other paths.

6. Softmax Layer (for classification)

A softmax layer is frequently employed as the last output layer in tasks involving categorization. In order to determine the likelihood that an input belongs to a specific class, Softmax transforms the raw output scores into probability values. When making a prediction, the most likely category is always used.

8.3.6 HYBRID DEEP LEARNING STRATEGY

An effective deep learning design, a hybrid CNN and LSTM model takes the best features of both Convolutional Neural Networks (CNNs) and Long Short-Term Memory (LSTM) systems. This integration makes it possible for the model to interpret details of space from pictures while also quickly processing and extracting characteristics from data that is sequential (including variables such as time series, video frames, or conversational sequences). The overall structure of the suggested model is seen in Figure 8.4.

The hybrid model typically involves two main components:

1. CNN for Feature Extraction

The CNN part of the hybrid model is responsible for processing static data, such as images. CNNs are adept at automatically learning hierarchical features from raw image data, making them well-suited for image-related tasks like object recognition, detection, and segmentation. The convolutional layers of CNN help to extract features, while the pooling layers help to downsample features and shrink the training set to a more manageable size.

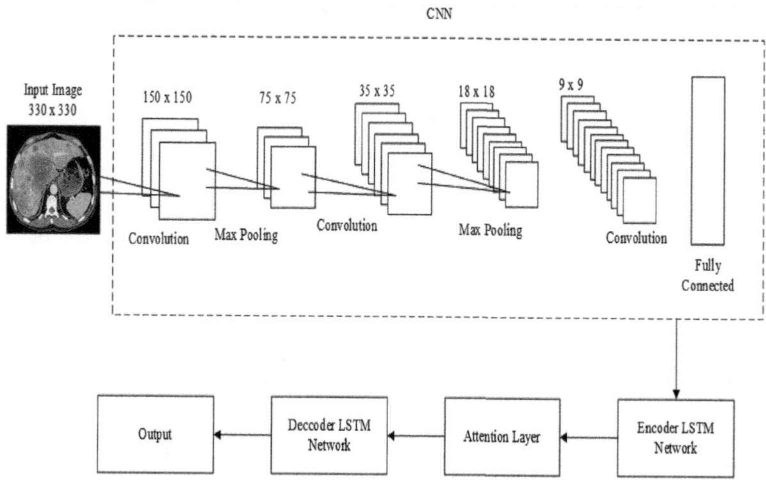

FIGURE 8.4 Architecture of proposed model.

2. LSTM for Sequence Modeling

The LSTM component of the hybrid model is optimized for handling sequential data like time series or text sequences. LSTM systems are often utilized in many fields, including NLP, recognition of voices, sentiment assessment, and more because of their exceptional ability to capture relationships that last in sequential data.

Hybrid CNN-LSTM models have demonstrated significant improvements in tasks that involve both spatial and sequential information. The combination of CNN's spatial processing and LSTM's temporal modeling enables more comprehensive feature extraction and context understanding in diverse real-world applications. A hybrid CNN and LSTM model can be a promising approach for liver disease detection, especially when dealing with medical image data and sequential patient records. Here's how such a model could be designed for liver disease detection:

1. Image Data (CNN part)

The CNN component of the hybrid model would be responsible for processing medical images, including computed tomography (CT) scans or MRI scans of the liver. The CNN layers would be used to extract relevant features from the images, capturing spatial patterns, and structures indicative of liver diseases.

2. Sequential Patient Records (LSTM part)

In addition to medical images, patient records can be crucial for diagnosing and predicting liver diseases. These records may include data such as patient demographics, medical history, blood test results, and other relevant clinical information. The LSTM part of the model would process this sequential patient data to capture temporal dependencies and long-term patterns that could be indicative of liver disease progression or risk factors.

3. Data Fusion

After processing both the image data and sequential patient records through their respective CNN and LSTM components, the outputs from these parts can be fused at a certain layer in the network. This data fusion step allows the model to combine spatial and temporal information to make more informed and accurate predictions about liver disease detection.

4. Fully Connected Layers and Output

Following the data fusion step, the combined features can be passed through additional fully connected layers for further processing and, finally, the output layer for binary or multiclass classification (diagnosis) of liver disease. The output layer would provide the probability of the presence of liver disease or the specific liver disease type for each input sample.

Overall, a hybrid CNN-LSTM model has the potential to provide more comprehensive and accurate liver disease detection by leveraging both spatial and temporal information, ultimately contributing to early diagnosis and more effective treatment strategies. However, it's essential to collaborate with medical experts and follow appropriate regulatory guidelines to ensure the model's safety and clinical relevance.

8.3.7 Antlion Optimization

Antlion Optimization (ALO) is a nature-inspired optimization algorithm inspired by the hunting behavior of antlions in nature. Antlions are insects that construct conical pits in sandy areas to trap ants, their prey. The key idea behind Antlion Optimization is to simulate the process of antlion foraging and trap construction to find the optimal solution to an optimization problem. The algorithm works by maintaining a population of potential solutions represented as antlions, and these antlions iteratively move toward better solutions in the search space. Antlion Optimization has been applied to various optimization problems, including function optimization, engineering design, and parameter tuning for machine learning algorithms. It is particularly suitable for continuous optimization problems with multiple local optima. While Antlion Optimization is a promising algorithm, its effectiveness depends on the specific problem and parameter settings. Like other metaheuristic optimization algorithms, it may require careful tuning and multiple runs to achieve good performance.

8.4 RESULTS AND DISCUSSION

For this project's implementation, we used Python's Jupyter Notebook. Considering hyperparameters are the major component of the model and have a significant impact on the learning process, they must be specified before the model is able to be trained. Finding the criteria may be done in a number of different ways. We use an 80%:20% split for training and testing when it comes to breast cancer ultrasound imaging. In machine learning, a batch size refers to the amount of training samples that are tallied in a single forward and backward pass. As the size of a batch increases, more RAM will be needed.

Our network's weights are updated in response to the loss gradient, and the learning rate is a hyperparameter that controls the magnitude of these changes. The lower the value, the slower we slide down the hill. In order to avoid missing any local minima, reducing the learning rate might be beneficial. However, this could cause the convergence process to drag on indefinitely, especially if we get stuck on a plateau. To describe the total number of times a machine learning algorithm has iterated over the whole training dataset, the term "epoch" is used. Most datasets (particularly those with a large quantity of data) are stored and processed in batches. Some people use the term "iteration" to refer to the process of running a model on a single batch. Training a neural network using sample data presents the significant challenge of overfitting. A model of neural networks learns characteristics that are specific to the sample information whenever more epochs are used during training than are strictly necessary. Stochastic gradient descent (SGD) was used in the training of DL models created by TL. The minibatch size we employed was 10, and the learning rate was set at 0.001. Every DL model was trained for 100 epochs before being utilized in the TL tests for recognizing and categorizing various types of BC, hence reducing the likelihood of overfitting.

8.4.1 PERFORMANCE EVOLUTION

In this research, we used accuracy, precision, recall, and F1-score to measure the efficacy of the models we employed. These may be computed in this way:

$$Accuracy = \frac{TPos + TNeg}{TPos + FPos + TNeg + FNeg} \tag{8.1}$$

$$Precision = \frac{TPos}{TPos + FPos} \tag{8.2}$$

$$Recall = \frac{FNeg}{FNeg + TPos} \tag{8.3}$$

$$F1 - Score = 2 \times \frac{Precision \times Recall}{Precision + Recall} \tag{8.4}$$

where TPos = True Positive, TNeg = True Negative, FPos = False Positive, and FNeg = False Negative

8.5 DISCUSSION

The detection capabilities of the suggested model are evaluated using CT scans in this experiment. Twenty percent of the data was used to evaluate the model, whereas 80% was utilized for training it in the present investigation. To be more specific, we consulted a total of 1034 CT images of liver disease (546 benign, 359 malignant, and 129 normal), split as follows: 376 for training, 252 for testing, and 95 each of benign, malignant, and normal individuals. All categories of liver illness are correctly classified with a high score, as shown in Figure 8.5 of the confusion matrix for the suggested model.

Identifying and categorizing liver diseases. Over the course of the 10 epochs, the suggested model was iterated a total of 100 times, or 10 times each epoch on average.

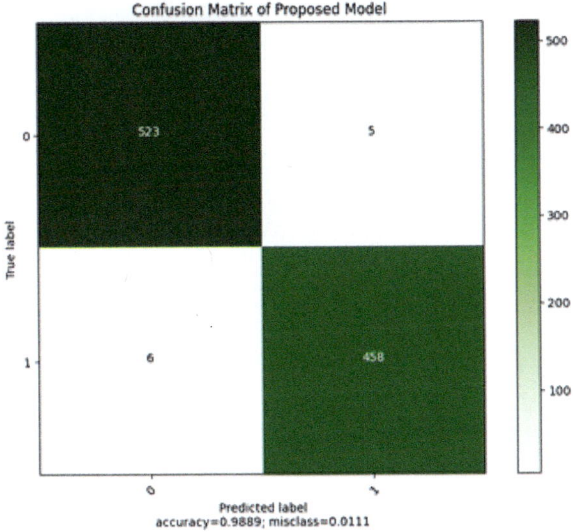

FIGURE 8.5 Confusion matrix of proposed model.

At epoch 100, the proposed model's classification accuracy, precision, recall, as well as F1-score values were as high as 98.89%, 98.59%, 97.69%, and 98.36%, respectively, proving the efficacy of our approach in identifying BC. Furthermore, in Figures 8.6 and 8.7, we present accuracy and loss to illustrate the robustness of the proposed technique throughout both training and testing. The loss function reveals the extent to which the framework accurately predicts the dataset. We find that our model is still superior to others in its ability to predict BC at epochs lower than 100, since both its loss and accuracy stay essentially constant after epoch 10.

To further prove the efficacy of the given method, we have trained the suggested framework using just 70% of the data for testing and 30% for training. Maximum values of 96.49% for accuracy in categorization, 97.23% for precision, 97.22% for recall, and 97.19% for F1-score were all attained by the suggested approach. Additionally, we made use of unique training settings, including a smaller minibatch size of 10 images and a slower learning rate of 0.01. In addition, the DL model used to detect and categorize BC subtypes was trained for 5 epochs. Maximum values of 96.88% for accuracy in categorization, 96.89% for precision, 97.03% for recall, and 96.69% for F1-score were all attained by the proposed model. That's why it's important to note that changing the data split and reducing the number of epochs both affect the suggested model's effectiveness.

This demonstrates how our proposed technique can boost the accuracy of liver disease diagnosis and categorization using CT images. These successes stem from our suggested method's prowess in extracting the best possible set of unique, powerful, and highly complex deep features to characterize the ultrasound picture, allowing for accurate and trustworthy identification.

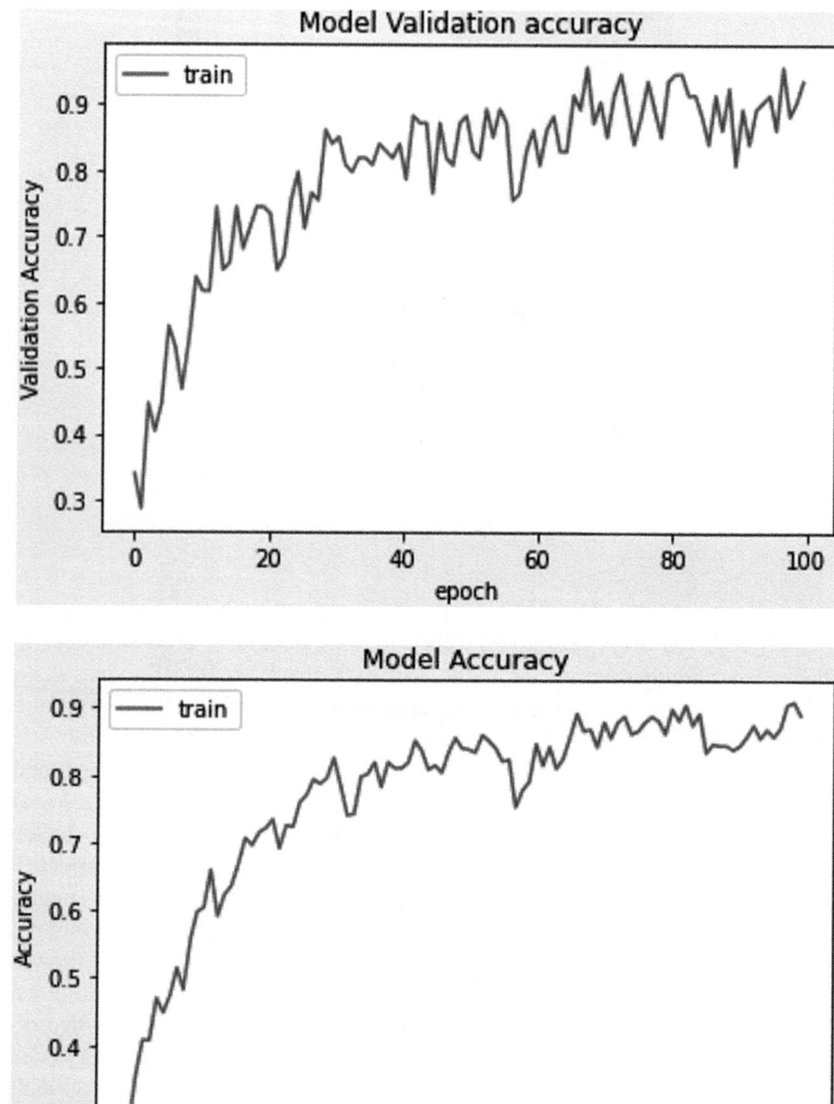

FIGURE 8.6 Model and validation accuracy.

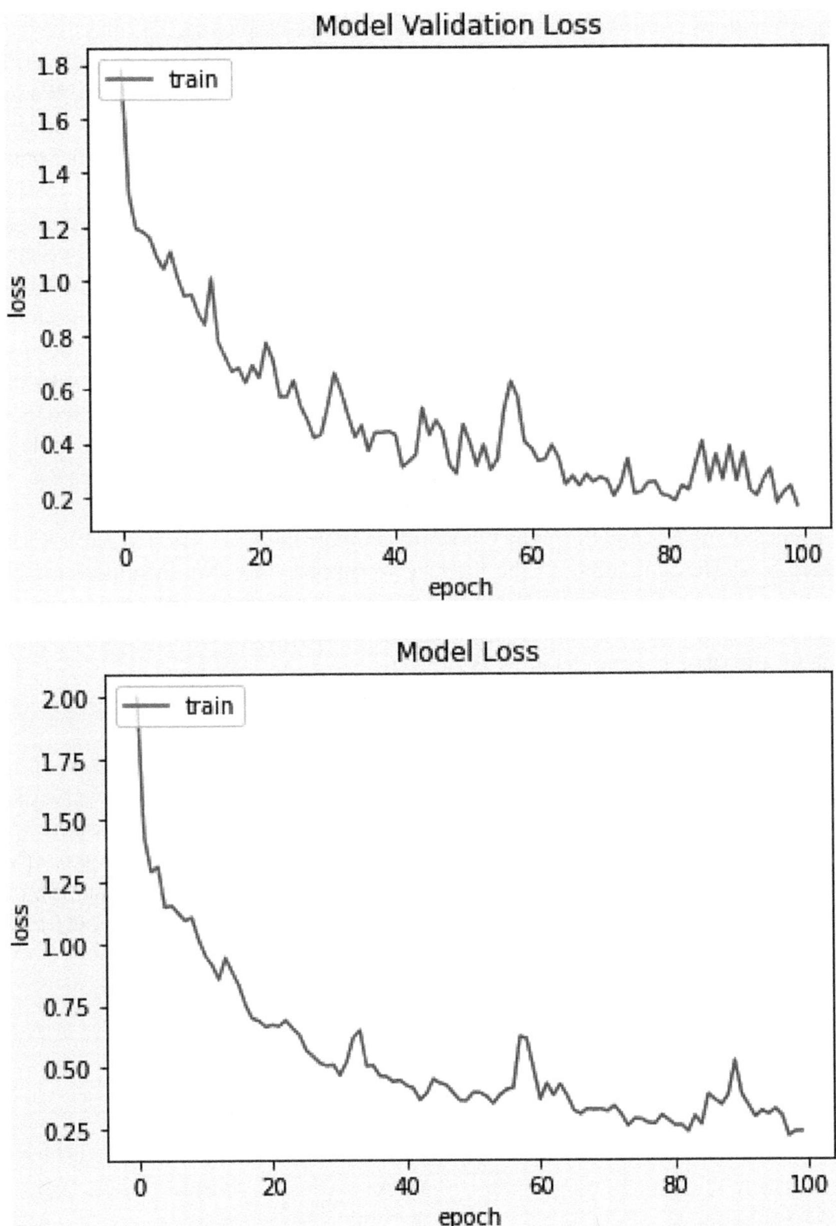

FIGURE 8.7 Model and validation loss.

8.5.1 COMPARISON WITH OTHER MODELS

Whenever testing through a smaller number of training and testing pictures, overfitting difficulties commonly occurred in DL methods; employing DL classifiers and precise tuning helps alleviate this issue. All DL models were trained and verified with the same variables for liver disease identification and categorization. We analyzed 1034 CT scans of the liver in order to spot cases of liver disease. Table 8.1 highlights the particular findings of numerous DL algorithms in categorizing photos of liver illness, demonstrating that all of them yield acceptable results. We analyzed and evaluated the TL methods by using standard metrics such as accuracy, precision, recall, and f-measure. The suggested research employed model-based categorization strategies such as AlexNet, MobileNet, CNN, Inception, ResNet50, and EfficientNet. The recommended model was seen to have the best accuracy (98.89%), the lowest accuracy (82.19%) being achieved by EfficientNet, and the second-lowest accuracy (82.16%) being achieved by MobileNet. An accuracy of 95.83% was reached by both Inception and ResNet50. Also, these results are superior to what was predicted by the baseline models. The models' classification results are also shown there in Table 8.1. In terms of accuracy, precision, recall, and F1-measure (as seen in Figures 8.8, 8.9, 8.10, and 8.11), the proposed model surpasses all the pre-trained models.

Names of models and how long it takes to compute them are listed in Table 8.2 and Figure 8.12. Here are some of the models we support: AlexNet, MobileNet, CNN, Inception, ResNet50, EfficientNet, and Proposed. The average calculation time for AlexNet is 13.77. A calculation in MobileNet takes 17.28 seconds. The computing time for the suggested model is 10.78 seconds.

8.6 CONCLUSION AND FUTURE SCOPE

Nonalcoholic fatty liver disease (NAFLD) is classified using an innovative deep learning model described in this work. In order to automatically diagnose liver illness from CT scan pictures, the model combines LSTM with a lightweight CNN. In order to make raw medical information acceptable for categorization, preprocessing plays a significant role in transforming them. Information imperfections

---

TABLE 8.1

Provides Experimental Findings from a Pre-Trained Model

Model	Accuracy	Precision	Recall	F1-Score
AlexNet	90.95%	97.32%	97.89%	97.63%
MobileNet	83.24%	98.34%	98.11%	98.25%
CNN	91.45%	97.78%	98.16%	97.52%
Inception	95.83%	97.58%	97.87%	98.12%
ResNet50	95.83%	98.77%	98.57%	97.45%
EfficientNet	82.19%	95.12%	93.25%	89.52%
Proposed	98.89%	99.25%	98.78%	98.89%

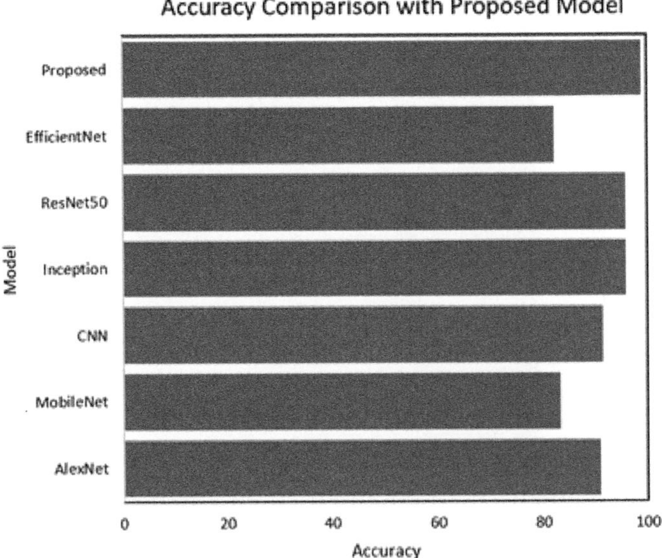

FIGURE 8.8 Evaluation of the proposed model's accuracy.

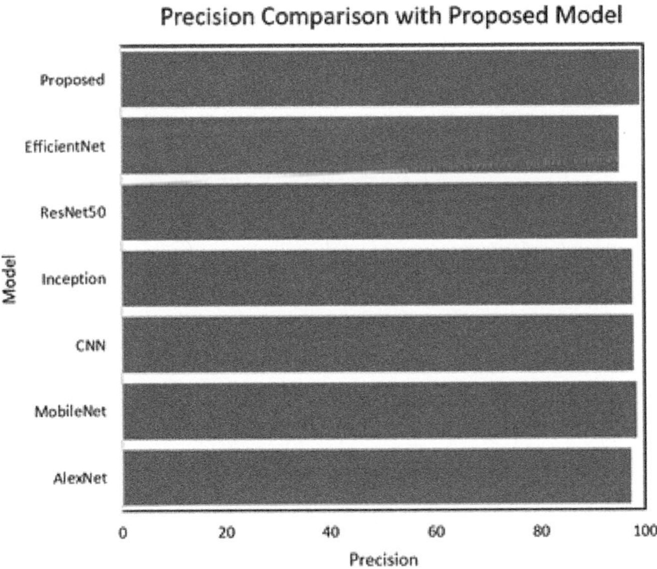

FIGURE 8.9 Evaluate the accuracy of the suggested model.

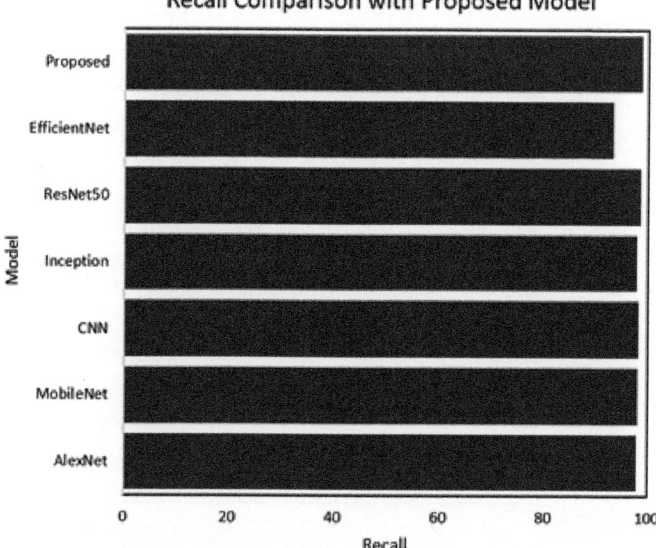

FIGURE 8.10 Model proposal recall and comparison.

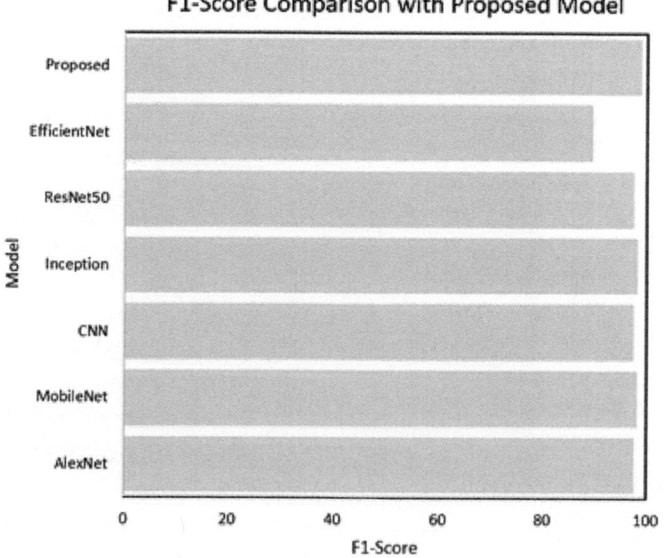

FIGURE 8.11 Analysis of proposed models using F1-scores.

TABLE 8.2

Computation Time for Various Models

Model	Computation Time
AlexNet	13.77
MobileNet	17.28
CNN	12.99
Inception	17.98
ResNet50	18.22
EfficientNet	24.34
Proposed	10.78

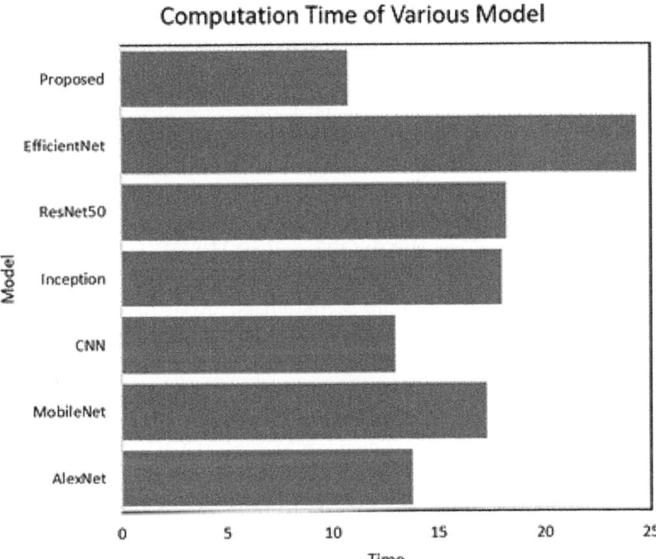

FIGURE 8.12 Different models' computation times.

and unwanted noise must be eliminated. The model is able to function with more accurate and pristine data when preprocessing procedures are used. An additional crucial stage in the classification of health records is the selection of features, in the same vein as selecting variables, attributes, or subsets of variables. In order to do this categorization process, we need to narrow down the collection of available qualities to only those that are most helpful. This research makes use of the Ant Lion Optimization (ALO) technique to pick features to analyze. As the results of the experiments show, the recommended method works. Nonalcoholic fatty liver disease classification accuracy for this model was a remarkable 98.89%. This level of precision shows that the LSTM-CNN model, when paired with ALO-based feature selection, can be an effective method for identifying and tracking liver disorders. As a whole, this research shows that a deep learning architecture can effectively classify NAFLD from CT scans. There is a lot of room for growth in the field of medical image analysis because of the combination of LSTM, CNN, and ALO-based feature selection, which together lead to excellent accuracy rates. Predicting liver illness using an ensemble of deep learning models is the scope of our study. The incorporation of additional data sources, the use of multiple machine learning techniques, and the training of algorithms using machine learning to estimate the possibility of liver disease among people according to their distinctive features are all potential future directions in enhancing the accuracy of liver disease forecasting and categorization models.

REFERENCES

[1] A. Touboul et al., "Unmixing multi-spectral electrical impedance tomography (EIT) predicts clinical-standard controlled attenuation parameter (CAP) for nonalcoholic fatty liver disease classification: A feasibility study," 2022 44th Annual International Conference of the IEEE Engineering in Medicine & Biology Society (EMBC), Glasgow, Scotland, United Kingdom, 2022, pp. 576–579, doi: 10.1109/EMBC48229.2022.9871313.

[2] A. J. M. Rani, S. Nishanthini, D. C. J. Josephine, H. Venugopal, S. G. Nissi and V. Jacintha, "Liver disease prediction using semi supervised based machine learning algorithm," 2022 3rd International Conference on Smart Electronics and Communication (ICOSEC), Trichy, India, 2022, pp. 1389–1392, doi: 10.1109/ICOSEC54921.2022.9952144.

[3] M. Byra et al., "Adversarial attacks on deep learning models for fatty liver disease classification by modification of ultrasound image reconstruction method," 2020 IEEE International Ultrasonics Symposium (IUS), Las Vegas, NV, USA, 2020, pp. 1–4, doi: 10.1109/IUS46767.2020.9251568.

[4] S. Ambesange, V. A, R. Uppin, S. Patil and V. Patil, "Optimizing liver disease prediction with random forest by various data balancing techniques," 2020 IEEE International Conference on Cloud Computing in Emerging Markets (CCEM), Bengaluru, India, 2020, pp. 98–102, doi: 10.1109/CCEM50674.2020.00030.

[5] J. Bayet, T. Hoogenboom, R. Sharma and E. D. Angelini, "Machine-learning on liver ultrasound to stratify multiple diseases via blood-vessels and perfusion characteristics," 2020 IEEE 17th International Symposium on Biomedical Imaging (ISBI), Iowa City, IA, USA, 2020, pp. 1351–1354, doi: 10.1109/ISBI45749.2020.9098700.

[6] L. Brausch, S. Tretbar and H. Hewener, "Identification of advanced hepatic steatosis and fibrosis using ML algorithms on high-frequency ultrasound data in patients with non-alcoholic fatty liver disease," 2021 IEEE UFFC Latin America Ultrasonics Symposium (LAUS), Gainesville, FL, USA, 2021, pp. 1–4, doi: 10.1109/LAUS53676.2021.9639128.

[7] R. T. Umbare, O. Ashtekar, A. Nikhal, B. Pagar and O. Zare, "Prediction and detection of liver diseases using machine learning," 2023 IEEE 3rd International Conference on Technology, Engineering, Management for Societal impact using Marketing, Entrepreneurship and Talent (TEMSMET), Mysuru, India, 2023, pp. 1–6, doi: 10.1109/TEMSMET56707.2023.10150135.

[8] R. Zhao, X. Wen, H. Pang and Z. Ma, "Liver disease prediction using W-LR-XGB Algorithm," 2021 International Conference on Computer, Blockchain and Financial Development (CBFD), Nanjing, China, 2021, pp. 245–248, doi: 10.1109/CBFD52659.2021.00055.

[9] S. Almeida, H. Mirghani and M. Edinburgh, "Convolutional neural network architectures for fatty liver disease detection," 2022 Sardar Patel International Conference on

Industry 4.0 — Nascent Technologies and Sustainability for 'Make in India' Initiative, Mumbai, India, 2022, pp. 1–5, doi: 10.1109/SPICON56577.2022.10180717.

[10] N. Gyorfi et al., "Development of bioimpedance-based measuring systems for diagnosis of non-alcoholic fatty liver disease," 2021 IEEE 15th International Symposium on Applied Computational Intelligence and Informatics (SACI), Timisoara, Romania, 2021, pp. 135–140, doi: 10.1109/SACI51354.2021.9465584.

9 Improvements in Analyzing Biomedical Signals and Medical Images Using Deep Learning

Manjula Nandi, Ngangbam Phalguni Singh, and Ashok Babu P.

9.1 INTRODUCTION

The use of digital image processing in medical diagnosis has increased in recent years as direct digital imaging technologies have been more accessible to the general public. In recent years, the imaging modalities endoscopy and radiography are only two examples of those that have transitioned to using digital sensors. Additional examples of digital technologies that were groundbreaking when they were originally invented are computed tomography (CT) and magnetic resonance imaging (MRI) [1]. The number of "picture elements" (a contraction of "picture" and "element") or "pixels" (a contraction of "picture" and "element") is the standard measurement used when assessing the quality of a digital photograph. Adjustments may be made on an individual basis to the hue, saturation, and brightness of each of these pixels. With the assistance of suitable communication networks and protocols, such as the Digital Imaging and Communications in Medicine protocol also Picture Archiving and Communication Systems, they are able to be processed rapidly, evaluated objectively, and made available in a number of locations all at the same time. The immense potential of digital image processing to be used in the medical field has been unlocked as a result of rapid improvements in imaging technology [2].

9.2 METHODS OF PROCESSING BIOMEDICAL SIGNALS

Methods of varying complexity are being developed to analyze the incoming biological information. Data collection, signal conditioning, feature extraction, and decision making are the four possible steps in the processing of a signal in a typical biomedical

DOI: 10.1201/9781032635149-9"

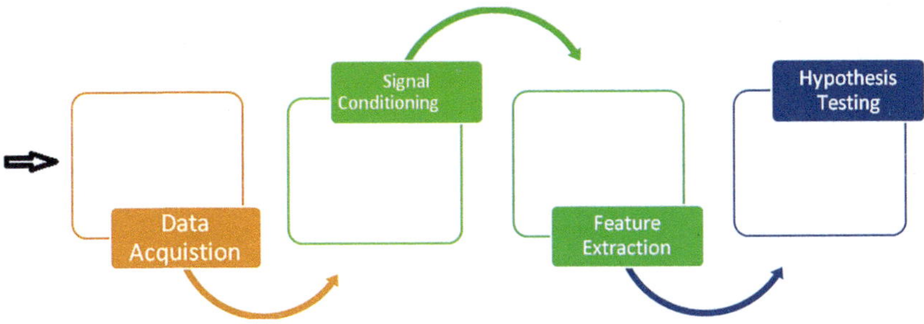

FIGURE 9.1 Processing steps for medical signals.

application (see Figure 9.1). Data acquisition is the process of gathering information and delivering it in a way that a computer can interpret and use. Preventing further signal data loss is now the highest priority. The goal of the process known as signal conditioning is the removal of noise and other undesired features of a signal. This is the desired end-state after carrying out signal conditioning.

The most popular approach is to use linear filters, while nonlinear operators are also commonly utilized instead. All through this presentation, the need to create filters with high signal-to-noise ratios was emphasized. The phrase "extracting features from a signal" refers to the procedure of selecting and quantifying a subset of a signal's qualities that are most indicative of the data of interest. There are a lot of crossovers between feature extraction and signal conditioning due to the fact that they both involve discarding extraneous data. The bulk of it consists mostly of one dimension. To facilitate storage, comprehension, and visualization, the extracted characteristics set should have much lower dimensionality than the conditioned output. The data may then be stored, interpreted, and displayed with little effort [3]. While conditioning may be approached in a generic way, feature extraction methods are often developed with a specific signal or use case in mind. The methods of conditioning are quite standard. The techniques of feature extraction discussed in these notes span from linear prediction in voice analysis to edge detection in image processing. Both of these are only two of the countless options out there. Decision making, which occurs at the conclusion of the signal processing pipeline and is also known as hypothesis testing, is given considerable weight in therapeutic applications. Questions such as "Does the patient show a specific pathology in heartbeats based on the electrocardiogram?" or "Does the patient have a tumor based on the results of the brain scan?" may be answered through this examination. These notes aim to provide a brief overview of many general statistical methods that may be used to make such judgments more reliable.

Digital image processing for the biomedical sciences is often referred to as "biomedical image processing," and this phrase is used to describe this service rather frequently. Figure 9.1 shows a possible division of the broad topic of digital image processing into its four main subfields.

- The creation of an image involves a number of steps, beginning with the act of snapping a photograph and continuing all the way through the creation of the digital picture matrix.
- Image visualization refers to techniques that improve upon an original image by manipulating this matrix, and the term is often used to include a wide range of techniques that achieve this goal.
- Quantitative measurements and abstract interpretations of biological pictures are only two examples of the types of processing that fall under the umbrella of "image analysis." These processes need highly abstracted a priori knowledge about the nature and content of the pictures to be put into the underlying algorithms. Due to the specialized nature of the process of image analysis, it is unusual for algorithms to be easily transferable to multiple application industries.
- "Image management" is the set of procedures that allows for efficient storage, sharing, transmission, and retrieval of visual content. The processes of storing, transmitting, and communicating fall under this category. As a result, telemedicine procedures are often incorporated as a part of image management.

On the other hand, high-level image processing encompasses activities such as picture analysis. These tasks, which may be carried out manually or mechanically and do not need any specific knowledge of the subject matter presented in the pictures, are categorized as "low-level" image processing. A description of the operations that may be carried out is provided by processing at a low level [4]. The use of these strategies yields consistent results when applied to a diverse assortment of visual data sources. You might try expanding the histogram in a radiograph the same way you would with vacation images in order to boost the contrast in the image. As a consequence of this, the majority of photo editing systems include some fundamental post-processing functions.

9.3   UNDERSTANDING DEEP LEARNING AND ITS APPLICATIONS IN HEALTHCARE

Deep learning is a branch of AI that involves teaching computer programs to scan large data sets for hidden patterns and draw inferences from those data sets. In recent years, deep learning has garnered a lot of attention and shown to be effective. One of the areas that it has been used to is healthcare, which is one of the many disciplines that it has been applied to. Particularly, deep learning has shown its potential usefulness in the field of medical diagnosis and therapy [5]. Because it is able to automatically acquire intricate patterns and representations from data, it is a valuable resource for tackling tough problems that arise in the medical field. This ability is one of its primary benefits. Some of the most important uses of deep learning in healthcare are detailed here.

Medical Imaging Analysis: X-rays, CT scans, MRI scans, and histopathology slides are only some of the medical imaging data that have been successfully analyzed by deep learning algorithms. Finding and labeling anomalies like cancers, fractures, and illnesses might help radiologists and physicians arrive at more precise diagnoses.

Disease Diagnosis and Prognosis: Electronic health records (EHRs), test findings, and medical histories are just some of the data that might be fed into a deep learning model and analyzed to aid in the diagnosis and prediction of medical conditions. These models may predict the onset or course of disease by analyzing patient data for patterns and risk factors.

Drug Discovery and Development: By making educated guesses about how chemicals and proteins will interact, deep learning is speeding up the process of discovering novel medicines. Large volumes of genomic data may be examined using this technology, which can lead to the discovery of new therapeutic targets and the enhancement of existing treatment choices.

Natural Language Processing (NLP) in Healthcare: Among the many uses for deep learning-based NLP methods are automated coding, medical transcribing, and sentiment analysis of patient ratings.

Predictive Analytics: Medical personnel may be able to make better use of available resources and offer better care for patients if they use deep learning models to predict patient outcomes, readmission rates, and potential medical concerns.

Virtual Health Assistants: Improvements in deep learning have made it possible to develop virtual health aides like chatbots that can communicate with patients and provide them basic medical advice.

Medical Robotics: Deep learning may be used in medical robot systems to increase their accuracy and level of automation during surgical procedures.

9.4 SIGNIFICANCE OF BIOMEDICAL SIGNAL AND MEDICAL IMAGE ANALYSIS

The study of biological signals and medical imaging are two of the most important applications of medical informatics in modern medicine [6]. Each of these subfields employs state-of-the-art strategies from signal processing and image processing with the ultimate objective of extracting useful information from large databases of medical records. Medical image analysis and biological signal analysis are discussed in further detail next.

Diagnosis and Disease Detection: Electrocardiograms, electroencephalograms, and electromyograms are only a few examples of the physiological signals investigated in the field of biomedical signal analysis. Just a few instances are shown earlier in the chapter. X-rays, CT scans, MRI, and ultrasound are just a few of the many imaging modalities that fall within the purview of medical image analysis. Both studies improve the speed and efficacy with which medical personnel can diagnose a wide range of illnesses and ailments, thereby benefiting the individuals who get care.

Treatment Planning and Monitoring: The study of biological signals and medical images may provide significant information about a patient's health and reaction to therapy. This information is used by clinicians in the process of creating individualized treatment plans and tracking the efficacy of therapeutic treatments as they are implemented. Medical personnel may make evidence-based judgments and fine-tune treatment plans by monitoring a patient's physiological signals or medical imaging during therapy.

Quantitative Assessments: Quantitative and objective measures are used in every field to enhance the diagnostic methods' validity and repeatability. It is essential, in order to make informed treatment decisions, to be able to assess and compare data not just across individuals but also throughout the course of time.

Telemedicine and Remote Monitoring: Wearable technology and other kinds of telemedicine may be used in conjunction with biomedical signal analysis to carry out patient monitoring at a distant location. Medical care providers, regardless of where they are physically located, have the potential to improve the efficiency of their collaboration by examining and interpreting medical pictures using software designed specifically for that purpose. This makes it possible to collaborate in a more productive manner and to disseminate specialized knowledge to a wider audience.

Development of Medical Devices and Technology: Modern medical imaging technologies and imaging equipment have been made possible by developments in signal and image processing methods. Improvements in diagnostic precision and turnaround time have resulted directly from advances in medical imaging, data collecting, and processing.

9.5 OVERVIEW OF BIOMEDICAL SIGNAL TYPES

Electrocardiograms, sometimes referred to as electrocardiograms (ECGs), are the biological signals that are used in clinical diagnostics of the heart to the greatest extent on the majority of occasions. The term "electrocardiogram" is a portmanteau word that was created by combining the prefix "electro," which means "electric signal," with the noun "cardio," which means "heart," and the verb "gramme," which means "recording." A recording of the electrical activity of the heart is what is meant by the term "electrocardiogram."

An electrocardiogram (ECG) may be used to determine whether or not a contraction of the heart muscle was caused by the activation of specific cells by an electric current. The depolarization causes the contraction of each muscle cell to quicken after it has already begun. This results in a higher rate of contraction overall. It's possible that the degree to which the electric activity going on within a cell is stimulated may be taken as an indicator of how effectively that cell is doing its role [7]. The depolarization of the heart muscle in a periodic and regulated manner is what causes an electrocardiogram to be recorded. It is feasible to analyze the pace at which electric depolarization occurs in cardiac muscle cells, which might potentially give insight into the effectiveness of the heart. By using this metaphor, medical professionals have a greater opportunity to locate the regions of the patient's heart that are not pumping blood as effectively as they should be. Analyzing the recorded signal of electric depolarization and looking for any deviations from what is regarded to be a normal electrocardiogram is the first step in arriving at a diagnosis of a particular heart issue.

A lot of territory was covered, from the basics of the biological cell through the electric potential across the cell membrane. There was a great distance to go. Our focus shifts to the heart's role as a pump in the following section of the essay [8]. Following this, we will talk about some of the more fundamental phenomena that are linked with the contraction process, as well as the electromagnetic impulses that are produced by the heart during each and every contraction. In the third and last segment of this multi-part series, we will discuss the history of electrocardiograms (ECGs), as well as how they are measured and processed.

The cardiac muscles of the heart refer to the component of the organ that is in charge of the circulation of blood throughout the body. The structural components of the heart's anatomy and its electrical conduction system are shown in Figure 9.2. The following is a list of the four primary functions of the heart: (1) drawing blood from all of the veins in the body; (2) transporting the blood to be cleaned to the lungs through pumping; (3) drawing blood that has been purified from the lungs; and (4) transporting the blood that has been purified to the rest of the body via pumping.

The fundamental structure of the human heart, which consists of two atriums and two ventricles, is seen in Figure 9.1. Together, the atrium and ventricle are responsible for the efficient pumping of blood. Because of a valve that only goes in one direction, blood cannot go backward from the veins into the atrium of the heart. Left atrium, on the other hand, receives its blood supply from the pulmonary veins,

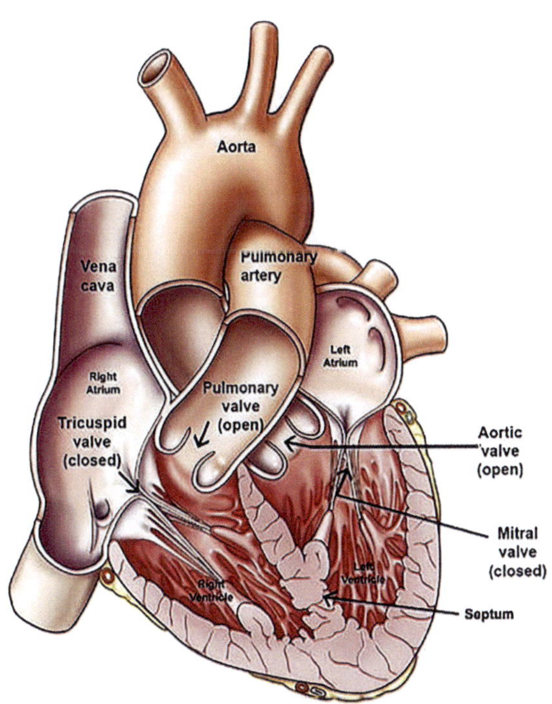

FIGURE 9.2 The heart's structure and the functions it performs.

in contrast to the right atrium, which receives its blood supply from the superior and inferior vena cava via the coronary sinus [9].

Blood that had been pooling in the atrium is pushed into the ventricle as the atrial contracts. The ventricle serves as the heart's lowest pumping chamber. The ventricle is the lower cardiac chamber. During normal cardiac function, the valve prevents blood from flowing backward from the atrium into the ventricle. In medical terms, this heart valve is called the atrioventricular valve. Blood is able to go from the right atrium to the right ventricle via a valve in the heart called the atrioventricular valve, also called the tricuspid valve. The mitral valve, also known as the bicuspid valve, is located between the left atrium and the left ventricle.

The volume of the ventricle grows as a result of the increased pressure created by the increased blood volume in the atrium. Because of an electric delay line connecting the ventricle's excitability to that of the atrium, ventricular contraction occurs at a time that is separate from atrial contraction. A one-way valve sits between the ventricle and the artery to ensure that blood only flows in one direction. The blood that has been pumped out of the ventricle and into the artery is then distributed throughout the remainder of the body. After being forced into the aorta, blood does not return to the left ventricle because of the aortic valve's ability to seal off this pathway. The fully oxygenated blood is distributed throughout the remainder of the body through the aorta. The pulmonary valve may be found in the right ventricle of the heart, and it has an opening that leads into the arteria pulmonalis. This valve allows blood that has to be filtered to leave the body via the pulmonary artery. One of the primary arteries that carries blood to and from the lungs is called the arteria pulmonalis.

The electrical depolarization and repolarization of cardiac muscle may be recorded and interpreted using an electrocardiogram, or ECG. Figure 9.3 depicts the structure of a single-period electrocardiogram recording, and Figure 9.3

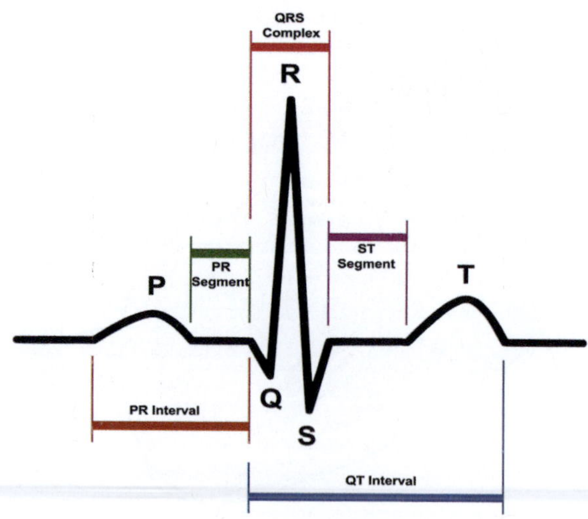

FIGURE 9.3 Periodic waveform typical of a normal electrocardiogram.

displays an example of a normal ECG signal. In an electrocardiogram, the letters P, Q, R, and S each represent one of the five most frequent peaks. In unusual circumstances, the sixth peak, which is represented by the letter U, may also be present. The P wave is produced as a consequence of depolarization occurring in the atrium, while the other waves are produced as a result of the ventricles contracting and filling with blood.

The brain controls and analyses data sent to it from the rest of the body. An electroencephalogram (EEG) or magnetoencephalogram (MEG) using electrodes or magnetic inductors may record electrical activity in the brain, which is generated by action potentials. Both electroencephalograms (EEGs) and magnetoencephalograms (MEGs) are often abbreviated by their initials. Electroencephalograms (EEGs) will be completely understood after reading the following materials.

Electroencephalograms (EEGs) are used to monitor electrical brain activity and are very similar to electrocardiograms (ECGs). The Greek en-kephale, "in the head," is the source of the suffix "-encephalo," which is the medical term for the brain. "encephalo" comes from the Greek for "head" or "brain." The third word, "gramme," refers to the method of recording itself. An EEG is a diagnostic tool used to capture brain electrical activity. "electroencephalogram" is the compound noun form of this phrase, and it describes this technique.

In 1929, a German scientist named Hans Berger attached electrodes to his daughter's head to test the theory that the brain creates electric activity. He kept an eye on his daughter's brain waves while she practiced mental arithmetic so he could observe how much progress she had made. He saw that she was becoming busier as she worked to solve a particularly challenging multiplication problem. This allowed him to conclude that the subject's brainwave patterns may be used to infer the subject's level of mental activity [10].

In this chapter, we'll talk about the science behind EEG and the clinical scenarios when it might be helpful as a diagnostic tool. Some disorders that need EEG testing for accurate diagnosis are also described. We also go through the several computational methods often used in EEG data processing.

The brain is an essential organ that must be healthy in order for the rest of the nervous system to function correctly. The brain is continually monitoring and controlling autonomic activities, such as breathing and digestion, among others, such as they are. Your brain is responsible for the majority of the voluntary acts that are carried out by your body. It is the part of your brain that is responsible for conscious processing, which includes activities such as acquiring new information and creating creative works of art. The picture of the head that is shown in Figure 9.4 is a cross-sectional view, and it displays the front of the brain as well as the base of the skull. This is seen in Figure 9.4, which shows the distribution of gray matter and white matter in the human brain. It is possible to draw parallels between the gray matter of the brain and the network of nerve cells that make up the skin since both include comparable components. When it comes to the processing of impulses in our bodies, it is the neurons in our brains that are responsible for the bulk of the work. The axons of the nerves are located in the white matter of the center of the brain, which is connected to the brain stem, the gray matter (cortex), and the parts of the periphery that are responsible for motor and sensory function. The gray and white

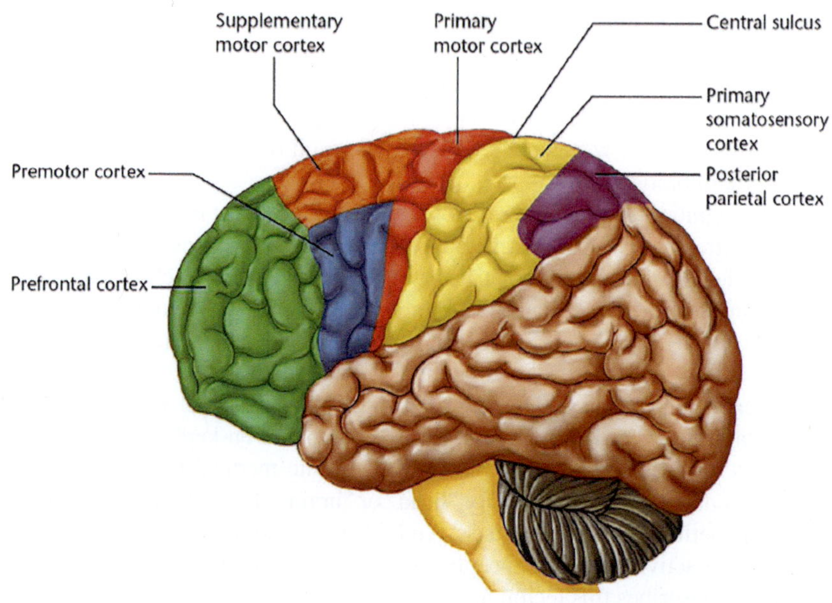

FIGURE 9.4 A simplified diagram of the brain's structure and function.

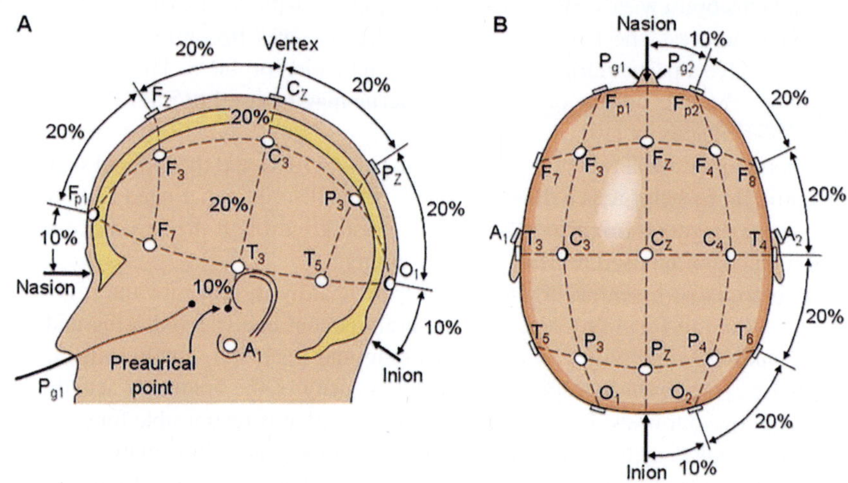

FIGURE 9.5 Positioning of EEG electrodes according to the international 10/20 system.

matter in the brain are both held together by connective tissue in the brain, which acts as a framework.

The bulk of electroencephalogram (EEG) readings are acquired via the use of the electrode configuration seen in Figure 9.5. EEG recordings of individuals who self-report having a medical or mental condition may now be repeated and compared, thanks to the establishment of this standard. It's possible that this will help doctors diagnose patients more accurately. In this technique, the electrodes are typically positioned in a hemispherical matrix across the sagittal plane of the skull at a distance of 20 degrees from one another and at a height that is about 10 degrees above the eyes. With the help of this method, one is able to record the electrical activity of the brain.

EEGs have the potential to identify a wide variety of neurological conditions, including tumors in the brain, head trauma, degenerative diseases, seizure disorders, and even death caused by brain damage. Research on the activity and function of the brain often makes use of the electroencephalogram. Evoked potentials (EPs) and event-related potentials (ERPs) are often recorded and analyzed with the use of electroencephalograms (EEGs). After observing how a person responds to an external stimulus (such as a sound or an image), EEG data are gathered. Electrophysiological (EP) and event-related potential (ERP) approaches may be used for the purpose of conducting research on the amount of time required by the brain to process different forms of information in reaction to a given stimulus. EPs are used extensively in research settings, where they are also utilized to examine subjects' levels of tension and attention. The following few sections of this chapter will focus on the clinical uses of EEG, including detailed explanations of EPs and ERPs.

9.6 ELECTROMYOGRAM

The name "electromyogram" is a portmanteau whose components stem from the prefix "electro," which refers to electric activity; the Greek word "myo," which means "muscle;" and the suffix "gramme," which is short for "recording." Together, these three words form the term "electromyogram." Electromyography, sometimes known as EMG, is the recording of the electrical activity that occurs in muscles.

As was said before, electrical activity is produced by each and every cell as a natural byproduct of the processes that take place inside them. There is no difference between muscle cells and any other kind of cell; the same concept applies to all. Electromyography, often known as EMG, is defined in part as a signal that captures the electric activity generated by the depolarization of muscle cells in response to nerve impulses that induce muscular contraction. This is one of the characteristics that gives EMG its name. Electromyography, or EMG for short, refers to the study of the electrical activity caused by the contraction of a muscle. Electromyography (EMG) may be interpreted as a signal that chronicles the electrical activity of the muscle when seen in this way.

Since its discovery in 1907 by Hans Piper, who recorded the action potentials produced by human muscular contraction, electromyography, more often referred to as EMG, has come to be acknowledged as an essential signal in the field of medicine. Electromyography, more often known as EMG, is a diagnostic technique that is used in modern medicine to evaluate a broad variety of neuromuscular conditions. In what follows, an investigation of the nature of this signal and the many computational methodologies that may be used to make use of it in the medical field will be presented. Let's begin this subject with a quick review of muscle, covering not just its structure but also the electrical activity in which it takes part. Through research into the anatomy and physiology of the muscle, it may be possible to identify the origin of the EMG signal.

A neuron may activate the fibers within a motor unit through the chemical mechanism shown in Figure 9.6. The fundamentals of this process are laid out in detail later in the chapter. In response to an external action potential, the axon of a nerve cell that ends in a synapse produces and secretes a chemical substance known as a neurotransmitter. Acetylcholine, sometimes known as ACh, is a neurotransmitter. When released by a nerve cell, this neurotransmitter goes to the muscle cell. ACh receptors, which are located on the postsynaptic membrane of muscle cells, bind ACh. The motor end plate is a part of the muscle that responds well to this ACh. At the membrane, on the exterior of the muscle cell, the neurotransmitter makes its first contact. When an acetylcholine (ACh) molecule binds to the motor end plate of the sarcolemma, the membrane that surrounds a muscle cell, the muscle cell becomes depolarized. Triggering the binding of the acetylcholine (ACh) molecule is the release of sodium anions across the sarcolemma. More details on the contraction procedure will be provided in the future section, which will be dedicated solely to that topic.

There are a number of ways to go about the electromyography (EMG) electrode recording technique. Electrode-equipped needles are inserted into the affected muscle as part of the second method.

The term "electromyography," which refers to the method of recording the electrical activity of different motor units through the skin, is occasionally used interchangeably with "electromyography." An electromyogram (EMG) signal is the sum of the electric activity of many motor units. Then, each motor unit's contribution is given a weight based on its distance from the electrode and the thickness of the skin and fat between the electrode and the sensor. Electrodes on the skin's surface may disclose how well distinct muscle groups are coordinating with one another, but they cannot offer information on the cells themselves. The purpose of this technique is to identify the sets of muscles responsible for performing a certain task. Unprocessed surface electromyographic data from the gluteus maximus is shown in Figure 9.7.

9.7 OTHER BIOMEDICAL SIGNALS

In the next part of our conversation about the electrocardiogram (ECG), we looked at the many components of the ECG and the functions that each of those components serves within the cardiovascular system. The monitoring of a patient's blood pressure is an essential component of clinical practices for the diagnosis and management of a wide variety of illnesses and ailments. Readings of the patient's systolic and diastolic blood pressure are often all that is required of the attending physician in these situations in comparison to the rest of the signal; the heart rate during diastole is seen later in the chapter. When balanced against the several other factors to be considered, when a reading of the patient's blood pressure is obtained, a large amount of ancillary data is also collected and made accessible.

Extravascularly and intravascularly are the two methods that are used most often in the process of blood pressure monitoring. In the same vein, it is customary to take a measurement of blood pressure that is taken outside of the arteries and veins. Methods that have been around since the beginning of time to measure blood pressure,

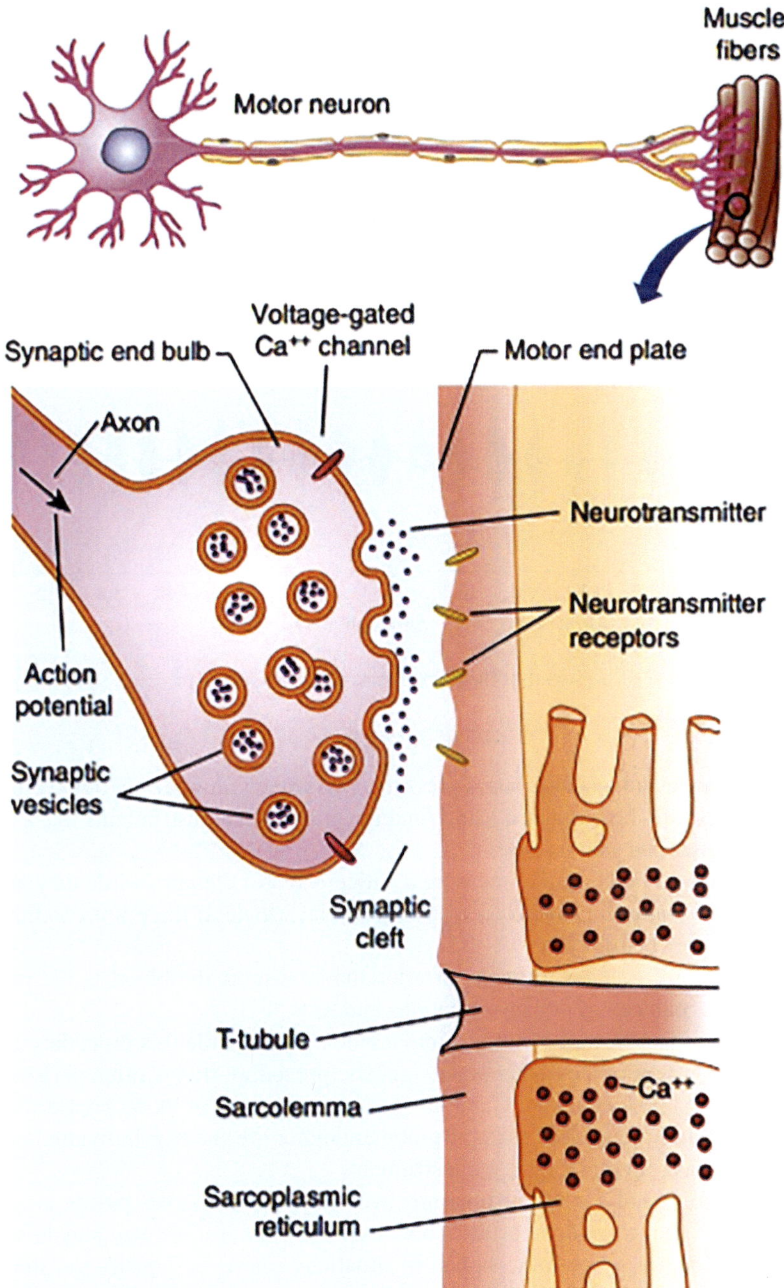

FIGURE 9.6 Motor units are composed of a nerve fiber, and the muscle fibers are innervated by this nerve fiber at the motor plate. The motor plate is a synapse junction that releases ACh in between the muscle fibers.

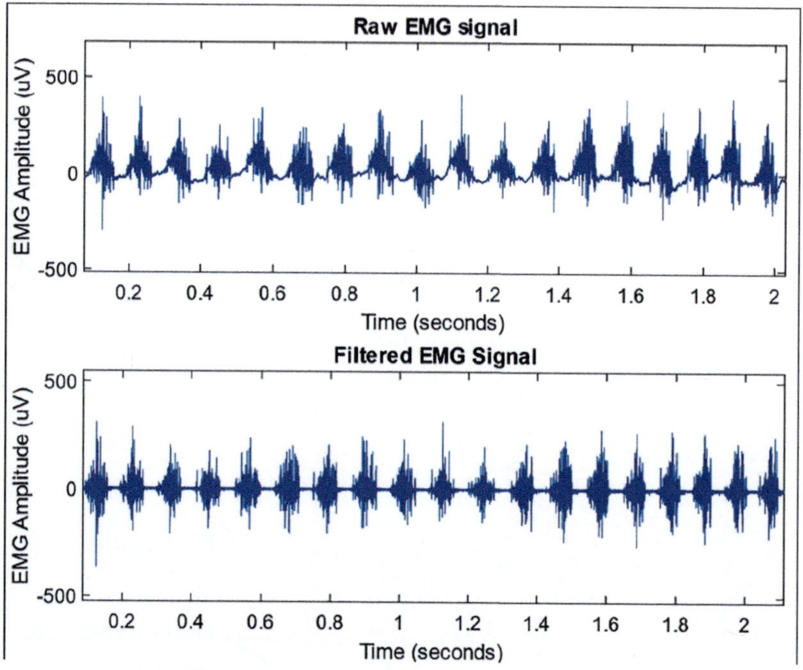

FIGURE 9.7 Raw EMG signal of the gluteus maximus.

The systolic and diastolic blood pressures of a patient are the only blood pressures that can typically be measured using fundamental medical instruments like a sphygmomanometer and stethoscope.

It is standard procedure to measure a patient's blood pressure while they are participating in some kind of physical exercise. Nevertheless, there are conditions in which this may be the case:

The pressure found within the arteries that transport the blood is the primary focus of the majority of our investigations and tests.

A catheter is now being inserted into a blood vessel while this procedure continues. The insertion of a catheter is a diagnostic procedure that is often performed to evaluate the signal as a whole, and not just the variations in blood pressure specifically. The stethoscope and the sphygmomanometer are the two individual components that make up this diagnostic instrument.

A typical signal for blood pressure over the course of two pulses is seen in Figure 9.8. The picture demonstrates how well the Fourier transform may be used to study this chaotic yet periodic signal. In situations where the Fourier transform (or, more accurately, the discrete Fourier transform) has been used for decomposition, the amplitude of the FT (or, in stochastic analysis of the signal, the poser spectrum) at six frequencies has been acquired and is now under investigation. When this happens, it follows the application of the Fourier transform (or, more precisely, the discrete Fourier transform). There are a total of six frequencies at play here: the fundamental (f0), the second (2f0) harmonic, the third (3f0) harmonic, the fourth (4f0) harmonic,

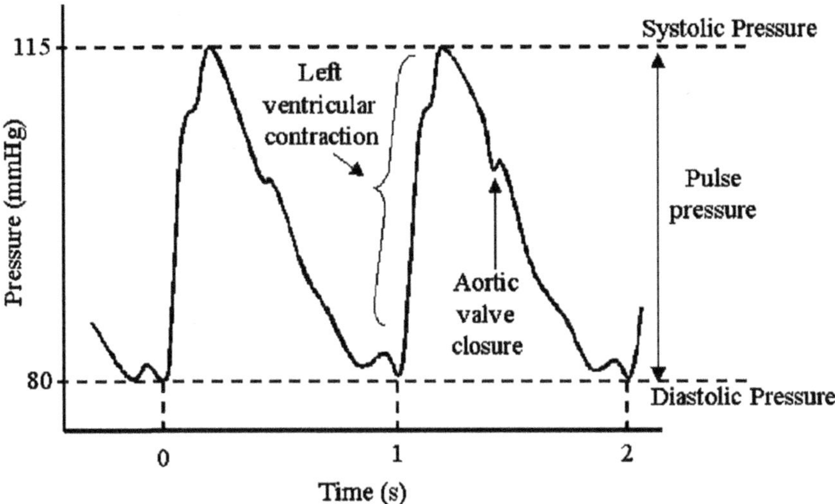

FIGURE 9.8 Typical blood pressure signal.

the fifth (5f0) harmonic, and the sixth (6f0) harmonic. These harmonics have come to the fore since they are responsible for transporting the bulk of the blood pressure signal's energy. Furthermore, the relative strength or weakness of certain harmonics is typically linked to a variety of disorders. If you've been wondering why Fourier analysis is so often used in the processing and analysis of blood pressure data, maybe this article has helped clear things up.

Blood pressure and the signal of blood flow are highly correlated. Accurately estimating blood flow requires knowledge of blood velocity at a given location. There are a number of methods that may be utilized to arrive at this estimate. The indicator dilution technique is one such approach; it involves injecting a drug or other substance into a patient's circulation and then monitoring the drug's concentration over time. There is a one-to-one relationship between the drug's dilution rate and the volume of blood flow. That is to say, the drug's dilution is a good indicator of blood flow. Since dilution data may be thought of as a signal, it can be evaluated using signal processing methods. In order to evaluate blood flow, a technique similar to thermal dilution might be utilized. This technique may be used to estimate blood flow by measuring the rise and fall in temperature of a substance injected into the body (often saline). The ultrasonic method, the electromagnetic flow approach, and the Fick method are among more ways for estimating blood flow. The rate of change in blood flow to a tissue over time may be indicative of the tissue's health.

9.8 CHALLENGES AND LIMITATIONS IN TRADITIONAL APPROACHES

Specialists in many different professions have, for a long time, relied on established methods and practices that are widely recognized within their fields when trying to solve problems. However, their attempts are delayed by a variety of obstacles. What follows is a more in-depth analysis of some of the most serious problems and limitations of the conventional approaches.

Subjectivity and Bias: The decisions that people make are often biased and vulnerable to subjectivity due to the fact that they are so frequently engaged in conventional procedures. When the prejudices, experiences, and points of view of the experts themselves are taken into consideration, the answers may be contradictory or inaccurate.

Limited Data Processing Capacity: In this day and age of big data, it's very possible that even time-tested procedures may be unable to cope with the enormous volumes of data that are at their disposal. It's possible that finishing the project on time will be impossible given the amount of time and effort needed to analyze and assess enormous datasets.

High Computational Complexity: Some classic algorithms, especially those designed to solve exceptionally difficult problems, may need a lot of computing power to perform. Therefore, they may need a great deal of time and computing resources, rendering them unusable for real-time applications requiring precision.

Lack of Adaptability: There are several well-established practices that are hard to change, even in the face of newly obtained knowledge or changing environmental factors. They are unable to adapt their strategy to accommodate new requirements, which is one of the reasons behind their poor level of output.

9.9 ADVANCEMENT IN DEEP LEARNING METHODS

There are limitations to the notability of medical data, notably images, despite the fact that the vast majority of deep learning approaches are geared toward supervised deep learning. This is especially accurate for visual information. There are a number of variables that contribute to this, such as the low incidence of a particular sickness or the absence of a trained expert in the region. The field of supervised deep learning has to make the transition from supervised learning to either unsupervised learning or semi-supervised learning so that it may get beyond the obstacle of a deficiency in huge volumes of data. It is consequently of the highest significance to understand the possibilities for unsupervised and semi-supervised techniques in healthcare, as well as the means by which we may make the transition from supervised learning to transformational learning without sacrificing the precision of our results. Since deep learning theories have not yet delivered full answers and there are still a large number of challenges that have not been addressed, we believe there is an infinite amount of space for progress.

9.10 MEDICAL IMAGE ANALYSIS USING DEEP LEARNING

The fundamental goal of medical image analysis is to let doctors see where on the body lesions are spreading so they can keep an eye on them. Preprocessing, segmentation, feature extraction, and pattern recognition or categorization are the steps that must be taken in order to process an image in Figure 9.9. During preprocessing, photos are checked for flaws and their data is enhanced before they are utilized in subsequent operations. Segmentation is both the name of the method and the name of the phrase defining the process of separating apart certain sections for the purpose of inspection, such as tumors or organs. To facilitate the detection of ROIs, a technique known as "feature extraction" might be used for the data. Based on the characteristics that were uncovered, the ROI may be sorted using classification.

Our bibliography focuses on studies that investigate the classification and labeling of medical pictures. Our research has resulted in a detailed summary of many methods that might be employed to enhance CNN's functional capabilities. Although deep learning networks allow for improved feature extraction, they are resource-intensive to execute. The model's greatest accuracy after testing on 3064 separate MRI images was 95.56% in a 10-fold cross-validation. With an error rate of just 22.7%, Rachapudi and Lavanya's proposed CNN design has been shown to be effective in identifying colorectal cancer in histopathology pictures. To reduce the possibility of overfitting, we employed five convolutional blocks, each of which had a dropout layer.

To use deep learning for picture segmentation, one needs both an encoder and a decoder. It is the job of the decoder to provide a segmentation mask, which is a representation of the object's shape, as the final output. The picture is filtered by the encoder so that information may be extracted from it, while the image itself is

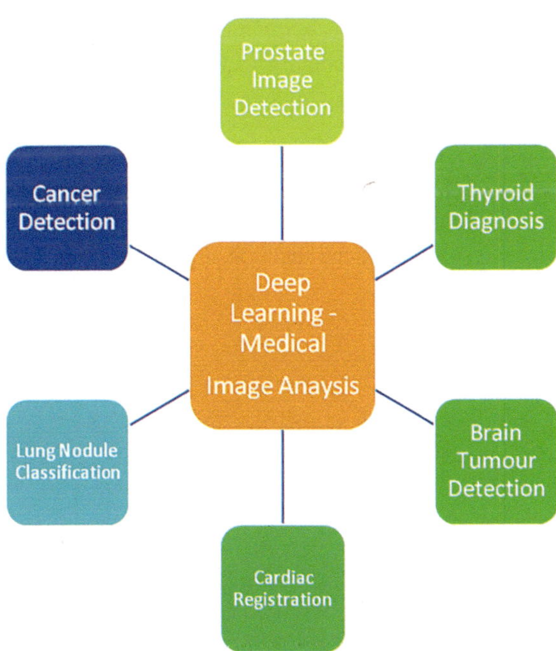

FIGURE 9.9 Medical image analysis using deep learning.

created by the decoder. In order to mimic the efficiency of fully connected layers in an encoder-decoder architecture, completely convolutional networks (FCNs) use 11 convolutions. Convolutions are utilized in place of deep layers to achieve this. Multimodal brain cancer images were segmented using a 3D FCNN-based model developed by Sun et al. The encoder extracted multiscale visual information through four separate paths. The whole map, comprising all four features, was then sent to the decoder. The model used a Dice-based technique to segment the 2019 Brain Tumour Segmentation Challenge Dataset before submitting it for experimental validation.

The results of medical imaging studies may be helpful in clinical decision making. This article reviews the latest advancements in deep learning techniques in detail. There are two goals for this discussion of DLA in the context of medical image analysis in Figure 9.10. First, we provide a high-level overview of the ideas and procedures fundamental to deep learning. We also want to provide a benefit of DLA for analyzing medical images, in brief. Before diving into our own neurological networks since the 1940s, we conclude with the most recent developments in DL's medical application algorithms. The first step is an investigation of several DL methods, both supervised and unsupervised, including the following:

Auto-encoders, convolutional neural networks, and limited Boltzmann machines are only a few of the tools used. Different magical featuresCaffe, TensorFlow, Theano, and PyTorch are all well-known frameworks and approaches in this field. Successes in DL-based medical picture classification, detection, and segmentation were then discussed. The advantages of using in the field of medical image analysis, RBM networks are represented in the literature survey. Prioritizing and CNN-based detection algorithms may be able to offer reliable results. Patients have more therapeutic options now than at any time in the past. But there are also a few questions that deep learning in the field of medical image processing can address. While DL is undoubtedly advancing, supervised approaches are still used by the vast majority of present applications.

Methods of learning without human intervention applied to real-world data identification and tracking of individuals. Clinical judgments made by radiologists of the future may benefit from DLA. The DLA is automated in radiologists' workflow and provides guidance to less-experienced medical staff in making important decisions.

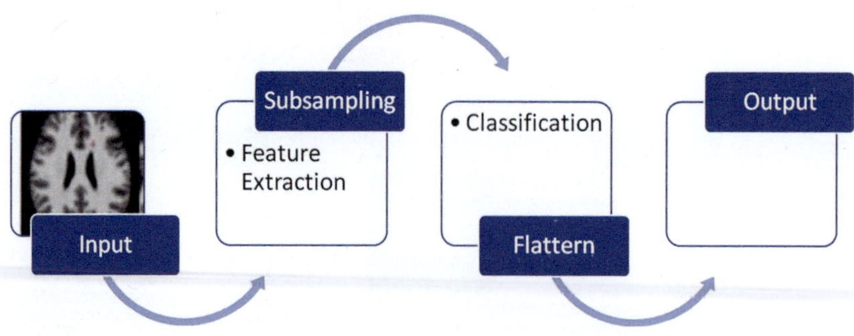

FIGURE 9.10 Proposed architecture for classification.

DLA is designed to help doctors; this software can spot and categorize lesions on its own higher levels of diagnostic accuracy. In principle, DLA might help doctors work faster and more accurately, hence reducing the number of times they make mistakes in clinical analysis of diagnostic images. In the next decades, DL-created medical pictures will be routinely employed in patient diagnosis and treatment. So, it's crucial that healthcare providers and researchers put in long hours to advance patient treatment. To aid the sufferer, try administering DLA. What may be gleaned from a patient's images depends directly on the topology of the networks used to access them. A baby is born by hand. Therefore, it is expected that Neural Network Search will be used in DL model construction to replace the existing cumbersome manual procedure. Equally important is the pursuit of knowledge and the development of practical talents. Cancer patients often get radiation therapy as part of their care. Different diagnostic imaging is being utilized to guide patient care. Radiological subspecialty high-throughput feature extraction is defined for use with medical pictures. According to the study, the use of deep learning in radionics analysis has shown promise as a method for advancing clinical investigation in future medication creation and treatment strategies for cancer patients, current patient outcomes, and historical data. To make up for deficiency applications of annotated medical records, reinforcement learning, semi-supervised learning, and unsupervised learning areas are only starting to emerge in deep learning research for analyzing medical images. In a broad sense, deep learning is a business, complete with all of its challenges and potential rewards, numerous medical uses may be found for medical imaging technology.

9.11   CONCLUSION

In this chapter, we discussed a broad variety of biological signals, each of which is significant in terms of both scientific research and medical treatment. Signals from the respiratory system, signals from the cardiovascular system such as blood pressure and heart sounds, and signals from the magnetoencephalographic (MEG) system are some examples of the types of signals that may be obtained. We may be able to use the same signal processing techniques that were created in earlier chapters for signals that are less frequent because of their similarities to signals that were described in earlier chapters in more depth. These similarities are due to the fact that less prevalent signals are more comparable to signals that are more common.

REFERENCES

[1] By Npatchett—Own work, CC BY-SA 4.0. (2020). https://commons.wikimedia.org/w/index.php?curid=39235282.

[2] File:2027 Phases of the Cardiac Cycle.jpg. (2017). Wikimedia Commons, the free media repository. Retrieved May 15, 2019, from https://commons.wikimedia.org/w/index.php?title=File:2027_Phases_of_the_Cardiac_Cycle.jpg&oldid=269849285.

[3] File:EKG leads.png. (2016). Wikimedia Commons, the free media repository. Retrieved May 15, 2019, from https://commons.wikimedia.org/w/index.php?title=File:EKG_leads.png&oldid=217149262.

[4] File:SinusRhythmLabels.svg. (2019). Wikimedia Commons, the free media repository. Retrieved May 15, 2019, from https://commons.wikimedia.org/w/index.php?title=File:SinusRhythmLabels.svg&oldid=343583368.

[5] Freeman, D. (2011) 6.003 signals and systems. Massachusetts Institute of Technology, MIT OpenCourseWare. https://ocw.mit.edu.

[6] Lee, G. et al. (2019). PyWavelets: A Python package for wavelet analysis. Journal of Open Source Software, 4(36), 1237. https://doi.org/10.21105/joss.01237

[7] Mallat, S. (2009). A wavelet tour of signal processing: The sparse way (3rd ed.) Elsevier.

[8] Mills, N. L. et al. (2008). Increased arterial stiffness in patients with chronic obstructive pulmonary disease: A mechanism for increased cardiovascular risk. Thorax, 63(4), 306–311.

[9] Puttagunta, M., Ravi, S. (2021). Medical image analysis based on deep learning approach. Multimedia Tools and Applications, 80, 24365–24398. https://doi.org/10.1007/s11042-021-10707-4

[10] Venegas, J., Mark, R. (2004). HST.542 J quantitative physiology: Organ transport systems. Massachusetts Institute of Technology, MIT OpenCourseWare. https://ocw.mit.edu

10 A Survey on Lung Cancer Diagnosis Using Deep Learning Techniques

Jiddu Krishnan O.P. and Dr. Pinki Roy

10.1 INTRODUCTION

This section is divided into three. First, we give a general idea about lung cancer, its types, and how they are diagnosed. The second briefly discusses the importance of Deep Learning over Machine Learning. In the last portion, an overview of DL techniques is portrayed.

10.1.1 OVERVIEW OF CANCER IN LUNGS

Cancer is a devastatingly severe disease that can prove fatal without the proper initial diagnosis. In a cancer patient, one could see abnormal growth of cells. This cell growth has immense potential to spread and invade other nearby organs [1]. These tumor growths are, in general, of two types. One that does not spread is called a benign tumor, and the other is a malignant tumor.

Of all the cancers existing today, lung cancers are among the deadliest, accounting for a significant share of the deaths caused by cancers. The significance of the health concern it brings is validated by the World Health Organization (WHO) study, which states that nearly 2.21 million deaths were reported in 2020 alone [2]. This study alone suggests the importance of figuring out methods for early detection and overall improved diagnostic techniques and approaches required to tackle this enormous threat.

Lung cancer is generally divided into Small Lung Cancer (SCLC) and Non-small Cell Cancer (NSCLC). Around 85% is accounted for by the NSCLC type of lung cancer, whereas the remaining by SCLC [1]. Both types behave and appear differently, making it necessary to have different treatment methods.

Cancer-causing substances or organisms are called carcinogens [2]. Exposure to these carcinogens contributes to lung cancer. The smoking of cigarettes has contributed primarily to carcinogens and tar, making it a significant cause of lung cancer. These carcinogens are found to damage both our DNA and lung tissues. This paves the way for cancerous cell growth. Apart from direct smoking, exposure to passive smoking is another major contributor. The remaining factors could range from various occupational hazards, genetic history of lung cancer, and even subjection to environmental pollutants.

DOI: 10.1201/9781032635149-10

Next, about lung cancer diagnosis, there are various parts to it. They mainly involve the combination of the following: clinical evaluation, acquiring the radiological images of the lung, and conduction of biopsies on the lung tissues. Here, radiological imaging modalities are X-rays, computed tomography (CT) images, magnetic resonance imaging (MRI), etc. This variety of images helps the oncologist ascertain the extensiveness of the tumor spread and helps them determine the most suitable treatment for the patient.

10.1.2 Role of Deep Learning in Medical Imaging

Medical imaging is vital in assessing medical conditions, especially in cancer treatment cases. Medical images are crucial in all the stages of a treatment plan, like detecting a medical state, the diagnosis imparted, the prognosis plan, and various other evaluation plans. Here, analyzing medical images can be tricky as it poses many challenges to doctors. Mainly, this is a time-consuming process. Moreover, the differences between healthy and cancerous tissue are very narrow. It requires highly skilled intervention almost all the time. In this regard, Deep Learning [5] has proven to be a great tool for analyzing cancerous tissues from medical images.

Deep learning is basically a subset of Machine Learning. It works with the idea of extracting the features from an image automatically instead of how it is traditionally done in machine learning methods [5]. In ML methods, we can see that the features are extracted manually, and then the important features among them are selected. After selecting features, it is passed to a classifier algorithm. These steps in ML are time-consuming and to deal with this, a substantial knowledge of the data is required. On the other hand, the feature extraction and selection part is done automatically when it comes to Deep Learning methods. This is done through various layers predominantly consisting of Convolutional Neural Networks (CNN) [6]. This multi-level automatic feature extraction works very well in identifying subtle patterns in the raw data that might not have been picked up by other methods. Here, a point to note is that, when compared to ML methods, DL methods require a huge amount of raw data to produce higher accuracy results.

Recently Deep Learning has gained wide acceptance in the medical imaging domain, predominantly in the classification of diseases. Across modalities like X-rays or CT scans, the impact deep learning has provided is very evident. Researchers across the globe have shown that the higher accuracy values yielded could help doctors provide reliable diagnoses.

Apart from just using Deep Learning as a classification or detection tool, other tasks like segmentation and tracking are also beneficial. Segmentation essentially means having a given image divided into different regions. In the case of lung images, the regions could represent various tissues. Deep Learning models can accurately segment medical images, helping medical practitioners identify the defects incurred relatively easily and further aid them in concentrating on the region of interest.

Tracking is about analyzing the changes involved in medical images over the course of time. A great example of the usage of tracking would be in prospective diagnosis methods that are usually undertaken by doctors. Tracking is helpful in the constant evaluation of disease progression. Here again, Deep Learning could provide clinicians with very important details of the changes incurred in the medical images, thereby helping them assess the situation.

To summarize, Deep Learning has an evidently critical role in the current and the future of medical imaging. The standout capability of DL models to directly and automatically extract the relevant features alone makes it a very powerful tool for detection, segmentation, or tracking purposes. With researchers across the globe working relentlessly to achieve greater accuracy with DL models, various applications are yet to be seen.

10.1.3 Deep Learning Techniques

As discussed in the previous section, DL works on the idea of automatic feature extraction. DL models require an abundant amount of data. The more data we have, the more accuracy we will get in comparison with ML-based models. Now, among plenty of available DL techniques, three of the commonly used techniques are discussed next:

Convolutional Neural Networks (CNNs): CNNs consist of multiple layers. They are primarily used in image processing tasks. The majority of the existing works on image processing are seen to be based on CNNs. CNN convolutional layers are used for extracting local spatial features of an image using a small-size filter, which generates the feature maps by incorporating non-linearity using various activation functions like—ReLu, Leaky ReLu, Swiss, and many more.

Generative Adversarial Networks (GANs): GANs are part of generative modeling, which automatically discovers existing patterns and replicates them. A GAN consists of two networks: a generator and a discriminator. The generator part creates random noise images from existing data, and the latter half, called the discriminator, attempts to distinguish it. Over iterations, the model gets better at distinguishing, and real fake images are generated.

Transfer Learning: Transfer learning uses the weights of pre-trained models while training new models. So, on bigger datasets, leveraging these weights helps the newer models to be efficient even with smaller datasets. This fine-tuning process can be extremely useful in obtaining better results on the models.

10.2 DEEP LEARNING APPROACHES IN LUNG CANCER DIAGNOSIS

10.2.1 Datasets Used

Over the years, there has been research on lung cancer detection done over various methods and techniques and a wide variety of datasets. Among all the work, only Lung Image Database Consortium and Image Database Resource Initiative (LIDC-IDRI) [4] and LUNA16 dataset-related papers are analyzed in this review work. Only these two datasets are large enough for DL models to perform reasonably.

The LIDC-IDRI dataset was published in 2011, consisting of 1018 annotated low-dose Lung CT scans. The LUNA16 consists of 888 annotated CT scans. The LUNA16 dataset is a part of the LIDC-IDRI dataset, with filtering made for images with slice thickness greater than 3 mm. These datasets are relatively huge compared to other available lung CT scan datasets. Additionally, the availability of proper annotation by various radiologists makes the datasets relatively even more robust for DL models.

10.2.1.1 Review of Papers

In this subsection, reviews of the selected papers are done. Two papers each from the year 2017 to 2023, which worked on either LUNA16 or LIDC-IDRI dataset, have been taken for review. Here, the evaluation metrics used are mostly that of a regular confusion matrix [3] and also Dice Coefficient Value (DSC) for segmentation-related works.

In the year 2017, Hamidian et al. [8] proposed a 3D CNN model. The authors trained the 3D CNN over the volume of interest taken from the LIDC dataset. They then converted them to a 3D Fully Convolutional Network (3D FCN). They found that their model gave them the results ten times faster. In this work, the authors obtained a sensitivity value of 80% but at a higher false positive per scan of 22.4.

In the same year, Nibali et al. [9] produced a work on the LIDC dataset. They created a model with ResNet as a base exploring how transfer learning, curriculum learning, etc., affect the accuracy of the classification. Ultimately, they obtained accuracy, specificity, sensitivity, and ROC values of 89.9%, 88.64%, 91.07%, and 0.9459, respectively.

Xie et al. [10], in the year 2018, published their work showcasing the effectiveness of a Multi-View Knowledge-based Collaborative approach. Here, they take three patches of images to fine-tune a set of pre-trained ResNet-50 models. They obtained a commendable accuracy of 91.6% and an AUC value of 95.7%. These results were way above average in comparison to the state-of-art methods.

Gruetzemacher et al. [11] did work on the LUNA16 dataset. Their model was a 3D Deep Neural Network architecture inspired by U-Net. Their model achieved substantial false positive rate reduction. For this they used the features extracted in their centroid computation as a threshold. They followed cross-validation techniques and obtained a sensitivity of 89.29% at a false positive per scan of 1.789.

Kasinathan et al. [12], in 2019, published a paper that uses Multiscale Gaussian distribution and an Enhanced CNN model. Their segmentation model combined the local image bias with an active contour model. They claim that the computational time for their model is relatively less. Further, they achieved 97%, 89%, and 91% accuracy, sensitivity, and specificity values, respectively.

Tran et al. [13] worked on creating a 15-layer novel 2D deep CNN model. The classification on the LUNA16 dataset was done to identify if the images were with a nodule or a non-nodule one. In order to get better accuracy, they applied a focal loss function to the training part. Even though the model required high computational resources to run, they obtained a high classification accuracy of 97.2%.

Masood et al. [14], in 2020, created a custom 3D deep CNN model. To select the region of interest, they applied median intensity projection and also a multi-Region Proposal Network (mRPN). They trained and validated their work on the LIDC dataset. They obtained an excellent sensitivity value of 98.7% with a false positive per scan of just 1.97.

El-Bana et al. [15] created a custom DeepLab-V3 model based on CNN. Their model had two stages, one for segmentation and the latter for classification. The authors analyzed the impact of multiple parameters and models. Finally, they obtained excellent results in both the segmentation and classification parts. The model achieved a DSC value of 0.8834 and an accuracy of 95.66%.

Sun et al. [16], in the year 2021, published a paper on attention embedded complementary stream (AECS) based CNN model. The system was of three parts. Intuitively an attention-guided mechanism for feature extraction, then another block for feature integration, and, finally, a classification block. Their model worked on the LUNA16 dataset and produced a sensitivity score of 92% with a false positive per scan of 4.

Neal Joshua et al. [17] proposed a 3D lightweight AlexNet-based model. They used the 3D CNN for automated classification, while 2D CNN was used for applying a multiview strategy. The complexity of the model was low, and they applied 10-fold cross-validation. The classification accuracy obtained was 97.17%.

Zhou et al. [18], in 2022, built a cascading framework featuring a YOLOv5 model. There are three parts to them. The first one is to locate the nodules on the slices. In the second part, they proposed an algorithm for candidate selection. And in the final stage, they do the segmentation. For the segmentation part, they obtained a DSC value of 86.75%.

Zheng et al. [19] worked on a two-stage nodule detection (TSND) model. Their primary aim was to reduce the FP rate. For this, they created a multi-scale feature selection network in the first stage. And in the second half, a novel candidate selection procedure was followed. On the LUNA16 dataset, for over a series of FP per scan values, the authors obtained a sensitivity value of 90.59%.

Ahmed et al. [20] in 2023, investigated the effectiveness of various models like Fast RCNN, SSD, and YOLOv3. The authors analyzed pulmonary nodules' classification problem as benign or malignant with these various deep learning models. An average accuracy range of 0.92 to 0.95 was obtained by them.

Jian et al. [21] proposed a custom 3DCNN model named 3DAGNet. This cascade model had parts, including an attention enhancement setup, a global search module, and a feature fusion part. When compared to other 3D DL models, they obtained a great sensitivity value of 88.08%.

10.3   CHALLENGES AND FUTURE SCOPE

From the review, we saw how well different DL models worked. But even then, the varied number of false positives is just an example showing there is huge room for improvement. On this note, this section discusses the challenges and future scope of using deep learning methods.

Challenges

1. Need for robust datasets: Annotated datasets like LUNA16 and LIDC-IDRI are available, as discussed in the previous sections. In comparison with other existing ones, these datasets definitely are more reliable. However, the uncertainties are still large with respect to the annotations given in them. Various radiologists have multiple opinions regarding a tumor's location in a particular CT Scan. This alone causes confusion among researchers working on the Artificial Intelligence domain regarding which label to follow. This is one of the major reasons for models producing varied amounts of

false positives in their results. The researchers may or may not pick the slice that actually has a nodule present. Hence, having a robust and larger dataset would immensely help researchers go further and help them validate the results with more reliability.

2. Need for explainability of models [7]: DL models are by large considered "black boxes." The reason is that we don't know what is happening inside a model. Unlike an ML model, where we alone pick or select the features, DL extracts the features independently and does all the steps up to classification. It is particularly important to know how a particular model works so that its shortcomings can be dealt with appropriately.

3. Issues regarding ethical clearances: Using any sort of patient-related data requires consent from the patient because of the potential breach that could happen to their privacy. And for this matter, following the regulatory standards or protocols is absolutely necessary. Only after the ethical committee standards are followed, can we either collect data or even use our models in real-time scenarios to see their effectiveness.

Future Scope

1. Synthetic Data Generation: One of the ways to counter the low availability of dataset is to generate them. The created images would look similar to the existing ones; this helps the researchers have more space to validate their models.

2. More collaborative research: Collaboration in research is very important. It scales in all ways, from data collection, data sharing, model creation, and execution. Effective collaboration between researchers, cancer centers, medical-tech companies, etc., helps evaluate DL-based CAD models in the real-time scenario.

3. Explainable AI [7]: This is a part of the recent advancement in the Artificial Intelligence domain. As said before, DL models, in general, are considered black box models. Explainable or interpretable AI was developed to explain how a particular model works and analyze its pitfalls. This, in general, would help researchers point out the issues in their model and help them achieve better results.

In conclusion, while challenges exist, the future of deep learning in lung cancer diagnosis and medical imaging is bright. Addressing data-related issues and promoting collaborative research will pave the way for AI-driven solutions that profoundly impact patient care, ultimately leading to earlier and more accurate diagnoses, personalized treatments, and improved overall outcomes.

10.4   TABULAR PRESENTATION OF THE PAPERS

In this section, a table of all the papers taken for review is created, listing the authors, year of publishing, the dataset used, techniques used, advantages, results achieved, drawbacks, and scope for improvement (Table 10.1).

TABLE 10.1

Tabular Representation of Papers Used in the Review

Author (s) and Year	Dataset (s) Used	Methodology Adopted	Advantages	Drawbacks/Scope for Improvement	Results Achieved
Hamidian et al. [8] (2017)	LIDC	3D FCN	FCN gives 10 times faster results.	Low sensitivity value. FP per case is too high.	Sensitivity of 80% for false positives per scan of 22.4
Nibali et al. [9] (2017)	LIDC	ResNet, transfer Learning, curriculum training	High classification accuracy.	A few of the performance measures could still be improved.	Accuracy = 89.90%, Specificity = 88.64%, Sensitivity = 91.07%, Precision = 89.35, and ROC of 0.9459
Xie et al. [10] (2018)	LIDC	Multi-View Knowledge-based Collaborative (MV-KBC) Deep Learning	Results are better than many state-of-the-art models, especially the AUC value.	Highly complex setup and requires higher processing power. Sensitivity could be improved.	Accuracy = 91.60%, Sensitivity = 86.52%, Specificity = 94%, and AUC = 95.70%
Gruetzemacher et al. [11] (2018)	LUNA16	U-Net-inspired DNN architecture	Achieved decent FP reduction. Cross-validation techniques were followed.	Sensitivity could be improved for lower FP/scan values.	Sensitivity of 89.29% at FP/scan = 1.789
Kasinathan et al. [12] (2019)	LIDC	Multiscale Gaussian distribution, Enhanced Convolutional Neural Network (CNN)	Excellent accuracy. Lower computational time.	Sensitivity could be improved without increasing the FPs/scan.	Accuracy = 97%, Sensitivity = 89%, Specificity = 91%
Tran et al. [13] (2019)	LUNA	15-layer 2D Deep Convolutional Neural Network	Exceptional classification accuracy was obtained.	The model requires higher computational resources.	Accuracy = 97.2%, Specificity = 97.3% and Sensitivity = 96%

(Continued)

TABLE 10.1 Continued

Author (s) and Year	Dataset (s) Used	Methodology Adopted	Advantages	Drawbacks/Scope for Improvement	Results Achieved
Masood et al. [14] (2020)	LIDC	3D Deep CNN	Excellent values of sensitivity for a lower FP/scan value.	The whole model setup is quite big. Detection accuracy for smaller nodules could be improved.	Sensitivity of 98.7 % with 1.97 FP/scan
El-Bana et al. [15] (2020)	LUNA16	DeepLab-V3 (a CNN model)	Excellent results in both segmentation and classification part.	Computational time could be improved.	DSC = 0.8834, Accuracy = 95.66%, Specificity = 97.24% and FP/Scan = 0.6
Sun et al. [16] (2021)	LUNA16	Attention Embedded Complementary Stream Convolutional Neural Network (AECS-CNN)	The results obtained were good.	Complexity of the model is high.	Sensitivity = 92% for FP/scan = 4
Neal Joshua et al. [17] (2021)	LUNA16	3D AlexNet with lightweight architecture	Lower model complexity. Application 10-fold-cross validation. High accuracy.	The model could be next experimented with for tracking purposes.	Accuracy = 97.17%
Zhou et al. [18] (2022)	LUNA16, LIDC	YOLOv5, candidate nodule selection (CNS), multi-size 3D-based fusion model	Well-defined cascade framework.	Model needs to be improved in terms of robustness.	CPM = 89.5% DSC = 86.75%
Zheng et al. [19] (2022)	LUNA16	Two-Stage Nodule Detection (TSND)	Commendable attempt at reducing false positive rate.	Scalability of the model is yet to be assessed.	Average sensitivity of 90.59% for various FP per scan values
Ahmed et al. [20] (2023)	LIDC	Fast RCNN, SSD, and YOLOv3	Analyses of these DL models were done.	More models could have been taken into consideration.	Accuracy range of 0.92 to 0.95 was obtained with these models
Jian et al. [21] (2023)	LUNA16	3DAGNet (a custom 3D CNN model)	A compact 3D CNN model.	The sensitivity score could still be improved.	Sensitivity = 88.08%

10.5 CONCLUSION

The integration of deep learning techniques into lung cancer diagnosis has got a bright future ahead. We have seen various works from 2017 to 2023. A quick go-through of these works shows us the improvement in the result parameters. The accuracy, specificity values, etc., are seen to be improved all the way from the 1980s to the 1990s. This alone shows us how impactful DL techniques have been in medical imaging. Initially, we could see that plenty of the models were concentrated on 2D images or slices of the CT scan of the LUNA16 or LIDC dataset. But, as time progresses, researchers have applied themselves to make compact 3D models with promising results. With the progression of time, the researchers' computational resources have also changed, hence their willingness to create complex models extensively for volumetric data.

In conclusion, the fusion of deep learning and medical imaging is poised to usher in a new era of precision medicine, where diseases like lung cancer are detected earlier and treated more effectively, and patient outcomes are vastly improved. As this field continues to evolve, it is the collaboration between medical experts, data scientists, and technology innovators that will drive us toward a future where healthcare is characterized by greater accuracy, efficiency, and compassion.

REFERENCES

[1] Rani, Ruchi, Jayakrushna Sahoo, and Sivaiah Bellamkonda. "Application of deep transfer learning in detection of lung cancer: A systematic survey." In *2022 OPJU International Technology Conference on Emerging Technologies for Sustainable Development (OTCON)*. IEEE, 2023.

[2] World Health Organization, Cancer: Key Facts, 2020, www.who.int/news-room/fact-sheets/detail/cancer.

[3] Advaitha, Vetagiri, Prottay Adhikary, Partha Pakray, and Amitava Das. 2023. CNLP-NITS at SemEval-2023 task 10: Online sexism prediction, PREDHATE!. In *Proceedings of the 17th International Workshop on Semantic Evaluation (SemEval-2023)*, pp. 815–822, Toronto, Canada. Association for Computational Linguistics.

[4] Samuel G. Armato. "The lung image database consortium (LIDC) and image database resource initiative (IDRI): A completed reference database of lung nodules on CT scans." *Medical Physics* 38 (2) (2011): 915–931.

[5] Rajesh, Sanapala, Nurul Amin Choudhury, and Soumen Moulik. "Hepatocellular carcinoma (HCC) liver cancer prediction using machine learning algorithms." In *2020 IEEE 17th India Council International Conference (INDICON)*. IEEE, 2020.

[6] Choudhury, Nurul Amin, and Badal Soni. "An efficient CNN-LSTM approach for smartphone sensor-based human activity recognition system." In *2022 5th International Conference on Computational Intelligence and Networks (CINE)*. IEEE, 2022.

[7] Xu, Feiyu, et al. "Explainable AI: A brief survey on history, research areas, approaches and challenges." In *Natural Language Processing and Chinese Computing: 8th CCF International Conference, NLPCC 2019*, Dunhuang, China, October 9–14, 2019, Proceedings, Part II 8. Springer International Publishing, 2019.

[8] Hamidian, Sardar, et al. "3D convolutional neural network for automatic detection of lung nodules in chest CT." In *Medical Imaging 2017: Computer-Aided Diagnosis*, Vol. 10134. SPIE, 2017.

[9] Nibali, A., He, Z. Wollersheim, D. Pulmonary nodule classification with deep residual networks." *International Journal of Computer Assisted Radiology and Surgery* 12 (10) (2017):1799–1808.

[10] Nibali, Aiden, Zhen He, and Dennis Wollersheim. "Pulmonary nodule classification with deep residual networks." *International Journal of Computer Assisted Radiology and Surgery* 12 (2017): 1799–1808.

[11] Gruetzemacher, Ross, Ashish Gupta, and David Paradice. "3D deep learning for detecting pulmonary nodules in CT scans." *Journal of the American Medical Informatics Association* 25 (10) (2018): 1301–1310.

[12] Kasinathan, Gopi, et al. "Automated 3-D lung tumor detection and classification by an active contour model and CNN classifier." *Expert Systems with Applications* 134 (2019): 112–119.

[13] Tran, Giang Son, et al. "Improving accuracy of lung nodule classification using deep learning with focal loss." *Journal of Healthcare Engineering* 2019 (2019).

[14] Masood, Anum, et al. "Cloud-based automated clinical decision support system for detection and diagnosis of lung cancer in chest CT." *IEEE Journal of Translational Engineering in Health and Medicine* 8 (2019): 1–13.

[15] El-Bana, Shimaa, Ahmad Al-Kabbany, and Maha Sharkas. "A two-stage framework for automated malignant pulmonary nodule detection in CT scans." *Diagnostics* 10 (3) (2020): 131.

[16] Sun, Wenqing, Bin Zheng, and Wei Qian. "Automatic feature learning using multichannel ROI based on deep structured algorithms for computerized lung cancer diagnosis." *Computers in Biology and Medicine* 89 (2017): 530–539.

[17] Joshua, Neal, Stephen, Eali, et al. "3D CNN with visual insights for early detection of lung cancer using gradient-weighted class activation." *Journal of Healthcare Engineering* 2021 (2021): 1–11.

[18] Zhou, Zhixun, et al. "A cascaded multi-stage framework for automatic detection and segmentation of pulmonary nodules in developing countries." *IEEE Journal of Biomedical and Health Informatics* 26 (11) (2022): 5619–5630.

[19] Zheng, Shaohua, et al. "A lower false positive pulmonary nodule detection approach for early lung cancer screening." *Diagnostics* 12 (11) (2022): 2660.

[20] Ahmed, Imran, et al. "Automated pulmonary nodule classification and detection using deep learning architectures." *IEEE/ACM Transactions on Computational Biology and Bioinformatics* 20 (4) (2023): 2445–2456.

[21] Jian, Muwei, et al. "3DAGNet: 3D Deep Attention and global search network for pulmonary nodule detection." *Electronics* 12 (10) (2023): 2333.

11 Content-Based Medical Image Retrieval Using CNN Feature Extraction and Hashing

Nepoleon Keisham and Arambam Neelima

11.1 INTRODUCTION

In the rapidly evolving landscape of modern healthcare, medical imaging has emerged as a cornerstone of diagnostic and treatment practices. With the advent of digital imaging technologies, vast amounts of medical images are being generated and stored in healthcare repositories worldwide. These images, ranging from X-rays and MRI scans to histopathological slides and ultrasound images, hold invaluable insights for medical professionals in their quest to provide accurate and timely patient care. Content-Based Medical Image Retrieval (CBMIR) stands at the intersection of medical imaging, computer vision, and information retrieval, offering a promising solution to the challenges posed by the growing volume and complexity of medical image data. CBMIR leverages advanced computational techniques to enable healthcare providers to efficiently and effectively search, retrieve, and analyze relevant medical images from vast archives based on their content characteristics [1].

Traditionally, medical image retrieval relied heavily on manual annotation and metadata tagging, which are often labor-intensive, error-prone, and limited in capturing the full spectrum of clinical information present in the images. CBMIR, on the other hand, obviates the need for exhaustive manual labeling by employing automated feature extraction, pattern recognition, and machine learning algorithms to analyze the inherent visual and structural attributes of medical images. This allows for the identification of intricate details, subtle patterns, and anomalies that might escape human perception. CBMIR techniques involve two main steps: first, extracting important features from images, and, second, comparing images based on these features to find similar ones [2]. Researchers have improved these systems over time to make them work better. They make upgrades during preprocessing or while extracting features [3]. A lot of research in medical image retrieval shows that using texture-based features is a popular choice for many researchers around the world [4]. But medical imaging is getting more advanced. It tries to gather as much information about the patient's body as it can. So, just using textures is not enough. There is a need for smarter CBMIR system that looks at different things like texture, edges, and shapes all together. In the context of CBMIR, a significant aspect revolves around the comparison of an image of interest with other images contained within a database. This procedure aids in the assessment of their degree of similarity, facilitating the identification of corresponding pairs [5]. The old-fashioned methods mostly look at basic features like colors, textures, shapes, and how features are arranged in the image. But sometimes, these basic features don't really capture what the image is about, so they don't work well for finding the right images.

To fix this, researchers are using a new approach. They use special deep learning models called deep convolutional neural networks (DCNN). These models are much better than the old methods. They've been doing really well in tasks like finding images or recognizing objects. These models understand images in a more detailed way and help improve how we find the right images. This chapter introduces a novel approach to CBMIR that harnesses Convolutional Neural Networks (CNN) for feature extraction and utilizes Hashing technique for data integrity verification and fast retrieval. The main contribution of the chapter is given as follows:

1. Through training on a comprehensive dataset of medical images, CNN (VGG-19) learns to extract discriminative and representative features effectively. This ability to capture intricate patterns and context in medical images enriches the feature representation, preserving essential diagnostic information.
2. After feature extraction, Hashing technique (SHA-256) is applied to convert the high-dimensional feature vectors into compact binary codes. This not only reduces storage requirements but also significantly speeds up retrieval times, making the proposed CBMIR system highly suitable for real-time applications.
3. In conclusion, the fusion of CNN-based feature extraction and Hashing technique presents a potent solution for Content-Based Medical Image Retrieval. The model's superior performance compared to existing methods demonstrates its effectiveness and highlights its potential to enhance medical image analysis and clinical decision-making processes.

The rest of the chapter is structured in a subsequent manner. The state of the art is detailed within the "State of the Art" section. The details of the Hashing technique used are found in the "Preliminaries" section. The methodology put forward is elucidated in the "Proposed Method" section. Descriptions pertaining to the framework employed for conducting experiments to assess the retrieval performance of both the proposed method and other comparative techniques can be found in the "Experimental Results" section. Ultimately, the "Conclusion and Further Studies" section encapsulates the final remarks and findings.

11.2 STATE OF THE ART

Researchers have extensively explored CBMIR methodologies to enhance medical image analysis, diagnosis, and treatment planning. Texture-based features have garnered widespread attention due to their efficacy in capturing distinct anatomical nuances. However, as medical imaging advances, the limitations of texture-centric approaches become evident, necessitating multi-dimensional retrieval systems encompassing diverse attributes like texture, edge, and shape. Traditional low-level feature extraction techniques, encompassing color, texture, form, and spatial structure analysis, have proved inadequate in accurately reflecting image semantics. Consequently, the emergence of deep learning, exemplified by pre-trained deep convolutional neural network (DCNN) models, marks a transformative leap. DCNN models exhibit superior performance in image retrieval and object recognition tasks, offering enriched semantic information and substantially elevating retrieval precision.

In [6], researchers discuss the utilization of convolutional neural networks (CNNs) in machine learning applications, exploring their effectiveness in generating proficient images through high-level feature descriptors. In [7], the researchers introduced a model that leverages the benefits of both local bit-plane decoded features and the accomplishments of deep learning in the field of CBMIR. The authors in [8] treat CNN filters as detectors of visual words, and through three inverse document frequency (idf) computation approaches and query expansion, it merges traditional term frequency-inverse document frequency (tf-idf) with modern CNN analysis, yielding potent image retrieval results across challenging datasets. In [9], the authors introduce a distinctive deep learning method to extract concise and discriminative features from medical images. Employing Residual Networks (ResNets), a renowned deep neural network, aids in capturing distinctive attributes. In [10], the authors proposed an approach, termed RbQE, for retrieving computed tomography (CT) and magnetic resonance (MR) images. RbQE utilizes the power of feature expansion and leverages pre-trained learning models like AlexNet and VGG-19 to extract compact, deep, and advanced attributes from medical images. RbQE involves two search phases: a rapid search and a final search. During the rapid search, the initial query is enhanced by incorporating top-ranked images from each class. These images help create new queries by calculating mean deep feature values. The final search employs the most similar new query, derived from the original, for precise retrieval from the image database. In [11], the authors proposed a CBMIR model by using a Siamese network along with the hash method. During the training phase, a loss function is formulated to enhance the distinctiveness of feature vectors, while an additional regularization component is introduced to promote alignment between actual real value outputs and the intended binary values. The authors introduced a model [12], termed Randomized Distributed Hashing (RDH), which employs a distributed framework utilizing Locality Sensitive Hashing (LSH). This technique distributes data randomly across cluster nodes, applying identical randomized hash functions to index local data on each node. During queries, the local search occurs across various nodes, capitalizing on parallelism to substantially enhance query time performance. In [13] the authors developed a model, employing transfer learning for feature extraction and incorporating a Locality Sensitive Hashing (LSH) index to expedite retrieval speed.

11.3 PRELIMINARIES

11.3.1 SECURE HASH ALGORITHM

SHA is a family of cryptographic hash functions that are widely used for various purposes in computer security and cryptography. The primary purpose of a hash function is to take an input (message, data, or file) and produce a fixed-size output, known as the hash value or digest. SHA-256 is a specific variant of the SHA-2 family. It produces a 256-bit (32-byte) hash value [14].

The overview of the SHA-256 algorithm:

1. Padding: The input message is padded to a fixed length to ensure that it is a multiple of the block size (512 bits for SHA-256).
2. Message Schedule: The padded message is divided into 512-bit blocks, and a message schedule of 64 words is generated from the block.
3. Initialize Hash Values: The hash values (eight 32-bit words) are initialized to specific constants.
4. Compression Function: The compression function operates on each block of the message schedule and updates the hash values through a series of logical and arithmetic operations.
5. Final Hash: The final hash value of 256-bit is obtained by concatenating the hash values from the compression function.

The main contributions of SHA-256 in CBMIR are as follows:

1. Data Integrity Verification: Employing SHA-256 to generate hash values enables individuals to validate the integrity of both the feature vectors and the original images. In cases where unauthorized alterations or corruption affect the feature vectors or images, distinct hash values will emerge, serving as an indication of possible data tampering.
2. Efficient Storage and Comparison: Storing and comparing hash values is more efficient than storing and comparing high-dimensional feature vectors. Hash values are compact and uniform in size, making them suitable for indexing and quick similarity calculations, which can enhance retrieval performance, especially for large datasets.

11.4 PROPOSED METHOD

The proposed method consists of several sequential stages, as shown in Figure 11.1, each comprising the following steps:

1. Pre-processing 2. Extracting the features 3. Converting the feature vectors in hash value 4. Similarity Measure.

11.4.1 PREPROCESSING

Initially, the medical database images undergo a pre-processing step that involves resizing images to a consistent size and normalization of pixel values.

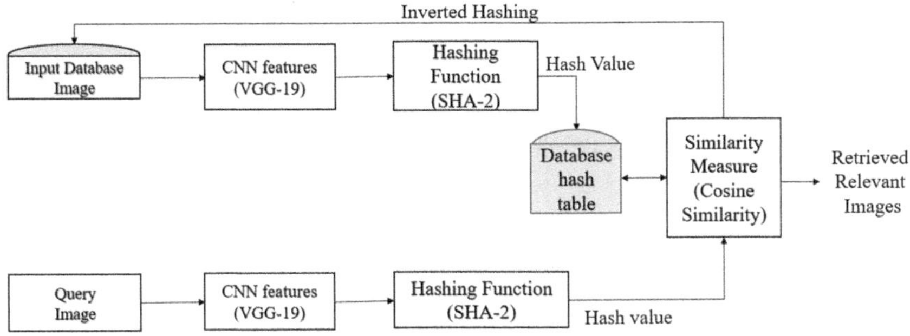

FIGURE 11.1 Block diagram of the proposed Hashing-based CBMIR.

11.4.2 Extracting the Features

Following this, the features inherent to the medical image database are extracted using a pre-trained deep learning model. Leveraging the capabilities of Deep Learning, especially the VGG-19 CNN architecture [15] for feature extraction offers a data-driven and impactful technique for capturing pertinent information from images, rendering it a robust choice for CBMIR applications. VGG-19 is a deep convolutional neural network architecture renowned for its simplicity and effectiveness. It consists of 19 layers, including convolutional layers with small receptive fields and max-pooling layers. The network is trained on a large dataset, enabling it to learn hierarchical and abstract features from images. The process commences by incorporating a pre-trained VGG-19 model that has undergone training on an extensive dataset, that is, ImageNet.

In the CBMIR system, the focus centers on feature extraction rather than image classification. Consequently, the fully connected layers situated at the VGG-19 model's culmination are omitted. This decision preserves solely the convolutional and pooling layers, shaping the model into a potent feature extractor.

Further consolidation of the extracted features and dimensionality reduction is achieved through the application of Global Average Pooling (GAP) to the final convolutional layer's output. GAP computes the mean value of each feature map, culminating in a standardized feature vector for each image. This step is pivotal to ensure that images with varying dimensions are transformed into feature vectors sharing the same dimensions.

In possession of the modified VGG-19 model, each medical image traverses the network. The outcome of the GAP layer serves as the feature vector extracted from the respective image. This feature vector encapsulates high-level depictions of the image's content, rendering it suitable for subsequent similarity comparisons.

11.4.3 Applying SHA-256

Nonetheless, it's important to acknowledge that the utilization of a deep learning model comes with the trade-off of heightened computational demands. To address these challenges, the next phase incorporates the utilization of the SHA-256 Hashing algorithm. The algorithm that is shown in Section 11.3.1 is applied to transform the extracted feature vectors into corresponding hash codes. The adoption of SHA-256 facilitates the establishment of hash values that serve to validate the integrity of both the original images and their associated feature vectors. Subsequently, any unauthorized alterations or instances of corruption affecting either the feature vectors or the images will lead to distinct hash values, thereby signaling the potential occurrence of data tampering.

Moreover, a crucial advantage of employing hash values lies in their operational efficiency for storage and comparison. As compared to the storage and comparison of high-dimensional feature vectors, hash values demonstrate enhanced efficiency. These hash values possess a compact and uniform size, rendering them apt for indexing and swift similarity calculations. This attribute, especially advantageous for extensive datasets, holds the potential to substantially amplify retrieval performance.

Additionally, it is noteworthy that the entire process described earlier is replicated for the query image, as elucidated in Figure 11.1. This ensures the holistic applicability and effectiveness of the method in retrieving similar images from the medical image database based on user queries.

11.4.4 SIMILARITY MEASURE

Cosine Similarity is used for finding the similarity between Hash values of query image and the database medical images. The mathematical equation for determining the Cosine similarity is given subsequently:

$$cosine\_similarity\left(\alpha, \beta\right) = \left(\alpha \cdot \beta\right) / \left(\|\alpha\| * \|\beta\|\right) \tag{11.1}$$

where α dot β is the dot product of vectors α and β, $\|\alpha\|$ is the Euclidean norm (magnitude) of vector α, $\|\beta\|$ is the Euclidean norm (magnitude) of vector β.

11.5 EXPERIMENTAL RESULTS

To analyze the proposed algorithm, the proposed scheme is tested using a publicly available standard dataset. The experiments are performed and the experimental results are given on the basis of *Mean Average Precision (mAP)*. *mAP* is computed by averaging the *Average Precision (AP)* values across multiple queries. The formula for mAP is as follows:

$$mAP = \frac{1}{Q}\sum_{q=1}^{Q} AP_q \tag{11.2}$$

where Q is the total number of queries APq stands for the Average Precision for query q.

$$AP = \frac{1}{N_{rel}}\sum_{k=1}^{N_{ret}} Prec\left(k\right) \times is\_rel_k \tag{11.3}$$

where N_{rel} signifies the total number of relevant images. N_{ret} indicates the total number of retrieved images. *Prec(k)* stands for the precision at rank k. is_rel_k is an indicator function that equals 1 if the image at rank k is relevant, and 0 otherwise.

11.5.1 EXPERIMENT ANALYSIS ON VIA/I-ELCAP DATASET

To analyze the proposed algorithm, the proposed scheme is tested using vision and image analysis group/international early lung cancer action program (VIA/I-ELCAP) dataset [16]. The experimental data are gathered through the collaboration of the Early Lung Cancer Action Program (ELCAP) and the vision and image analysis (VIA) research groups. In this dataset [16], there are 12,645 images of whole-lung computed tomography (CT) scans. The CT scans were acquired during a single uninterrupted breath-holding period, using a slice thickness of 1.25 mm. Each image had dimensions of 512×512 pixels. After removing blurry and duplicated images, a total of 12,000 images remained. Some of the images from the dataset are selected randomly and shown in Figure 11.2.

For training and testing purposes, the images in the dataset are sub-grouped into two parts. Ninety percent of images from the image dataset are used for training and 10% of images from the image dataset are used for testing. The proposed method is tested by retrieving the top k images. The values of k used for testing are 10, 20, 30, and 40. One example of retrieving the top 10 images using a particular query is shown in Figure 11.3.

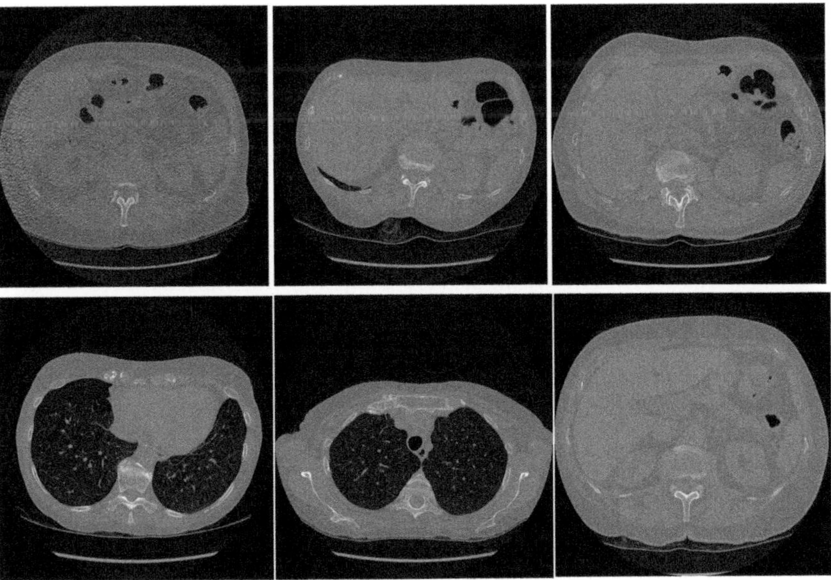

FIGURE 11.2 Sample images from VIA/I-ELCAP dataset.

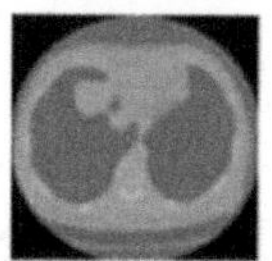

Query Image

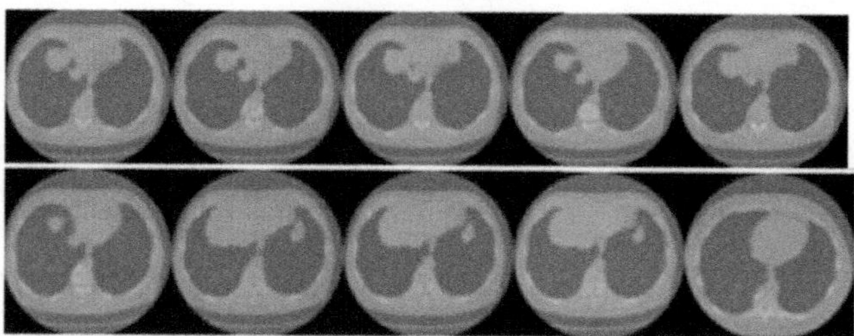

Retrieved Images

FIGURE 11.3 Top 10 images retrieved from VIA/I-ELCAP dataset.

TABLE 11.1

Comparison of Proposed Model with Various State-of-the-Art Model

Model	mAP (k = 10)	mAP (k = 20)	mAP (k = 30)	mAP (k = 40)
Proposed	0.89	0.86	0.85	0.83
CNNSH [11]	0.88	0.86	0.84	0.83
DH [17]	0.81	0.79	0.76	0.75
KSH [18]	0.74	0.71	0.68	0.66
MLH [19]	0.67	0.64	0.63	0.62
SH [20]	0.62	0.60	0.56	0.55

The proposed method is compared with the existing state of the art and the result is shown in Table 11.1. All the models are compared with various values of k. The accuracy of the models decreases gradually when the value of k increases. It is clearly shown that the proposed model gives a better retrieval rate when compared with DH [17], KSH [18], MLH [19], and SH [20]. But the proposed model is slightly better than CNNSH [11] when the value of k = 10 and k = 30. But it is almost the same when the value of k = 20 and k =40.

11.6 CONCLUSION AND FURTHER STUDIES

The proposed model introduces a novel approach to CBMIR that harnesses Convolutional Neural Networks (CNN) for feature extraction and utilizes SHA-256 for Data Integrity Verification and fast retrieval. Through training on a comprehensive dataset of medical images (VIA/I-ELCAP dataset), CNN learns to extract discriminative and representative features effectively. This ability to capture intricate patterns and context in medical images enriches the feature representation, preserving essential diagnostic information. After feature extraction, SHA-256 Hashing technique is applied to convert the high-dimensional feature vectors into compact binary codes. This not only reduces storage requirements but also significantly speeds up retrieval times, making the proposed CBMIR system highly suitable for real-time applications. In conclusion, the fusion of CNN-based feature extraction and Hashing technique presents a potent solution for Content-Based Medical Image Retrieval. The model's superior performance compared to existing methods demonstrates its effectiveness and highlights its potential to enhance medical image analysis and clinical decision-making processes.

In future, various deep learning models will be used along with different Hashing techniques to increase the efficiency of the retrieval system and will compare it with various standard datasets.

REFERENCES

[1] A. Kumar, J. Kim, M. Fulham, and D. Feng, Content-based medical image retrieval: A survey of applications to multidimensional and multimodality data, Journal of Digital Imaging, Vol. 26, 2013, pp. 1025–1039.

[2] M. Owais, Effective diagnosis and treatment through content-based medical image retrieval (CBMIR) by using artificial intelligence, Journal of Clinical Medicine, Vol. 8 (4), 2019, p. 462.

[3] A. Shinde, A. Rahulkar, and C. Patil, Content based medical image retrieval based on new efficient local neighborhood wavelet feature descriptor, in Biomedical Engineering Letters, Springer, Vol. 9, 2019, pp. 387–394.

[4] A. W. Smeulders, M. Worring, S. Santini, A. Gupta, and R. Jain, Content-based image retrieval at the end of the early years, IEEE Transactions on Pattern Analysis and Machine Intelligence, Vol. 22 (12), 2000, pp. 1349–1380.

[5] J. Ahmad, M. Sajjad, I. Mehmood, S. Rho, and S. W. Baik, Saliency-weighted graphs for efficient visual content description and their applications in real-time image retrieval systems, Journal of Real-Time Image Processing, Vol. 13, 2017, pp. 431–447. 1996.

[6] S. ur Rehman, S. Tu, M. Waqas, Y. Huang, O. ur Rehman, B. Ahmad, and S. Ahmad, Unsupervised pre-trained filter learning approach for efficient convolution neural network, Neurocomputing, Vol. 365, 2019, pp. 171–190.

[7] S. R. Dubey, S. K. Roy, S. Chakraborty, S. Mukherjee, and B. B. Chaudhuri, Local bit-plane decoded convolutional neural network features for biomedical image retrieval, Neural Computing and Applications, Vol. 32, 2020, pp. 7539–7551.

[8] N. Kondylidis, M. Tzelepi, and A. Tefas, Exploiting tf-idf in deep convolutional neural networks for content based image retrieval, in Multimedia Tools and Applications, Springer, Vol. 77, 2018, pp. 30729–30748.

[9] M. Rashad, I. Afifi, and M. Abdelfatah, Content-based medical image retrieval based on deep features expansion, in 2022 5th International Conference on Computing and Informatics (ICCI), IEEE, 2022, pp. 331–336.

[10] M. Rashad, I. Afifi, and M. Abdelfatah, An efficient method for content-based medical image retrieval based on query expansion, Journal of Digital Imaging, 2023, pp 1–14.

[11] Y. Cai, Y. Li, C. Qiu, J. Ma, and X. Gao, Medical image retrieval based on convolutional neural network and supervised hashing, IEEE Access, Vol. 7, 2019, pp. 51877–51885.

[12] O. Durmaz, and H. S. Bilge, Fast image similarity search by distributed locality sensitive hashing, in Pattern Recognition, Elsevier, Vol. 128, 2019, pp. 361–369.

[13] M. Parola, A. Nannini, and S. Poleggi, Web image search engine based on LSH index and CNN Resnet50, arXiv preprint arXiv:2108.13301, 2021.

[14] H. Handschuh, H. C. van Tilborg, and S. Jajodia, Sha-0, sha-1, sha-2 (secure hash algorithm) in Cryptologia, Brian Journal of Winkel, Vol. 24, 2000, p. 2.

[15] K. Simonyan, and A. Zisserman, Very deep convolutional networks for large-scale image recognition, arXiv preprint arXiv:1409.1556, 2014.

[16] *VIA/I-ELCAP Database*. Accessed: Aug. 2023. [Online]. www.via.cornell.edu/databases/lungdb.html

[17] R. Xia, Y. Pan, H. Lai, C. Liu, and S. Yan, Supervised hashing for image retrieval via image representation learning, Association for the Advancement of Artificial Intelligence, Vol. 28, 2014.

[18] A. Krizhevsky, I. Sutskever, and G. E. Hinton, Imagenet classification with deep convolutional neural networks, Advances in Neural Information Processing Systems, Vol. 25, 2012.

[19] W. Liu, J. Wang, R. Ji, Y. G. Jiang, and S. F. Chang, Supervised hashing with kernels, in 2012 IEEE Conference on Computer Vision and Pattern Recognition, IEEE, 2012, pp. 2074–2081.

[20] M. Norouzi, and D. J. Fleet, Minimal loss hashing for compact binary codes in MIJ, Citeseer, Vol. 1, 2011, p. 2.

12 Experimental Evaluation of Deep Learning-Assisted Brain Tumor Identification with Advanced Classification Methodology

*Neelaveni P., Gayathry S. Warrier, Tamilarasi K.,
Gopila M. and Thandaiah Prabu R.*

12.1 INTRODUCTION

A brain tumor is any tumor that affects the central nervous system, as defined by the World Health Organization (WHO) in its 2016 reclassification. Brain tumors are described as clusters of abnormally proliferating brain cells. Tumors of this sort expose brain tissue to a size decline, which in turn causes extensive harm to the brain's neuronal network and affects its function. The brain, the most important part of the human nervous system, and the spinal cord are what make up the CNS. The brain is responsible for evaluating, integrating, organizing, determining, and commanding the bulk of the body's processes [1]. There is a great deal of complexity in the human brain's anatomy. Stroke, infection, brain tumors, and headaches are all examples of CNC illnesses that are notoriously hard to diagnose, evaluate, and find an effective therapy for.

Cancer is a major health problem that poses a serious threat to individuals today. Brain tumors are the most terrifying and life-threatening kind of malignancy. Synapses and the billions of cells that make up the human brain make it the most complicated organ in the body. The human brain acts as the body's neural control hub, regulating every bodily function. Therefore, having a brain abnormality is extremely detrimental to human health. Cancer's wide range of symptoms, low survival rate, and generally destructive behavior make it the deadliest and most debilitating illness known to man [2]. Misdiagnosis of a brain tumor can lead to inefficient medical therapy, decreasing the patient's odds of survival. The pituitary, glioma, lymphoma, Medulloblastoma, malignant, and auditory neuroma are all distinct forms of tumors

DOI: 10.1201/9781032635149-12

with distinct textures, locations, and shapes. Brain tumors are the most common kind of brain illness. A proliferation of brain cells that is out of control. Tumors can be classified as benign (slow-growing and not invasive) or malignant (extremely aggressive and spreading to other parts of the body).

It takes a lot of time and expertise on the part of the radiologist to diagnose a brain tumor. The sheer volume of data necessitated by the expansion in the patient population has rendered the use of conventional methods impractical and prohibitively expensive. Problems arise because brain tumors of the same kind can vary greatly in size, form, and severity, as do analogous indications of other diseases [3]. Misdiagnosis of a brain tumor has serious repercussions and decreases a patient's chance of survival. There has been a recent uptick in research and development efforts aimed toward automating image processing in order to circumvent the shortcomings of human-run alternatives. Recently, many computer-aided design systems have been developed to automatically detect and diagnose brain cancers.

Depending on which part of the brain the tumor is pressing on, it can cause a wide range of symptoms. Headaches, seizures, visual issues, vomiting, mental disturbances, memory lapses, loss of balance, etc., may be among the prominent symptoms. Brain tumors can develop for several reasons, including heredity, ionizing radiation from cell phones and other electronic devices, extremely low-frequency magnetic fields, chemicals, physical damage to the head, infections, and other immunological variables. Malignant tumors, also known as cancerous tumors, can begin in the brain (primary tumor) or elsewhere in the body (secondary tumor) and then move to the brain. CT scans, MRIs, tissue biopsies, etc., are just a few of the many diagnostic tools available.

Medical professionals have relied heavily on Magnetic Resonance Imaging (MRI) to diagnose brain cancers due to the high tissue contrasts it provides in each imaging modality. Brain tumor structural MRI scans must still be manually segmented and analyzed by trained neuroradiologists, which is a laborious and time-consuming process. Therefore, the identification and treatment of brain tumors will be greatly improved by an automated and strong segmentation of these lesions. The initial identification of neurological diseases including Alzheimer's disease (AD), schizophrenia, and dementia is another potential benefit. As radiologists work to improve patient outcomes by tailoring treatment based on tumor characteristics such as volume, location, and shape, an automated method for Lesion segmentation can be a valuable resource. Size, bias field (undesirable artifact owing to the poor picture capture), position, and form are only a few examples of how a tumor and its normal adjacent tissue (NAT) differ, all of which reduce the efficiency of segmentation in medical imaging analysis [4]. In the medical imaging field, several models have been created to better detect the border curves of brain tumors. As a result of its adaptability, deep learning is becoming a popular method for analyzing MRI scans of the brain in the pursuit of tumor identification. In many applications of machine learning, such as medical picture segmentation, deep learning is the superior and more resilient method. It corrects the flaws in human brain tumor prediction. The MRI scan of a brain tumor is displayed in Figure 12.1.

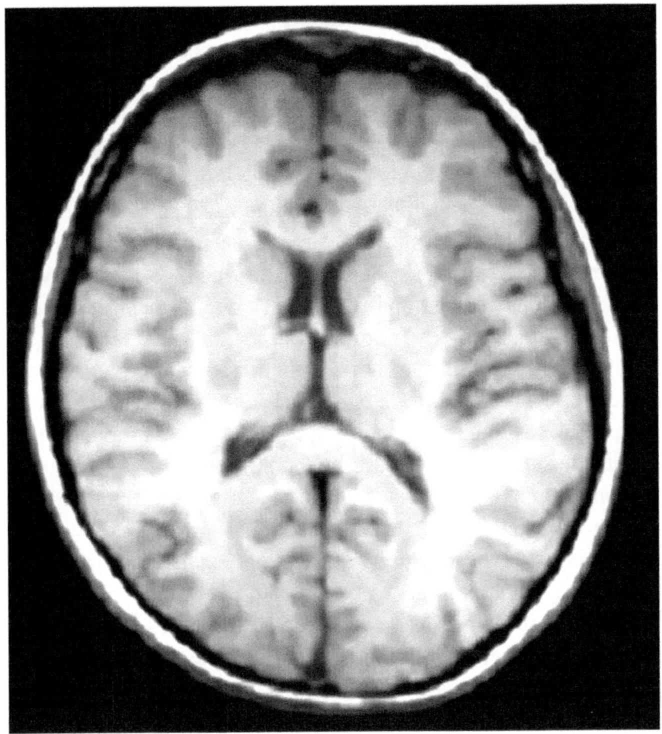

FIGURE 12.1 MRI brain tumor image.

Oncologists typically use diagnostic imaging procedures like MRI and CT scans to first assess brain malignancies. Changes in brain anatomy may be readily observed in the detailed pictures produced by these two modalities. However, a surgical sample from the suspicious tissue (tumor) is essential for a complete diagnosis by the expert if the doctor has reason to suspect a brain tumor and wants to know more about its nature. Over the past several years, many technologies have improved brain tissue imaging by increasing picture contrast and resolution, allowing the radiologist to detect even tiny lesions and so obtaining greater diagnostic accuracy. The accuracy of identifying brain tumors in the field of artificial intelligence (AI) for applications related to computer vision can be improved by fusing (combining) the images acquired from different imaging modalities and incorporating (integrating) AI with these imaging modalities to construct a computer-aided diagnosis (CAD) system. A higher rate of successful early cancer identification may be achieved with the use of such technologies, which can be of great assistance to doctors. These days, AI methods like artificial neural networks (ANNs), support vector machines (SVMs), and convolutional neural networks (CNNs) are being used to identify and categorize brain cancers.

Medical imaging patterns may now be recognized and categorized, thanks to recent developments in machine learning, especially deep learning. As a result of progress in this field, it may soon be possible to learn not from experts or scientific literature but rather by obtaining and extracting knowledge from data. Machine learning is quickly emerging as a useful tool for enhancing the efficiency of many medical applications across a wide range of domains, such as illness prognosis and diagnosis, molecular and cellular structure identification, tissue segmentation, and picture categorization. Since Convolutional Neural Networks (CNNs) contain many layers and a high diagnostic accuracy if the quantity of input pictures is high, they are currently the most effective approaches employed in image processing [5]. Autoencoders are a form of unsupervised learning that uses neural networks to learn representations. Surprisingly, some deep learning and machine learning algorithms have been utilized to detect cardiovascular stenosis and diagnose cancers (including lung tumors). In addition, their diagnostic accuracy is quite good, as evidenced by performance assessments. The identification of brain tumors using different approaches and models has been the subject of several investigations. Some of these research, nevertheless, have had a number of flaws, such as not comparing the suggested model's effectiveness to that of more conventional machine learning techniques. One study's model suggested was computationally intensive. Most relevant research has excluded healthy patients while developing classification models for three subtypes of brain cancers.

Deep learning is a type of machine learning that teaches computers to behave and think in the same ways that humans would. A computer model may do categorization tasks from pictures, sounds, or texts using deep learning. It's not uncommon for deep learning methods to outperform humans. Artificial neural networks, which consist of a network of simulated neurons, are among the most often used types of neural networks. Each neuron functions as a node, and the links between them form a network. A new method was developed in this research to detect and isolate tumors in the brain using 2D MRI scans. This technique uses a pre-trained GoogLeNet model with deep transfer learning to derive informative characteristics from MRI scans of the brain. Because of this, the model can accurately detect and categorize malignant brain tumors. A streamlined version of the U-Net architecture was used to carry out the segmentation. The U-Net framework has a stellar reputation for precision when segmenting surgical pictures. The model is able to precisely outline brain tumors in MRI scans by integrating the feature extraction skills of GoogLeNet with the U-Net architecture. In addition, a deep learning model and the Moth Flame optimization (MFO) method are used to classify the tumor segments. The retrieved characteristics are used by the deep learning model to categorize the tumors. However, MFO is used to fine-tune the classification model's settings and boost its overall efficacy. This method provides a comprehensive solution for successfully recognizing and categorizing brain tumors from MRI images by merging deep transfer learning, U-Net segmentation, and MFO-based classification. The findings of this research add to the growing body of work in computer-assisted medical picture analysis and show promise for enhancing brain tumor patients' access to accurate diagnoses and effective treatment plans.

12.2   RELATED WORKS

Tumor segmentation using MR images is a time-consuming and complex procedure performed by doctors. In this study, we present a totally automated and effective method for detecting and segmenting brain tumors, one that is based on picture registration and classification methodologies. We use two common methods for altering MRI images before feature extraction—intensity normalization and contourlet transform—as part of our feature extraction strategy. We replace the standard Laplacian pyramids with Pyramid transforms in our improved contourlet substitution in [6], substantially enhancing the effectiveness of the proposed technique. After applying a genetic algorithm to the acquired data, MRI scans of the brain are classified using a neuro-fuzzy inference technique based on attributes that may be utilized to locate tumors. The proposed procedure is put through a rigorous quantitative evaluation to extract useful measures such as specificity, segmentation accuracy, sensitivity, precision, and the dice similarity coefficient.

Tumors are collections of cancerous cells that can occur in any part of the body, including the brain and its surrounding tissues. Several variables may affect a person's susceptibility to developing a brain tumor. Among these include genetic defects, exposure to radiation, and heredity. When looking for cancer in the brain, an MRI scan is the gold standard. This approach, while labor-intensive, is fraught with error due to human error, especially in the first phases of tumor development. This emphasizes the need for a prompt and accurate identification of a brain tumor [7]. Increasing the speed and precision with which brain tumors are detected is intended to lower death rates, increase access to healthcare in low-resource areas, and inspire patients to lead better lifestyles. Using a dataset of 251 photos, the authors of this publication train a convolutional neural network model to detect brain cancers. When a dataset lacks sufficient source information, data augmentation can be used to fill in the gaps. The suggested CNN model's predictions were evaluated with respect to their accuracy, F1-score, precision, and recall. The model achieves an average accuracy of 85%. Thus, it has been demonstrated that, with no additional effort or cost, deep learning CNN models may accurately detect brain tumors.

A brain tumor develops because brain cells multiply inappropriately. A fatal illness that radiologists have trouble identifying. Unfortunately, most malignancies are incorrectly identified because of the wide variety and complexity of lesions, reducing patients' chances of survival. It is challenging to use computer vision algorithms for the diagnosis of brain cancer. Traditional segmentation or feature extraction is now used to diagnose brain tumors; however, it is a laborious process prone to human mistakes. In [8], the author explores the possibility of employing Deep Learning (DL) as well as Machine Learning (ML) for multiclass classification of brain tumors. End-to-end image categorization of brain MRI images is initially performed using Convolutional Neural Network (CNN) algorithms that include ResNet-18 and GoogLeNet. The deep features gleaned from the CNN models are also applied to categorization using Support Vector Machine (SVM). The proposed method, which relies on a CNN-SVM-based methodology, achieved 98% accuracy on a dataset consisting of 15,320 MRI scans utilized for both training and assessment. Our proposed technique is superior to existing methods of brain tumor detection and can benefit doctors in both the identification and management of these diseases.

The prognosis of a patient with a brain tumor might be greatly improved by a timely diagnosis. Currently, MR imaging is the most advanced imaging method for diagnosing brain tumors. Brain tumors can be difficult to diagnose, but there has been a lot of effort invested into developing computer-aided diagnostic models, both manually and via deep learning. However, identifying BT is complicated by the fact that MR images display a wide range of contrast and distortion. Each of the various pretrained networks (InceptionNet, VGG19, VGG16, Xception, ResNet101, ResNet152V2, and DenseNet121) is used to create the ExRAN model. In contrast to the single network's weak generalization and convergence, the stacked single networks employed by ensemble methods yield more resilient and generalizable features. The deep discriminative feature is selected from a pool of various pre-trained deep learning models using an ensemble ExRAN model, as described by researchers [9, 10]. The purpose of this research is to verify the accuracy of the proposed ExRAN model using a publicly available MR imaging dataset.

The dawn of the era of big data in medicine is upon us, thanks to the lightning-fast development of medical technology. This data mining and analysis will have immediate and far-reaching consequences for the prediction, monitoring, diagnosis, and treatment of tumor-related disorders. Most people agree that brain tumors are the deadliest and most disabling disease there is because of their unique combination of characteristics, poor prognosis, and aggressive behavior. It has been suggested that the challenges of identifying and treating brain cancer can be overcome with the help of deep learning. The goal of this study is to address the issue of centralized data collection through the application of FL to the problem of identifying brain tumors in MRI scans. The goal of this research was to create a CNN model structure for the problem of recognizing brain tumors utilizing the Visual Geometry Group (VGG 16), as well as discover the factors to train the technique. Our approach might be used to examine the MR images for signs of brain cancer. The results of the tests demonstrated that the algorithm was superior to the currently utilized approaches for detecting brain cancers.

12.3 METHODOLOGY

12.3.1 Image Preprocessing

The clarity of the pictures, the removal of noise, and the highlighting of vital characteristics for correct diagnosis and segmentation all benefit greatly from proper image preprocessing, which is an essential part of brain tumor image analysis. Preprocessing seeks to normalize data, enhance visual contrast, and remove artifacts so that analysis may be performed with confidence. To guarantee uniformity throughout the collection, the brain tumor photos should be resized to a consistent resolution. Cropping can be used to zero in on the target area (the brain) and eliminate distractions. Fix image illumination issues such as uneven intensity distribution. This is crucial for enhancing the efficiency of image analysis algorithms by eliminating brightness and contrast differences throughout the image. Images of brain tumors would benefit from increased contrast so that anomalies and critical structures might be better seen. For this, you can utilize histogram equalization or adaptive histogram equalization. Accurate and trustworthy evaluation of brain tumor pictures requires careful preparation. The specifics of the dataset and the needs of the analytic algorithms mean that the selection and sequence of preprocessing processes might vary. Brain

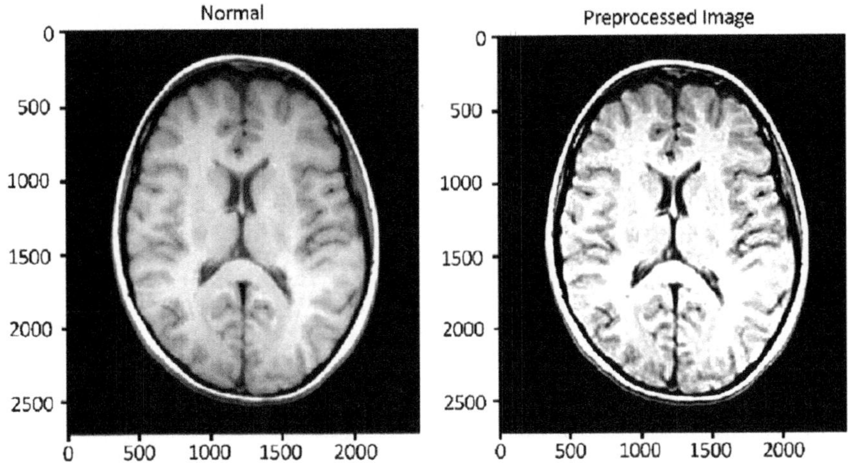

FIGURE 12.2 Normal and preprocessed image.

tumor image analysis also requires domain experience and an understanding of medical imaging to guide the selection and execution of preprocessing approaches. In Figure 12.2, we see the original, unedited picture.

12.3.2 IMAGE AUGMENTATION

The original brain tumor pictures are transformed using a data augmentation approach called image augmentation, which is intended to improve the variety and quantity of the training dataset. To better analyze and classify brain tumor images, researchers are turning to machine learning models, namely Deep Neural Networks (DNNs). Data diversification helps the model adapt to new circumstances and prevents it from being overfit. It is essential to make sure that the enhanced pictures retain their semantic significance and accuracy while using image augmentation. When using an augmentation technique, care must be taken to prevent the introduction of artificial artifacts or distortions that might confuse the model during training. Built-in image augmentation functions are available in many deep learning frameworks and libraries like TensorFlow and PyTorch, making it simple to include these methods in the training pipeline. The model is strengthened by expanding the training dataset so that it can analyze and diagnose brain tumor pictures from a wider variety of patients and under a wider range of imaging settings. Figure 12.3 displays both the original and enhanced versions of the photograph.

12.3.3 IMAGE SEGMENTATION—UNET

When it comes to medical image analysis, the U-Net architecture is frequently employed as a CNN for semantic segmentation tasks. Its encoder and decoder form a distinctive U shape, thus the term "U-Net architecture." It's meant to help with

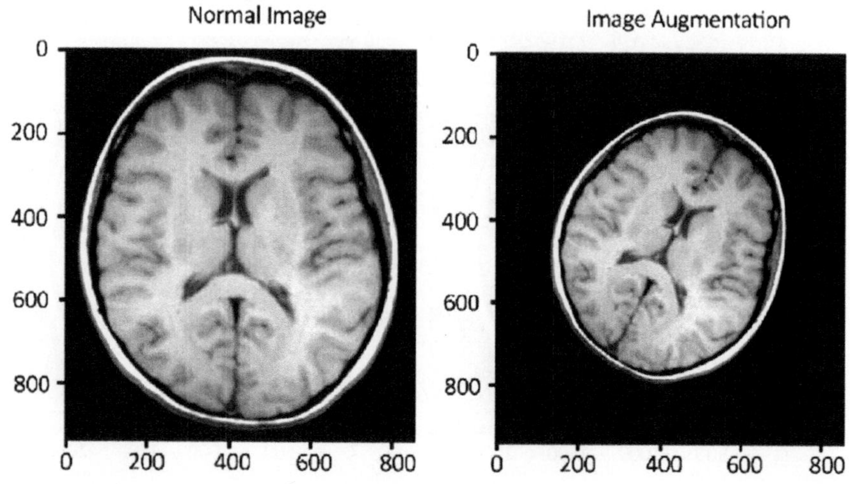

FIGURE 12.3 Normal and augmented image.

downsampling (pooling) pictures, which can cause CNNs to lose spatial information and make it difficult to properly segment objects or structures of interest. The overall structure of the suggested model is depicted in Figure 12.4.

Encoders are used to record simplified, abstract models of input images. Non-linearity is often introduced into the model by placing an activation function (such as ReLU) after each convolutional layer. The bottleneck is the hub of the U-Net and connects the encoder and decoder. The number of filters in its convolutional layers is usually rather low. The bottleneck does not employ pooling or striding processes to preserve spatial information, in contrast to the encoder and decoder. This design decision aids in maintaining the granularity of space.

The decoder is a reflection of the encoder, with upsampling (transposed convolution) layers placed before the convolutional layers. The decoder's job is to restore the spatial resolution that was sacrificed during the encoder's downsampling processes. The feature maps' spatial resolution is improved while the number of channels is decreased by using upsampling layers, which are also known as deconvolution or transposed convolution layers. To prevent checkerboard effects and further enhance the feature maps, a convolutional layer with a small kernel size is often used after each upsampling layer.

Detailing the segmentation results using spatial information obtained from the encoder's concatenated feature maps. U-Net is efficient at object segmentation while preserving spatial accuracy, thanks to the skip links' ability to communicate both local and global contextual information. Following the U-Net's 1 × 1 convolutional output layer is an activation function that adjusts itself to the specific segmentation job at hand. It is common practice to utilize a softmax activation function to derive pixel-wise class probabilities for multi-class segmentation applications like semantic segmentation with multiple classes. To create pixel-wise binary masks for tumor versus non-tumor segmentation, a sigmoid activation function is commonly utilized.

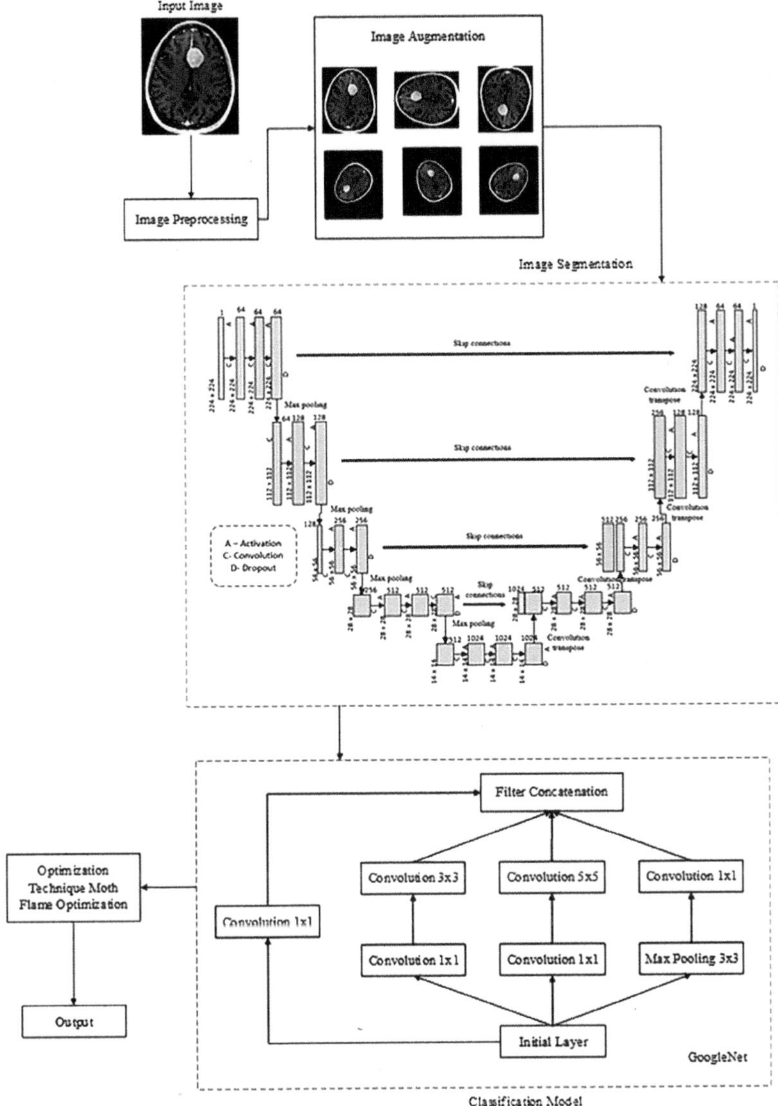

FIGURE 12.4 Architecture of proposed model.

When it comes to semantic segmentation tasks, where it's necessary to precisely delineate items of interest in an image, the U-Net architecture is built to handle the difficulties. Because of the skip links, the model can take advantage of both local and global knowledge to produce very accurate and comprehensive segmentation results. Accurate segmentation is crucial for diagnosis and treatment planning, and the U-Net has become a popular choice for numerous medical picture segmentation applications due to its efficacy and speed.

12.3.4 GoogLeNet

GoogLeNet, or Inception v1, is a deep CNN structure first described in a 2014 article titled "Going Deeper with Convolutions" by Google researchers. Problems in training extremely deep networks while keeping computational efficiency in check inspired the creation of GoogLeNet. Its groundbreaking "Inception" module captures data at several scales by simultaneously employing filters of varying sizes. While this design is effective for general image categorization tasks, it may not be the best fit for brain tumor classification due to the unique problems posed by medical pictures. Nevertheless, a specific architecture for categorized brain tumors may be designed using the ideas of GoogLeNet and its inception modules.

There were problems with disappearing gradients and computing needs as deep neural networks became deeper before GoogLeNet was developed. GoogLeNet intended to improve its general effectiveness by fixing these problems and designing a more robust architecture. The Inception component is the backbone of GoogLeNet. For multi-scale data collection, it employs parallel convolutional filters of varying sizes (1×1, 3×3, and 5×5). The depth dimension is used to chain these parallel filters together, giving the network the ability to learn several abstraction layers. There is also a max-pooling layer for gathering data at the 1×1 level. This component encourages feature extraction that works well across several scales.

GoogLeNet incorporates reduction blocks after various Inception modules to manage the processing needs of a deep architecture. These reduction blocks minimize the number of feature channels and the spatial dimensions by using a mix of 3×3 and 1×1 convolutions and max pooling. This aids in lowering the computational burden and keeping a healthy equilibrium between efficiency and thoroughness. During training, GoogLeNet adds supplementary classifiers to the network at intermediate levels. These classifiers use 1×1 convolutions, then pool across global averages, and finally finish with fully linked layers. These supplementary classifiers are used to combat the vanishing gradient problem, especially in deeper layers, by supplying additional gradients during training. To compress feature maps into a uniform representation, GoogLeNet uses global average pooling in its deepest layers. Next, a softmax activation is used for classification, followed by fully linked layers. In its original incarnation, GoogLeNet competed successfully in the ImageNet Large Scale Visual Recognition Challenge. GoogLeNet proved that computationally friendly, high-performance architectures are possible. Its Inception module paved the way for future developments in deep learning architectures due to its ability to record multi-scale information simultaneously.

We begin by capturing low-level information from the input brain tumor photos using a series of convolutional and pooling layers. Edges, textures, and even high-level forms may be identified with the aid of these additional layers. Create parallel convolutional filters of varying sizes to collect multi-scale data, like in the inception algorithm. Brain tumor-related traits should be a primary focus in the development of these modules. Computational complexity can be better handled using these building elements. Convert feature maps to a fixed-size representation as the final step in your design using global average pooling. The next step is to classify tumors and normal cells using completely linked layers and a softmax activation. To avoid overfitting and boost generalization in your models, use regularization strategies like dropout and batch normalization. To train your model, pick an optimizer and a loss function (such as categorical cross-entropy). Make sure the loss function works for your categorization problem.

12.4 MOTH FLAME OPTIMIZATION

An algorithm called Moth Flame Optimization (MFO) was developed with inspiration from the natural behavior of moths and flames. The phenomena of moths flying into lit candles served as the inspiration for MFO. The technique may be used to solve optimization issues by mimicking the flight patterns of moths as they seek out fires. Modeling the behavior of moths and their interactions with flames, MFO seeks optimal solutions by repeatedly changing a population of viable solutions. A summary of the algorithmic workings behind Moth Flame Optimization is as follows:

1. Initialization

A pool of candidates (moths) for the problem is produced at random. Each moth stands for a potential answer to the optimization issue.

2. Flame Creation

Multiple synthetic fires are ignited in the search volume. These sparks stand for promising approaches to the issue at hand. The fitness rating of each fire determines how powerful it will be.

3. Moth Movement

There are three natural moth behaviors that inform how each moth moves during each iteration: Moths flock to lights (best practices). Moths orient themselves toward the light source. Moths look for food by making seemingly random movements. When on the move, moths strike a balance between probing and exploiting. Some of the moths fly closer to the flames, while others fly away to discover new territory.

4. Flame Intensity Update

Depending on the moths' fitness ratings, the fire's ferocity (the optimal solution) is adjusted. Stronger flames with higher fitness scores are more likely to attract moths.

5. Iteration

The stages of updating the moth's position and the flame's intensity keep happening until a halting requirement is fulfilled.

6. Solution Extraction

At the conclusion of the optimization procedure, the optimal moth is chosen from the population.

Using a population-based approach, MFO seeks optimum or near-optimal solutions to optimization issues by balancing exploration and exploitation. The engineering, economic, and scientific communities have all benefited from its application to their own unique challenges. MFO is a metaheuristic algorithm that, like many others, does not provide a global optimum but does give a means of avoiding being stuck in a rut and successfully probing the search space.

12.5 RESULTS

The recommended system was built with the help of the scikit-learn machine learning technology in Python. Data scientists rely heavily on scikit-learn because it provides a full suite of resources for all their machine learning needs. The system includes not only scikit-learn but also additional well-known libraries like pandas, NumPy, matplotlib, and seaborn. These libraries provide further features for doing numerical calculations, visualizing data, and manipulating data. The system explores the potential of a pre-trained GoogLeNet in tandem with UNET Segmentation to improve the classifier's efficiency. GoogLeNet are well-suited to jobs like picture categorization because of its sophisticated feature extraction capabilities. The classifier's major responsibility in this setup is to recognize typical ROIs. The system's goal is precise regional classification and the ability to reliably identify normal and abnormal photos by utilizing the strengths of the GoogLeNet model.

To prevent overfitting, the GoogLeNet Model's two convolution layers employ a dropout normalization of 25%. Kernels of either 32 bits or 64 bits are used in these convolution layers. A thick layer is added after the image has been flattened. In contrast to the TanH activation used in the remainder of the network, the output layer instead uses the sigmoid activation function. The effectiveness of various models is compared by evaluating Linear Regression (LR), K-Nearest Neighbor (KNN), ANN, and CNN against one another and state-of-the-art models. The suggested model outperforms a baseline conventional artificial neural network by 4% in terms of accuracy. The goal of this approach is to improve model generalization by reducing the effects of overfitting, and it achieves comparable accuracy outcomes in relation to other models. Table 12.1 and Figure 12.5 compare the performance of several models in terms of accuracy.

The provided framework was built effectively using 64 batches across 10 epochs. This model has a training loss of 0.31 and a validation accuracy of 0.96. Accuracy of 0.85 is reached by LR (Linear Regression). As a simple prediction method, LR relies on linear associations between variables. The accuracy of KNN is 0.90. KNN is a clustering algorithm that uses the majority class labels of a data point's k closest

TABLE 12.1

Comparison of Models' Reliability

Model	Accuracy
LR	0.85
KNN	0.90
ANN	0.93
CNN	0.94
Proposed Model	0.98

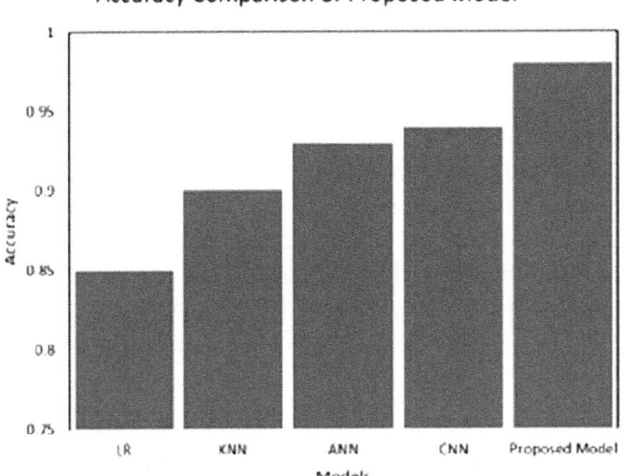

FIGURE 12.5 Accuracy evaluation of various models.

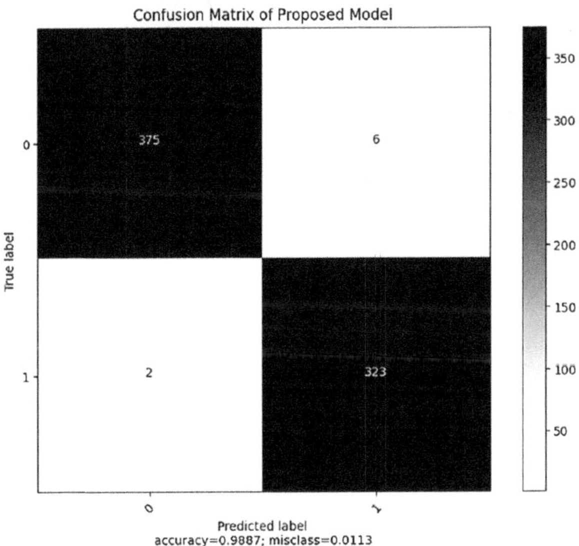

FIGURE 12.6 Confusion matrix of various models.

neighbors to determine what class that data point belongs to. ANN achieves a 0.93 accuracy rate. In terms of precision, CNN achieves 0.94. By capturing spatial hierarchy with its convolutional and pooling layers, CNN performs exceptionally well in image identification tasks. The proposed model excels with a remarkable precision of 0.98. Among these models, the suggested model obtains the maximum accuracy with the help of the potentially cutting-edge methodologies we outlined before. Model misunderstanding is depicted in Figure 12.6.

In classification, precision is a crucial parameter since it assesses how well a model does at making correct positive predictions. It determines how many instances were correctly predicted as positive as a percentage of all forecasts. Accuracy, in mathematical terms, may be written as:

If the model has a high accuracy score, then its positive predictions are likely to be accurate and have a small number of false positives. Whenever the model predicts a favorable outcome, it is usually accurate. If the model's optimistic predictions have a low accuracy score, it's likely that such forecasts are erroneous. The model may be too optimistic in its predictions, which increases the likelihood of false positives. The accuracy of several models is compared in Table 12.2 and Figure 12.7.

The sensitivity of a model may be evaluated by the number of true positives that it successfully predicts. It determines how many times a forecast was correct relative to the overall number of correct predictions. Sensitivity may be written as a mathematical expression:

$$Precision = \frac{True\ Positives}{True\ Positives + False\ Positives}$$

TABLE 12.2

Precision Evaluation of Various Models

Model	Precision
LR	0.86
KNN	0.89
ANN	0.92
CNN	0.94
Proposed Model	0.97

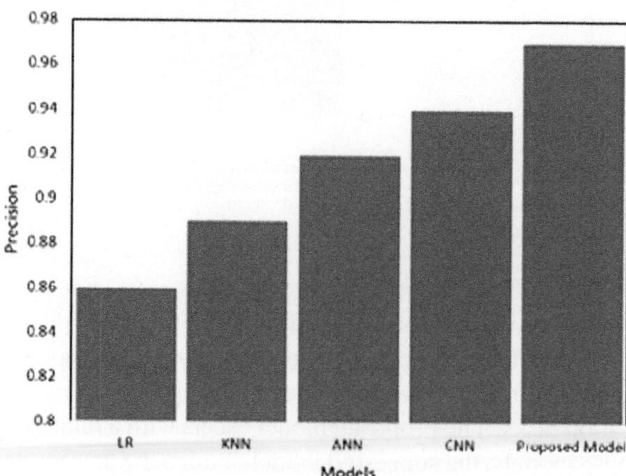

FIGURE 12.7 Precision model evaluations.

Sensitivity measures how well the model can detect positive situations while reducing the possibility of false negatives. Sensitivity is essential in medical diagnosis because it prevents false-positive results from being ignored. Specificity quantifies how well a model is at excluding false positives. Table 12.3 and Figures 12.8 and 12.9 compare the various models' sensitivities and specificities, respectively. The mathematical definition of specificity is:

The suggested model has a training accuracy of 98.50% and a validation accuracy of 98.10%. With a peak accuracy during training of 92.13%, CNN was able to reach a validation accuracy of 91.32%. ANN was able to attain a 90% validation accuracy and a 91.04% training accuracy. Figure 12.10 depicts the training as well as validation reliability of the suggested model, though Figure 12.11 shows the training as well as validation loss. With the Adam optimizer, we set the epochs to 200 and the batch size to 32 when putting the models into action. The suggested model outperformed the others in the accuracy graph analysis since its validation accuracy had a

TABLE 12.3
Sensitivity and Specificity Evaluation of Various Models

Model	Sensitivity	Specificity
LR	0.84	0.87
KNN	0.88	0.89
ANN	0.91	0.92
CNN	0.93	0.95
Proposed Model	0.98	0.97

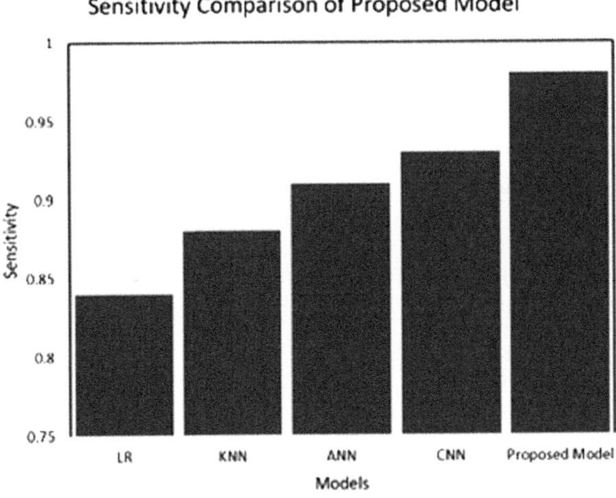

FIGURE 12.8 Model evaluation for sensitivity.

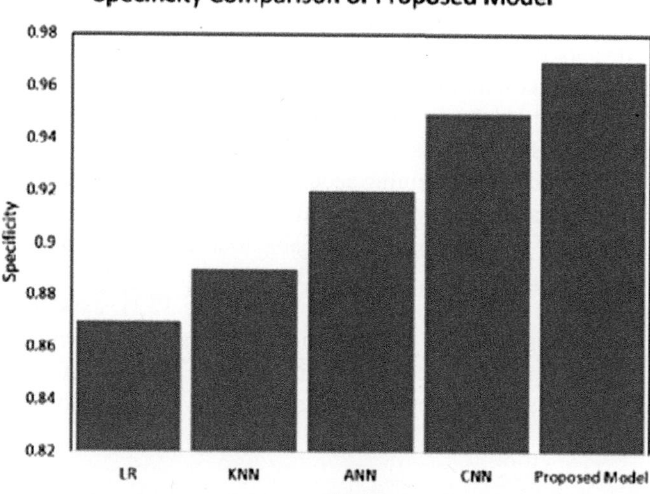

FIGURE 12.9 Comparison of model specificity

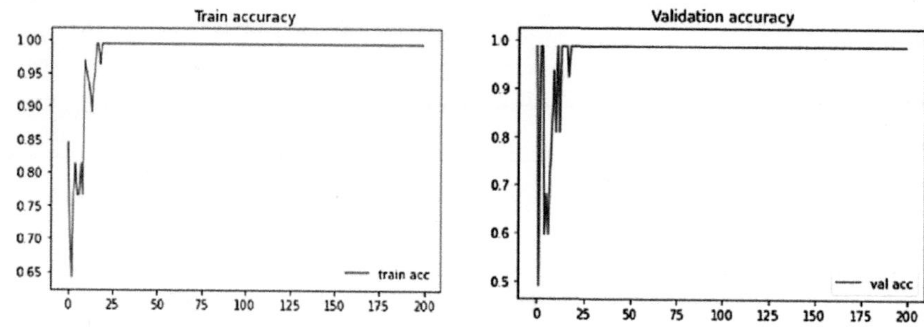

FIGURE 12.10 Validation and training suggested model's accuracy.

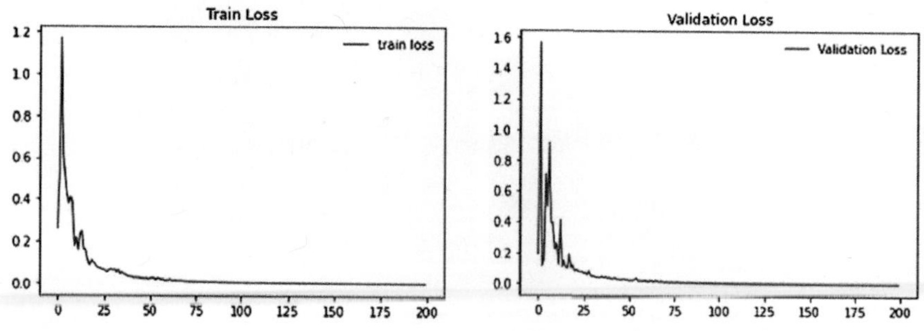

FIGURE 12.11 Methods of instruction and verification loss of the suggested model.

strong output curve relative to its training accuracy, and there were no instances of over-fitting or under-fitting.

12.6 CONCLUSION AND FUTURE SCOPE

Preventing a worldwide increase in death rates due to brain tumors requires its diagnosis at an early stage. Correct identification of brain cancers remains extremely difficult because of the tumor's shape, size, and structure. For the first time, we provide a unique method for the segmentation of brain tumors using 2D MRIs of the brain that makes use of deep transfer learning. The approach employs a GoogLeNet that has already been trained to extract characteristics from MRI scans of the brain. A streamlined version of the U-Net Architecture was used for the segmentation of brain tumors. A deep learning model and the Moth Flame Optimization (MFO) method are combined for the classification process. The earlier method is superior to other methods now in use due to its superior mean categorization accuracy of 98%, sensitivity of 96.58%, and specificity of 97.83%. The results of the study prove that the proposed technique is far superior to the alternatives. The success may be traced back to the use of carefully crafted training functions, accurate feature extraction, and painstakingly optimized preprocessing methods. All of these critical elements come together to give the proposed method its remarkable performance. A disadvantage of our study was that the training method was time-consuming because the CNN had several layers and the computer lacked a powerful GPU. It will take more time to train if the dataset is huge, such as having a thousand photos. We were able to shorten the training period by optimizing our GPU hardware. Using individual patient data acquired from any source, more research may be done to improve the proper identification of brain tumors.

REFERENCES

[1] L. J. Ahmed, P. M. Bruntha, S. Dhanasekar, V. Chitra, D. Balaji and N. Senathipathi, "An Improvised Image Registration Technique for Brain Tumor Identification and Segmentation Using ANN Approach," 2022 6th International Conference on Devices, Circuits and Systems (ICDCS), Coimbatore, India, 2022, pp. 80–84, doi: 10.1109/ICDCS54290.2022.9780846.

[2] A. Chakraborty and D. Vetrithangam, "ExRAN: Deep Ensemble Majority Voting using Transfer Learning for Brain tumor Identification from Magnetic Resonance Imaging," 2023 International Conference on Inventive Computation Technologies (ICICT), Lalitpur, Nepal, 2023, pp. 130–134, doi: 10.1109/ICICT57646.2023.10134332.

[3] H. Kibriya, M. Masood, M. Nawaz, R. Rafique and S. Rehman, "Multiclass Brain Tumor Classification Using Convolutional Neural Network and Support Vector Machine," 2021 Mohammad Ali Jinnah University International Conference on Computing (MAJICC), Karachi, Pakistan, 2021, pp. 1–4, doi: 10.1109/MAJICC53071.2021.9526262.

[4] J. K. Periasamy, B. S and J. P, "Comparison of VGG-19 and RESNET-50 Algorithms in Brain Tumor Detection," 2023 IEEE 8th International Conference for Convergence in Technology (I2CT), Lonavla, India, 2023, pp. 1–5, doi: 10.1109/I2CT57861.2023.10126451.

[5] K. S. Rani, K. M. Kumari, T. Nireekshna, D. V. Shobana, N. Kavitha and B. B. Sri, "Identification of Brain Tumors using Volume rendering Techniques," 2021 International

Conference on Artificial Intelligence and Smart Systems (ICAIS), Coimbatore, India, 2021, pp. 1080–1087, doi: 10.1109/ICAIS50930.2021.9395828.

[6] B. Saju, L. Thomas, F. Varghese, A. Prasad and N. Tressa, "Deep Learning-Based Brain Tumor Classification Prototype Using Transfer Learning," 2023 International Conference on Advances in Intelligent Computing and Applications (AICAPS), Kochi, India, 2023, pp. 1–7, doi: 10.1109/AICAPS57044.2023.10074201.

[7] R. Sankaranarayaanan, M. S. Kumar, B. Chidhambararajan and P. Sirenjeevi, "Brain tumor detection and Classification using VGG 16," 2023 International Conference on Artificial Intelligence and Knowledge Discovery in Concurrent Engineering (ICE-CONF), Chennai, India, 2023, pp. 1–5, doi: 10.1109/ICECONF57129.2023.10083866.

[8] A. Sarkar, M. Maniruzzaman, M. S. Ahsan, M. Ahmad, M. I. Kadir and S. M. Taohidul Islam, "Identification and Classification of Brain Tumor from MRI with Feature Extraction by Support Vector Machine," 2020 International Conference for Emerging Technology (INCET), Belgaum, India, 2020, pp. 1–4, doi: 10.1109/INCET49848.2020.9154157.

[9] R. Singh, N. Sharma and R. Gupta, "Proposed CNN Model for Classification of Brain Tumor Disease," 2023 International Conference on Distributed Computing and Electrical Circuits and Electronics (ICDCECE), Ballar, India, 2023, pp. 1–5, doi: 10.1109/ICDCECE57866.2023.10151070.

[10] R. Setyawan, R. B. Asrori, G. Fajar Shidik, A. Z. Fanani and R. Anggi Premunendar, "Brain Tumor Identification using FCM Threshold Method and Morphological Area Selection," 2020 International Seminar on Application for Technology of Information and Communication (iSemantic), Semarang, Indonesia, 2020, pp. 560–566, doi: 10.1109/iSemantic50169.2020.9234223.

13 Study of Biomedical Segmentation Based on Recent Techniques and Deep Learning

Jogendra Haobam and Palungbam Roji Chanu

13.1 INTRODUCTION

With the introduction of electronic mediums, particularly computers, society has become increasingly reliant on computers for information processing, storage, and transmission. Computers play an essential role in all aspects of life and society in modern civilization. As men grow more involved with computers, a new era has dawned in which humanity has entered a new world known as the technological world. Nowadays, computer plays a vital role in the medical field. From open-heart surgeries to X-rays to other clinical diagnostics, everything is now computerized. Diagnostics imaging is an individual tool in medicine. MRI (Magnetic Resonance Imaging), CT (Computed Tomography), and digital mammography, and other imaging modularity are effective means for non-invasively mapping the anatomy of the human body [1]. With the help of medical imaging, the doctor can diagnose a patient's condition accurately and quickly based on the reports provided by the patient and other relevant information [2]. Image segmentation is regarded as one of the most important and primary tasks to be performed in computer vision. Image segmentation is the process of dividing an image into many nonoverlapping, connected sections that are homogeneous and share some common attributes, such as tone, color, brightness, texture, and boundary continuity [3]. Imaging has advanced significantly as device computing power has increased, storage and transmission devices have become more readily available, and the cost of storage and transmission devices has decreased. For image segmentation, there are various techniques and methodologies such as threshold-based, graph-based, morphological-based, edged-based, clustering-based, neural network-based, and so on [4–6]. All these methods have their own set of benefits and drawbacks; thus, one must choose the algorithm depending on their requirements.

DOI: 10.1201/9781032635149-13

13.2 OVERVIEW OF TECHNIQUES USED IN BIOMEDICAL SEGMENTATIONS

13.2.1 SEGMENTATION TECHNIQUES

Various popular, essential, and commonly utilized segmentation techniques are recognized by scientists and researchers, which are listed as follows:

1. Thresholding-based segmentation
   a. Local thresholding
   b. Otsu's method
   c. Gaussian mixture method
2. Region-based segmentation
   a. Region growing
   b. Region merging and splitting
3. Edge-based/Boundary-based segmentation
   a. Prewitt edge detection
   b. Laplacian of Gaussian
   c. Watershed
4. Clustering method
   a. K-means algorithm
   b. Fuzzy c-means algorithm
   c. Expectation maximization algorithm
5. Model-based algorithms
   a. Markov Random field
   b. Atlas-based approach
   c. Artificial neural networks

13.3 THRESHOLDING-BASED SEGMENTATION

Thresholding is regarded as one of the simplest, most widely used, and fastest segmentation techniques. Here the image is divided into regions based on intensity values or properties of the value. It attempts to distinguish between the image's backdrop and foreground. In this thresholding-based segmentation, an assumption is made such that an image is composed of multiple gray level regions. Even though it is very simple and fast, it ignores an image's spatial characteristics. As a result, the thresholding method is susceptible to noise and intensity inhomogeneity and leads to a shading effect shown in Figure 13.1 [7].

The Thresholding technique is determined by the characteristics of the image [8]. The thresholding technique converts the multilevel image into a binary image to select an appropriate threshold "T" and to separate objects from the backdrop or background by dividing the image pixel into various areas or regions. This threshold "T" can be defined as a minimum between the two peaks in a bimodal histogram. Let us consider any pixel F (x, y). When F (x, y) $\geq$ T, that is, the intensity of the pixel is greater than or equal to the threshold then the image is in the foreground (F) otherwise it is in the background (B) [9–10].

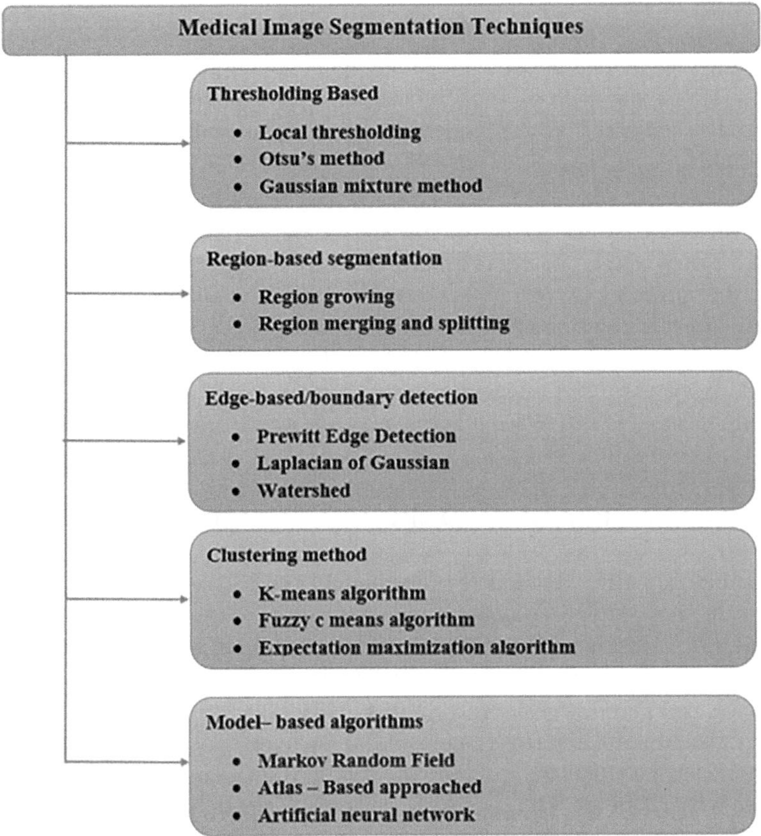

FIGURE 13.1 Medical image segmentation techniques.

a) Local thresholding

Images that do not have a consistent backdrop or have variability in between the objects cannot be efficiently segmented using global thresholding, and the results will be unsatisfactory. When there are a variety of backgrounds or objects in an image, local thresholding is a good option [11]. For the local thresholding technique, each pixel has its threshold. This threshold is computed based on local statistics namely mean, range, and a combination of mean and standard deviation variance Local thresholding is a useful approach for images with a diverse range of backgrounds and objects [12]. They help us determine distinct threshold levels of images partitioned into several sub-images or areas. Sub-images are combined when each threshold value is calculated. Local thresholding is time-consuming so a hybrid approach that uses both the local thresholding and global thresholding methods was used, as well as morphological operators.

b) Otsu's method

Nobuyuki Otsu created this method, and that's one of the numerous binarization algorithms. This approach works by calculating an optimal threshold value for image segmentation. Otsu mainly determines the image pixel values and chooses the best spot in which the two sets of classes can be separated into two by minimizing the difference between the histograms. Typically, this approach yields adequate results in bimodal images. Considering the image as bimodal reduces the intra-class variance of the image [13]. The intra-class variance is calculated by adding the weighted total of the variances of each cluster. Each class's probability is represented by the weights. After the intra-class variance is determined the mean value for each class is calculated. And then the individual class variance is determined. The optimal threshold is the value that maximizes between-class variation [14]. The selection of the ideal threshold value, on the other hand, significantly increases completion time as the degrees of thresholds raise.

c) Gaussian mixture (GM) approach

An initialization-free method developed in 2012 by Nicole and Alexander enables the estimation of component amounts, means, and covariances sequentially [15–16]. The posterior probability, as well as maximum likelihood, is determined, given the number of features or components in an image, as well as their respective mean, covariance, and mixing coefficients, in this image segmentation approach. Starting with a single mixture component and splitting incrementally throughout the expectation maximizing steps, the method begins with a single mixture component covering the whole data set. An effective GM approach can only be demonstrated after numerous tests [17].

13.4   REGION-BASED SEGMENTATION

The term "region" refers to a group of connected pixels that have similar characteristics. It is possible to compare pixels based on their brightness, color, and other characteristics. In this sort of segmentation, pixels must conform to certain established rules to be grouped into related pixel regions. This segmentation approach is being used to precisely locate regions or areas of the image. It is incredibly convenient and divides image regions or areas based on similarity [18], but they are immune to noises [8, 19].

a) Region growing

This segmentation technique is used for extracting a particular location from an already existing image based on certain criteria, such as edges of an image or intensity level inhomogeneity [20]. Start with a certain pixel called the seed pixel [21] and then examine the nearby pixels. If the nearby pixel follows the predetermined rules, then the pixel is added to the seed pixel and continuous until no similarity is left and they are selected to grow the region [22]. Since region growth can be susceptible to noise, continuous gaps may occasionally occur in extracted regions [23]. There may also be a unification of several separate regions because of it. This segmentation technique follows the bottom-up approach.

b) Region splitting and merging

Based on some criteria, an image can be separated into unconnected parts and then merged again [8, 28]. That is, it comprises two steps: splitting as well as merging. This method is quick and efficient, producing little or no noise, and is completely noise-free [24]. Four-branch quad trees form the basis of this strategy. Quad-branches are used to represent sub-images [25]. This is accomplished by splitting the image region into four branches. These branches are then blended back together until no further splitting is possible.

13.5   EDGE-BASED/BOUNDARY DETECTION

This segmentation approach is concerned with finding and locating image boundaries, such as edges. These edges are the image intensity levels. This approach is useful for detecting, revealing, and segmenting image artifacts [26]. Edge detectors are filters or masks that are overlaid on an image to identify boundaries or discontinuities [27]. It is vital for medical imaging to identify human organs as objects using edge detection.

a) Prewitt Edge Detection

It was claimed in 1970 by Prewitt and J. M. that using the Prewitt edge detector, one can determine the size and orientation of edges [29]. In the case of edge detection using a differential gradient, orientation is determined from the magnitudes in the x and y direction, which is time-consuming while in edge detection using compass, orientation is determined directly from the kernel with the highest response. It turns out that even though the Prewitt operator only can handle eight different orientations [30], most direct orientation estimates aren't very accurate.

b) Laplacian of Gaussian

Developed in 1980 by Marr and Hildreth, this filter is also called the Marr-Hildreth operator. It turns out that even though the Prewitt operator only can handle eight different orientations, most direct orientation estimates aren't very accurate. Machine vision seldom uses this approach. Berzins in 1984; Shah, Sood, and Jain in 1986; and Huertas and Medioni in 1986 were researchers who continued this methodology [31–32]. This algorithm uses an adaptive and differential operator that is adjustable to suit different applications [33]. This technique is mostly used for detecting jagged edges and finely focused details in images.

c) Watershed

As a result of S. Beucher and F. Meyer's work in 1990, they introduced a segmentation technique called Watershed. It enables overlapping items to be distinguished.

When analyzing natural images, too much segmentation occurs. This method was developed to address this issue. Using mathematical morphology, this technique segments images by distinguishing overlapping objects [34]. This method utilizes both the watershed transform and homotropy modification. This approach is used when dealing with gray-level images. As well as being quick, straightforward, and easy to use, it contributes to the global segmentation of an image [35]. According to this theory, low-intensity pixels are perceived as valleys, whereas high-intensity pixels are perceived as hills [36]. There are several problems with regular watershed algorithms, but power watershed algorithms fix them, resulting in the best results possible [37]. A marker-controlled watershed algorithm and a distinctive feature combination were used to extract tumors from brain MR images [38].

13.6 CLUSTERING METHODS

In clustering methods, objects are grouped into established classes. Clusters occur when objects have similar properties, and these objects must be identical to one cluster but different from the others to achieve effective clustering [39]. They are mainly used when classes are predefined or known. Aiming to maximize intraclass similarity and minimize interclass similarity is the objective [40]. This method falls under unsupervised learning and training the data is not required and doesn't rely upon predefined classes and utilizes unsupervised learning to categorize training data. This is done by increasing iterations [41]. Various algorithms and techniques were proposed by the researchers, but the most widely used are k means, fuzzy c means, expectation-maximization algorithm, etc.

a) K-means algorithm

K-means algorithm is an unsupervised learning algorithm, and this type is among the simplest and most popular algorithms. Iteratively, it places the "n" datasets in clusters based on k clusters. Using k-means clustering, a data set is categorized into k-number groups [42–43]. This was first proposed by Kaus et al. in 2004 [44]. The mean intensity is calculated for each cluster, and then the pixels are classified accordingly with the closest mean values. To reduce the number of clusters and the variability of clusters this approach is used [45]. This algorithm is also called an iso-data algorithm.

b) Fuzzy C-Means algorithm

Fuzzy c-means algorithm is also an unsupervised learning algorithm and it is nothing but a generalized k-means algorithm; the only difference between K-means and Fuzzy c-means is that in fuzzy c-means data are classified based on the degree of membership. Using the fuzzy c-means algorithm, a given collection of data can be divided into similar groups that are different from each other [46–47]. Developed in 1981 by Bezdek, this approach aids in soft segmentation and is based on Zadeh's fuzzy set theory. Due to its ease of use and capacity to extract more relevant information from the data, it is becoming more and more popular in medical image segmentation.

By considering, fuzziness vagueness, and ambiguity [48], the data classification process may sometimes be enhanced by the introduction of a higher-order fuzzy set to address hesitations and uncertainty. Statistical analysis of multivariate data based on fuzzy clusters is essential for unsupervised pattern recognition, which is regarded as one of the most important subfields of statistics [49–50]. A growing number of fields have benefited from the application of fuzzy cluster analysis in recent years, such as pattern recognition, data mining, computer vision, and fuzzy control [51]. By using fuzzy c-means segmentation based on hidden Markov models, decent segmentation is produced with smooth segmentation boundaries, minimal image noise, and strong robustness [52].

c) Expectation maximization algorithm

The expectation-maximization algorithm is an image segmentation technique that is based on clusters [53–54], and they are classic algorithms that have diverse applications. Two steps comprise the Expectation-Maximization algorithm [55], that is, the Expectation process and Maximization process. In the first step, the expectation of the likelihood of the probability function is calculated, and in the second step, the maximum likelihood of the parameters is calculated. When the parameters are calculated, they are applied in the expectation process and these processes are repeated until the outcome converges. As a result of iterating several times, the algorithm computes the posterior probabilities and maximum likelihood estimates [56]. Due to the lack of spatial modeling in this clustering method, intensity inhomogeneity and noise are generated during the image processing. Karim Katli and Mohamed Ali Mahjoun [57] have proposed an EM algorithm that takes advantage of adaptive distances.

13.7 MODEL-BASED ALGORITHMS

Model-based algorithms are defined as the process of assigning labels to the pixel, which is done by comparing the image data to the previously identified object model. This model is nothing but the generalization of the classical segmentation, where the deterministic label is assigned to the pixel using just low-level criteria like discontinuity and homogeneity. This model-based approach is the ideal image analysis technique to be used with a model.

a) Markov Random field

Inspired by the Ishing model [58], a model system for particles interacting in a two- or three-dimensional lattice was created in the early 20th century and utilized in statistical Markov Random field model mechanics. This model involves a stochastic process, in which the distribution of future states depends simply on the current state not on how it got to the current condition. Segmentation of images by MRF methods is widely used, and the image is revamped since the edges are protected by parameters [59]. The Hidden Markov random field (HMRF) [60] is based on the notion that random processes can be created using a Markov random field model, whose way of arrangement cannot be seen directly but can be viewed through an investigation. In terms of computing complexity, it was found that the PRF (Pickard random fields) model is more effective than the standard MRF.[61]

b) Atlas-based approach

Atlas-based segmentation, in contrast to previous image segmentation techniques, could very well segment images without clearly established correlations among regions as well as pixel intensities. Atlas-guided techniques are accessible in the parametric and nonparametric approach types. Parametric approaches combine new and trained images to create an atlas, whereas all the photos are processed individually for training in the non-parametric technique. Atlas maps require image registration to be created [62]. Atlases play a crucial role in the partition precession, and image enrolment plays a key role in it. The neighborhood assessment weights have been dimensionally adjusted to restrict the Atlas labels for the earmark presentation. There is a wide variation in the form and size of human organelles. Due to the diversity of the population, portraying these images can become challenging. Atlases can provide an effective uniform template allowing photographers to take into account this heterogeneity in their work [63].

c) Artificial neural networks

Frank Rosenblatt first described a neural network (ANN) as a self-learning computing system in 1958 [64]. It can be also defined as a mathematical representation of neurons that is modeled after a biological neural network. The node is a copy of a neuron that can be coupled with functional units, and communication between these nodes is facilitated by synaptic weights. A categorization or identification process is carried out by the activation function based on the input of synaptic weights [65].

13.8 EVALUATION OF DIFFERENT MEDICAL IMAGE SEGMENTATION METHODS

THRESHOLDING TECHNIQUES

	Advantages	Disadvantages
Local thresholding	Neither prior knowledge nor complicated implementation is required.	It creates edges that are noisy and fuzzy.
Otsu's Method	Ensures that intra and interclass differences are reduced to a minimum. Histogram shapes were not considered prior. Multi-level thresholding is an option that could be extended.	With increasing threshold levels, the complexity of the regions increases. Regions can be combined or mixed.
Gaussian Mixture Approach	It is used to solve histogram issues. Reduces the likelihood of categorizing errors for small classes. Iterative process.	This model is not appropriate for all histograms and results intensities that are non-negative and finite. Flat models find it difficult to cope with it.

REGION-BASED SEGMENTATION

	Advantages	Disadvantages
Region growing	With the simultaneous consideration of several criteria and minimal noise, excellent outcomes are produced	Over-segmentation occurs when there are noises or changes in intensity, making it difficult to distinguish genuine images from fakes and consuming a great deal of power.
Region Merging and Splitting	The linkage of regions is assured. While merging, the improved quadtree eliminates lengthy neighbor issues.	Image orientation and position can lead to blocky final segmentation. As a result of regular division, excessive segmentation occurs

EDGE-BASED/BOUNDARY DETECTION

	Advantages	Disadvantages
Edge detection approaches	Edge detection works well for images with good contrast between regions since humans perceive objects through their edges.	It doesn't work well with photos with a lot of edges or poorly defined edges In comparison with other methods, this method is less noise-proof.
Prewitt edge detection	The ability to recognize edges and their orientations, as well as the simplicity of the process	Lack of accuracy and noise sensitivity
Laplacian of Gaussian	Edges can be located in their proper locations. A larger area around the pixel can be tested.	There is malfunctioning in corners, curves, and places where the Gray level intensity function fluctuates. The Laplacian filter does not allow one to determine the edge orientation.
Watershed	In noise-filled images, they perform better. Speedy and reliable output	The seed point must be specified. In addition, it can be easily over-segmented. This is a time-consuming process and is only useful for gradients

CLUSTERING METHODS

	Advantages	Disadvantages
K-Means	It is quick and easy to implement. This method is more efficient than hierarchical clustering. Optimizes cluster variability as well as cluster number.	The number of output clusters must be determined before the user begins classifying the data. Random centroids determine the outcome. Inability to display clustering data

(Continued)

CLUSTERING METHODS

Fuzzy C-Means algorithm	Clearly explained and easy to understand. Unsupervised and vague. The unpredictable nature of an image.	It is unknown what is the optimal solution. Initialization entails some risk. Images with noisy pixels are the least compatible.
Expectation-Maximization (EM) algorithm	Unsupervised iterative processes and reduced sensitivity	Intensity-inhomogeneity and noise are produced. Convergence is slow. Computed costs are high

MODEL-BASED ALGORITHMS

	Advantages	Disadvantages
Markov Random field models	Safeguard the edges by approximating parameters.	Computational complexity.
Atlas-based approached	Transfer of labels occurs during segmentation. Structures suitable for the study population Fast in terms of computation.	Nonlinear registration methods pose a challenge to the accurate segmentation of complex structures.
Artificial neural networks	Simple implementation. Suitable for a variety of problems.	There is no strong theoretical basis for ANNs. It is difficult to choose the best architecture and black box problem.

13.9   CONCLUSION

A survey of existing methods of image segmentation is provided in this chapter, including prior methods and current techniques. There are advantages and disadvantages to each segmentation method discussed here, and it is not advisable to establish a single benchmark for comparison. A comprehensive categorization of the segmentation of medical images has been presented in this chapter. It is, therefore, appropriate to refer to this article as a source of information. A comparison of the new segmentation methods with the pre-existing methods has demonstrated that they perform well. In medical imaging, where segmentation accuracy is crucial to making crucial decisions, such as detecting tumors, segmentation accuracy remains a major concern. A future focus should be on improving the precision, and accuracy, and reducing the amount of manual intervention in segmentation algorithms.

REFERENCES

[1] Wang, Y.H., 2010. *Tutorial: Image segmentation* (pp. 1–36). National Taiwan University, Taipei.

[2] Lee, L.K., Liew, S.C. and Thong, W.J., 2015. A review of image segmentation methodologies in medical images. *Advanced Computer and Communication Engineering Technology*, pp. 1069–1080.

[3] Kang, W.X., Yang, Q.Q. and Liang, R.P., 2009, March. The comparative research on image segmentation algorithms. In *2009 First international workshop on education technology and computer science* (Vol. 2, pp. 703–707). IEEE.

[4] Wahba, M., 2009. An automated modified region growing technique for prostate segmentation in trans-rectal ultrasound images (Master's thesis, University of Waterloo).

[5] Aurdal, L., 2006. Image Segmentation beyond thresholding. *Norsk Regnescentral, 10*, pp. 102–113.

[6] Ma, Z., Tavares, J.M.R., Jorge, R.N. and Mascarenhas, T., 2010. A review of algorithms for medical image segmentation and their applications to the female pelvic cavity. *Computer Methods in Biomechanics and Biomedical Engineering, 13*(2), pp. 235–246.

[7] Rajchl, M., Baxter, J.S., McLeod, A.J., Yuan, J., Qiu, W., Peters, T.M. and Khan, A.R., 2016. Hierarchical max-flow segmentation framework for multi-atlas segmentation with Kohonen self-organizing map-based Gaussian mixture modeling. *Medical Image Analysis, 27*, pp. 45–56.

[8] Feng, Y., Zhao, H., Li, X., Zhang, X. and Li, H., 2017. A multi-scale 3D Otsu thresholding algorithm for medical image segmentation. *Digital Signal Processing, 60*, pp. 186–199.

[9] Zhou, C., Tian, L., Zhao, H. and Zhao, K., 2015, June. A method of two-dimensional Otsu image threshold segmentation based on an improved firefly algorithm. In *2015 IEEE international conference on cyber technology in automation, control, and intelligent systems (CYBER)* (pp. 1420–1424). IEEE.

[10] Greggio, N., Bernardino, A., Laschi, C., Dario, P. and Santos-Victor, J., 2012. Fast estimation of Gaussian mixture models for image segmentation. *Machine Vision and Applications, 23*(4), pp. 773–789.

[11] International conference on cyber technology in automation, control, and intelligent systems, 2015 (pp. 1420–1424). Greggio, N., et al., 2012. Fast estimation of Gaussian mixture models for image segmentation. *Machine Vision Applications* (Special Issue: Microscopy Image Analysis for Biomedical Applications), 23(4), pp. 773–789.

[12] Kumar, D., Pramanik, A., Kar, S.S. and Maity, S.P., 2016, June. Retinal blood vessel segmentation using matched filter and Laplacian of Gaussian. In *2016 International conference on Signal Processing and Communications (SPCOM)* (pp. 1–5). IEEE.

[13] Hore, S., Chakraborty, S., Chatterjee, S., Dey, N., Ashour, A.S., Van Chung, L. and Le, D.N., 2016. An integrated interactive technique for image segmentation using stack-based seeded region growing and thresholding. *International Journal of Electrical & Computer Engineering (2088–8708)*, 6(6).

[14] Zhang, H., Fritts, J.E. and Goldman, S.A., 2008. Image segmentation evaluation: A survey of unsupervised methods. *Computer Vision and Image Understanding, 110*(2), pp. 260–280.

[15] Chang, Y.L. and Li, X., 1994. Adaptive image region-growing. *IEEE Transactions on Image Processing, 3*(6), pp. 868–872.

[16] Singh, K.K. and Singh, A., 2010. A study of image segmentation algorithms for different types of images. *International Journal of Computer Science Issues (IJCSI), 7*(5), p. 414.

[17] Taori, A.M., Chaudhari, A.K., Patankar, S.S. and Kulkarni, J.V., 2016, August. Segmentation of macula in retinal images using automated seeding region growing technique. In *2016 International Conference on Inventive Computation Technologies (ICICT)* (Vol. 2, pp. 1–5). IEEE.

[18] Javadpour, A. and Mohammadi, A., 2016. Improving brain magnetic resonance image (MRI) segmentation via a novel algorithm based on genetic and regional growth. *Journal of Biomedical Physics & Engineering, 6*(2), p. 95.

[19] Hancer, E. and Karaboga, D., 2017. A comprehensive survey of traditional, merge-split, and evolutionary approaches are proposed for the determination of cluster numbers. *Swarm and Evolutionary Computation, 32*, pp. 49–67.

[20] Kelkar, D. and Gupta, S., 2008, July. Improved quadtree method for split merge image segmentation. In *2008 First international conference on emerging trends in engineering and technology* (pp. 44–47). IEEE.

[21] Sakamoto, R., Yakami, M., Fujimoto, K., Nakagomi, K., Kubo, T., Emoto, Y., Akasaka, T., Aoyama, G., Yamamoto, H., Miller, M.I. and Mori, S., 2017. Temporal subtraction of serial CT images with large deformation diffeomorphic metric mapping in the identification of bone metastases. *Radiology*, *285*(2), p. 629.

[22] Anand, A., Tripathy, S.S. and Kumar, R.S., 2015, February. Improved edge detection using morphological Laplacian of Gaussian operator. In *2015 2nd International conference on signal processing and integrated networks (SPIN)* (pp. 532–536). IEEE.

[23] Zhang, Y.J., 2006. An overview of image and video segmentation in the last 40 years. *Advances in Image and Video Segmentation*, pp. 1–16.

[24] Prewitt, J.M., 1970. *Object enhancement and extraction* (Vol. 75). Academic Press, New York.

[25] Chaple, G.N., Daruwala, R.D. and Gofane, M.S., 2015, February. Comparison of Robert, Prewitt, Soand bel operator-based edge detection methods for real-time uses on FPGA. In *2015 International Conference on Technologies for Sustainable Development (ICTSD)* (pp. 1–4). IEEE.

[26] Albovik, 2000. *Handbook of image and video processing*. Academic Press, New York.

[27] Haralick, R.M. and Shapiro, L.G., 1992. *Computer and robot vision* (Vol. 1, pp. 28–48). Reading: Addison-Wesley, Boston.

[28] Yang, Y., Tong, S., Huang, S. and Lin, P., 2014. Log-Gabor energy-based multimodal medical image fusion in NSCT domain. *Computational and Mathematical Methods in Medicine, 2014*.

[29] Kwon, G.R., Basukala, D., Lee, S.W., Lee, K.H. and Kang, M., 2016. Brain image segmentation using a combination of expectation-maximization algorithm and watershed transform. *International Journal of Imaging Systems and Technology, 26*(3), pp. 225–232.

[30] Husain, R.A., Zayed, A.S., Ahmed, W.M. and Elhaji, H.S., 2015, December. Image segmentation with an improved watershed algorithm using radial bases functions neural networks. In *2015 16th International conference on sciences and techniques of automatic control and computer engineering (STA)* (pp. 121–126). IEEE.

[31] Pavlidis, T., 2012. *Algorithms for graphics and image processing*. Springer Science & Business Media, Berlin.

[32] Arabnia, H.R., 2010. *Advances in computational biology* (pp. 4–18). Springer Science Business Media, Berlin.

[33] Benson, C.C., Lajish, V.L. and Rajamani, K., 2015, August. Brain tumor extraction from MRI brain images using marker-based watershed algorithm. In *2015 International Conference on advances in Computing, Communications, and Informatics (ICACCI)* (pp. 318–323). IEEE.

[34] Dehariya, V.K., Shrivastava, S.K. and Jain, R.C., 2010, November. Clustering of image data set using k-means and fuzzy k-means algorithms. In *2010 International conference on computational intelligence and communication networks* (pp. 386–391). IEEE.

[35] Abdel-Maksoud, E., Elmogy, M. and AlAwadi, R., 2015. Brain tumor segmentation based on a hybrid clustering technique, Egypt. *The International Journal of Information Management, 16*(1), pp. 71–81. https://doi.org/10.1016/j.eij.2015.01.003

[36] Ajala Funmilola, A., Oke, O.A., Adedeji, T.O., Alade, O.M. and Adewusi, E.A., 2012. Fuzzy kc-means clustering algorithm for medical image segmentation. *Journal of Information Engineering and Applications*, 2(6), pp. 21–32.

[37] Celebi, M.E., Kingravi, H.A. and Vela, P.A., 2013. A comparative study of efficient initialization methods for the k-means clustering algorithm. *Expert Systems with Applications, 40*(1), pp. 200–210.

[38] Dhanachandra, N., Manglem, K. and Chanu, Y.J., 2015. Image segmentation using K-means clustering algorithm and subtractive clustering algorithm. *Procedia Computer Science, 54*, pp. 764–771.

[39] Kaus, M.R., Von Berg, J., Weese, J., Niessen, W. and Pekar, V., 2004. Automated segmentation of the left ventricle in cardiac MRI. *Medical Image Analysis*, 8(3), pp. 245–254.

[40] Sharma, M., Purohit, G.N. and Mukherjee, S., 2018. Information retrieves from brain MRI images for tumor detection using the hybrid technique K-means and artificial neural network (KMANN). In *Networking communication and data knowledge engineering* (pp. 145–157). Springer, Singapore.

[41] Amiya, H., Soumajit, P. and Arindam, K., 2011. Dynamic image segmentation using Fuzzy c-means based genetic algorithm. *International Journal of Computer Application*, 28(67).

[42] Ali, A.M., Karmakar, G.C. and Dooley, L.S., 2008. Review on fuzzy clustering algorithms. *Journal of Advanced Computations*, 2(3), pp. 169–181.

[43] Meena Prakash, R. and Shantha Selva Kumari, R., 2017. Spatial fuzzy C means and expectation maximization algorithms with bias correction for segmentation of MR brain images. *Journal of Medical Systems*, 41(1), pp. 1–9.

[44] Wen, F., Wu, N. and Gong, X., 2020. China's carbon emissions trading and stock returns. *Energy Economics*, 86, p. 104627.

[45] Geng, Q., Zhou, Z. and Cao, X., 2018. Survey of recent progress in semantic image segmentation with CNNs. *Science China Information Sciences*, 61(5), pp. 1–18.

[46] Feng, Y., Lu, H.Q. and Hong, Y., 2017. Fuzzy C-means clustering image segmentation method based on multi- chain quantum bee colony algorithm. *Computer Science & Engineering Apps*, 53(24), pp. 8–14.

[47] Xu, R., 2022. Fuzzy C-means clustering image segmentation algorithm based on hidden Markov model. *Mobile Networks and Applications*, pp. 1–9.

[48] Frank, D., 2002. *The expectation-maximization algorithm, college of computing* (pp. 982–103). Georgia Institute of Technology, APRI, Springer.

[49] Do, C.B. and Batzoglou, S., 2008. What is the expectation maximization algorithm? *Nature Biotechnology*, 26(8), pp. 897–899.

[50] Tatiraju, S. and Mehta, A., 2008. Image Segmentation using k-means clustering, EM, and normalized cuts. *Department of EECS*, 1, pp. 1–7.

[51] Huang, K.W., Zhao, Z.Y., Gong, Q., Zha, J., Chen, L. and Yang, R., 2015, August. Nasopharyngeal carcinoma segmentation via HMRF-EM with maximum entropy. In *2015 37th annual international conference of the IEEE Engineering in Medicine and Biology Society (EMBC)* (pp. 2968–2972). IEEE.

[52] Mahjoub, M.A., 2012. Image segmentation by adaptive distance based on EM algorithm. *arXiv preprint arXiv:1204.1629*.

[53] Kindermann, R., Snell, J.L., 1980. *Markov random fields and their applications* (1st ed., (pp. 1–147). American Mathematical Society, Providence, Rhode island.

[54] Held, K., Kops, E.R., Krause, B.J., Wells, W.M., Kikinis, R. and Muller-Gartner, H.W., 1997. Markov random field segmentation of brain MR images. *IEEE Transactions on Medical Imaging*, 16(6), pp. 878–886.

[55] Zhang, Y., Brady, M. and Smith, S., 2001. Segmentation of brain MR images through a hidden Markov random field model and the expectation-maximization algorithm. *IEEE Transactions on Medical Imaging*, 20(1), pp. 45–57.

[56] Goubalan, S.R., Goussard, Y. and Maaref, H., 2016, September. Unsupervised malignant mammographic breast mass segmentation algorithm based on Pickard Markov random field. In *2016 IEEE International Conference on Image Processing (ICIP)* (pp. 2653–2657). IEEE.

[57] Phellan, R., Falcao, A.X. and Udupa, J., 2014, September. Improving atlas-based medical image segmentation with a relaxed object search. In *International symposium computational modeling of objects represented in images* (pp. 152–163). Springer, Cham.

[58] Iglesias, J.E. and Sabuncu, M.R., 2015. Multi-atlas segmentation of biomedical images: A survey. *Medical Image Analysis*, 24(1), pp. 205–219.

[59] Ian, G., et al., 2016. *Deep learning*. Book in preparation for MIT Press. www.deeplearningbook.org.

[60] Barot, V., Kapadia, V. and Pandya, S., 2020. QoS enabled IoT-based low-cost air quality monitoring system with power consumption optimization. *Cybernetics and Information Technologies*, 20(2), pp. 122–140.

[61] Singh, V. and Misra, A.K., 2017. Detection of plant leaf diseases using image segmentation and soft computing techniques. *Information Processing in Agriculture*, 4(1), pp. 41–49.

[62] Egmont-Petersen, M., de Ridder, D. and Handels, H., 2002. Image processing with neural networks—a review. *Pattern Recognition*, 35(10), pp. 2279–2301.

[63] Zheng, X., Lei, Q., Yao, R., Gong, Y., and Yin, Q., 2018. Image segmentation based on adaptive K-means algorithm. *EURASIP Journal on Image and Video Processing*, 2018(1), pp. 1–10.

[64] Singh, T.R., Roy, S., Singh, O.I., Sinam, T. and Singh, K., 2012. A new local adaptive thresholding technique in binarization. *arXiv preprint arXiv*:1201.5227.

[65] Yadav, N.K. and Saraswat, M., 2022. A novel fuzzy clustering based method for image segmentation in RGB-D images. *Engineering Applications of Artificial Intelligence*, 111, p. 104709.

14 Deep CNN in Healthcare

*Farooq Shaik, Rajesh Y., Noman Aasif Gudur,
and Jatindra Kumar Dash*

14.1 INTRODUCTION

Deep Learning (DL) [1] is a subset of Machine Learning (ML) and the broader field of Artificial intelligence (AI). It involves training artificial neural networks with multiple layers (hence the term "deep") to analyze and learn patterns from large datasets. These networks are inspired by the structure and function of the human brain and are designed to automatically learn representations of data through a process of trial and error. DL has had tremendous growth in recent years due to the advancement of computational power in terms of GPU and the availability of large data sets; machines are able to understand and manipulate massive amounts of data, including images speech, and languages. Healthcare tends to benefit from deep learning because of the sheer amount of data generated every day through medical devices and medical record systems.

In contrast to conventional programming, which relies on a linear sequence of instructions, machine learning (ML) algorithms function by mapping input data to corresponding output data. These algorithms leverage statistical techniques driven by data to decipher and learn the underlying relationships or functions that connect input and output data, as exemplified by Esteva et al [2]. Nevertheless, ML algorithms necessitate skilled engineers and domain experts to extract meaningful features from raw data, transforming it into a format compatible with machine processing. On the other hand, deep learning presents a distinctive approach. When employing deep learning models, raw data is directly inputted, and the intricate architecture of the deep learning framework adeptly identifies intricate patterns within the data for subsequent processing.

DL architecture is composed of layers that are stacked over each other, where each layer performs non-linear operations such that the output of a layer is fed to its next layer as data flow though layers so that complex functions can be learned that map raw input data to output. DL systems can deal with multiple types of data as relevance to heterogeneous data available in the healthcare system. Most DL systems are supervised where data with output or label are used to train the system where the system learns a function to map betwcen input and output.

DL plays a tremendous role in computer vision where the task is to mimic human visual systems to understand video and images; it includes tasks such as object recognition, segmentation, and classification tasks. For example, examining radio graph of a patient and determining whether the patient has cancer or not. Convolutional neural network (CNN) is a type of deep neural network that is used for processing images. In medical imaging, a variety of modalities are employed, including Magnetic Resonance Imaging (MRI), Computed Tomography (CT) Scans, and X-rays (Radiography).

Ultrasound Imaging, Positron Emission Tomography (PET) Scans, Nuclear Medicine Scans, Endoscopy, Mammography, Fluoroscopy, Dermoscopy, Ophthalmic Imaging, and Electroencephalography (EEG). These medical images can be used to train Deep CNN to learn patterns in images and perform tasks such as the classification of disease and detection of tumors or infections. The general structure of deep learning models is shown in Figure 14.1 [2].

14.1.1 Different Types of CNN

As mentioned, CNN has revolutionized computer vision tasks performing at human-level accuracy. There are different architectures some of them as follows LeNet-5, an early CNN architecture that was crafted specifically for the recognition of handwritten digits. Its structure encompasses convolutional layers succeeded by fully connected layers. AlexNet [3], unveiled during the ImageNet Large Scale Visual Recognition Challenge, played a key role in popularizing deep CNNs. This architecture incorporates numerous convolutional and fully connected layers, integrating methods such as "dropout" to achieve regularization. VGGNet is recognized for its straightforwardness, featuring a consistent design of successive convolutional layers coupled with max-pooling layers. This profound architecture empowers it to acquire intricate features effectively. However, VGGNet is preferred over AlexNet for certain tasks due to its deeper architecture and ability to capture more intricate features. GoogLeNet, also referred to as InceptionNet, pioneered the concept of inception modules.

These modules involve the parallel combination of filters of varying sizes, enabling the network to effectively grasp multi-scale features. This approach allows GoogLeNet to achieve a deeper network architecture while maintaining manageable

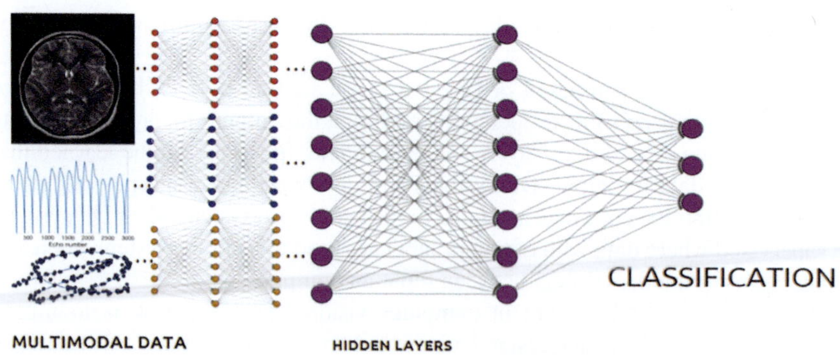

FIGURE 14.1 Deep learning can learn from variety of data types.

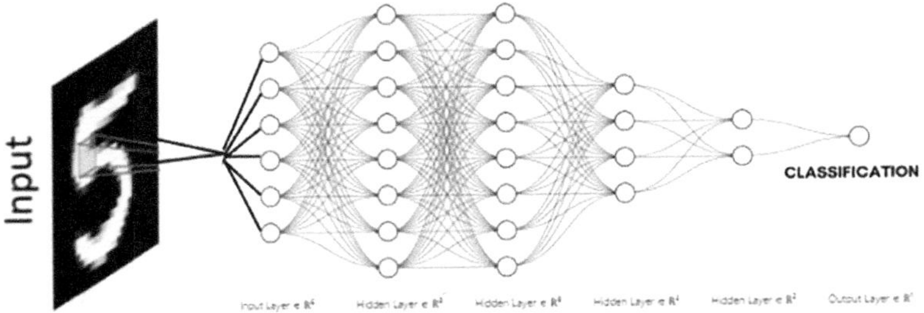

FIGURE 14.2 CNN architecture.

computational complexity. In contrast, while VGGNet is known for its simplicity and uniform architecture ResNet (Residual Networks) introduces a novel concept through its residual blocks, where layers learn residual mappings. This unique architecture facilitates the training of exceptionally deep networks by effectively addressing the challenge of vanishing gradients. DenseNet stands out with its emphasis on feature reuse through dense connections, ensuring that each layer receives inputs from all preceding layers. This approach promotes efficient gradient flow, enhances parameter efficiency, and leads to heightened accuracy. MobileNet is tailored for mobile and embedded devices, utilizing depth-wise separable convolutions to substantially decrease parameter count while upholding accuracy. The typical CNN network will look like the image shown in Figure 14.2 [2].

14.2   IMPORTANCE OF DEEP CNN

The significance of Deep Convolutional Neural Networks (CNNs) in healthcare is profound and multi faceted, owing to their transformative capabilities and potential to revolutionize various aspects of medical practice. Here are some key reasons illustrating the importance of Deep CNNs in the realm of healthcare.

- **Feature Extraction**

Deep CNN has the ability to extract both low-level features such as texture edges and high-level features such as objects and contexts. This makes them highly effective for tasks like image and video classification.

- **State-of-the-Art Performance**

Deep CNNs have consistently achieved top-tier performance on benchmark datasets, surpassing traditional methods in various image-related tasks. This includes tasks like image classification, where models like AlexNet, VGG, ResNet, and Inception have achieved unprecedented accuracy.

- **Transfer Learning**

Deep CNNs can be pre-trained on large datasets, enabling transfer of knowledge from one task to another. This significantly reduces the need for extensive labeled data, making it easier to develop models for specific applications.

- **Medical Imaging**

Deep CNNs have revolutionized medical image analysis by aiding in early disease detection, accurate diagnosis, and treatment planning. They can analyze medical images (X-rays, MRIs, CT scans) to identify anomalies and assist healthcare professionals.

- **Natural Language Processing (NLP)**

CNNs, originally developed for images, have been adapted for NLP tasks like sentiment analysis, text classification, and machine translation. This demonstrates their versatility beyond visual data.

14.3 CHALLENGES OF DEEP CNN

Deep CNN has promised results; however, there are some challenges [4] that need to be addressed. Some key highlights are as follows.

14.3.1 VOLUME OF DATA

From a healthcare standpoint, comprehending diseases and their associated variations in features presents a greater complexity than tasks like image classification and speech recognition. In the context of healthcare, consider ECG data that can vary in duration from 30 minutes to 1 hour per recording. If we were to analyze recordings from 200 patients, the accumulated time could reach one to two hundred hours. This extensive amount of data has the capacity to substantially prolong the training process, increase computational complexity, and necessitate specific hardware resources [5].

14.3.2 QUALITY OF DATA

Healthcare data exhibit a diverse and intricate nature, marked by elements of heterogeneity, noise, incompleteness, and ambiguity. Consider ECG data, which often suffers from artifacts stemming from eye blinks, lateral eye movements, and muscle interference. Medical records encompass a spectrum of formats, including frequency domain representations and electromagnetic images, contributing to their inherent heterogeneity. The presence of missing values, attributed to equipment malfunctions or instrumental discrepancies, further contributes to data incompleteness. At times, medical data may be subject to voltage fluctuations, while in other instances, these fluctuations may be negligible, leading to potential ambiguity. The endeavor to train a deep learning model on this vast and diverse array of datasets poses significant challenges. Addressing concerns such as data redundancy, missing values, and sparsity becomes pivotal in this context.

14.3.3 TEMPORALITY

Infections are constantly progressing and changing over time in an unpredictable manner. However, most current deep learning models, including those designed for medical applications, rely on static vector inputs that do not naturally account for the temporal aspect. Developing deep learning methods capable of handling time-dependent healthcare data is crucial and calls for innovative solutions [6]

14.3.4 DOMAIN COMPLEXITY

In contrast to other domains like image and speech analysis, biomedical and healthcare fields present more intricate challenges. Diseases exhibit significant heterogeneity, often lacking a comprehensive understanding of their causes and progression. Additionally, the availability of patients for study is usually limited within real clinical settings, preventing us from accessing a vast number of patients as needed [7].

14.3.5 INTERPRETABILITY

Despite the success of deep learning models in various applications, they often operate as black boxes. While this might not pose an issue in other more deterministic domains such as image labeling (since end users can objectively verify assigned labels), in healthcare, it's crucial not only to assess the quantitative algorithmic performance but also to understand the rationale behind the model's functioning. In fact, this model interpretability (i.e., identifying the driving factors behind predictions) is essential to convince medical professionals about the recommendations made by the predictive system [8], like prescribing a specific medication or identifying a high risk of developing a certain illness.

14.4 APPLICATIONS OF DEEP CNN IN HEALTHCARE

14.4.1 MEDICAL IMAGE ANALYSIS

Deep learning techniques play a significant role in the realm of Medical Imaging through four primary approaches: classification, segmentation, generation, and detection. These techniques have notably advanced the analysis of medical images, making a substantial impact within the realm of medical imaging.

14.4.1.1 Image Classification

Classification of Medical images was an early adopter of Deep Learning technology. This technique is mainly used for categorizing images into different classes, particularly in multiclass scenarios. Within the medical imaging community, there has been a notable focus on techniques like Stacked Autoencoders (SAEs), Deep Belief Networks (DBNs), and Restricted Boltzmann Machines (RBMs). Often with an emphasis on unsupervised pre-training. The initial use of these models for multiclass classification dates back to around 2013, particularly within the realm of neuroimaging. For example, Suk et al. [9], Brosch et al. [10], and Plis et al [11] employed SAEs and DBNs to classify data from Alzheimer's disease patients based on MRI scans.

In more recent times, Convolutional Neural Networks (CNNs) have become widely renowned for their effectiveness in image classification. In the span between 2015 and 2017, a substantial volume of research publications emerged, particularly centered around multiclass classification. These models exhibit a wide range of applications, encompassing fields such as brain MRI, CT SCANS, X-rays, and other medical images.

14.4.1.2 Image Detection

In medical image processing, tasks like segmentation and therapy planning often involve localizing anatomical objects (such as organs and landmarks) within images. Detecting and localizing these objects is crucial for simplifying subsequent segmentation work or clinical workflows. Parsing 3D volumetric data is a necessity in medical image analysis. To overcome the complexity of handling 3D information through deep learning models, several strategies have been devised. A commonly used method involves treating collections of orthogonal 2D planes as if they were virtual 3D spaces. For instance, Yang et al. [12] utilized regular CNNs to identify landmarks on the surface of the distal femur by processing three separate sets of 2D MRI slices. The 3D position of a landmark is determined by the intersection of three 2D slices with the highest classification outcomes. Nonetheless, tackling the direct identification of objects and landmarks within 3D images remains an ongoing challenge. Zheng et al. [13] simplified localization detection for carotid artery bifurcation using a decomposition of 3D convolutions into three 1D convolutions on Computed Tomography. Ghesu et al. [14] proposed a sparse adaptive DNN approach fueled with marginal space learning for localizing the aortic valve in 3D transesophageal echocardiograms, addressing data complexity. Convolutional Neural Networks (CNNs) are renowned for recognizing scan planes or pivotal frames in temporal datasets. One way to employ CNNs to recognize standardized scan planes from video frame information, particularly for mid-pregnancy fetal scans. In the context of high-dimensional medical videos with temporal information, Recurrent Neural Networks (RNNs), specifically Long Short-Term Memory (LSTM) networks, are employed to capture temporal patterns. Chen et al. [15], for instance, used LSTM-RNNs to incorporate temporal information from consecutive ultrasound videos aiding in the detection of standard fetal planes.

14.4.1.3 Image Segmentation

The process of delineating and identifying organs and other structures within medical images is crucial for performing quantitative analyses of clinical parameters like volume and shape, especially in areas like cardiac or brain analysis. This segmentation step is also vital in computer-aided detection systems. Segmentation involves identifying the specific set of voxels that constitute the interior or boundary of the object of interest. This task has been a focal point for applying Deep Learning (DL) to medical images, leading to a wide range of methodologies. A recent trend in segmentation involves Recurrent Neural Networks (RNNs), which have gained popularity. For instance, Xie et al. [16] employed a spatial RNN clockwork to segment the perimysium in HE-histopathology images. In the realm of medical imaging, segmentation has witnessed a surge in DL methods. Specialized networks are designed for image segmentation tasks directly, yielding promising results that often rival or even surpass outcomes achieved with Convolutional Neural Networks (CNNs). This demonstrates the significant potential of DL in advancing medical image segmentation techniques.

14.4.1.4 Image Registration

Medical image registration aligns and matches different medical images of the same anatomy. It finds a transformation to link points between images, ensuring spatial alignment. The aim is to merge or compare information from diverse images for better analysis. This is typically done using an iterative framework with predefined metrics (e.g., L2-norm) for optimization. While lesion detection and segmentation are important areas for deep learning; nevertheless, researchers have discovered that deep learning can also yield remarkable outcomes for image registration. In the literature, two predominant strategies have come to the forefront. The initial approach involves employing deep learning networks to calculate a measure of similarity between images, which guides an iterative optimization process. The second method directly forecasts transformation parameters by utilizing deep regression techniques. Wu et al [17], Cheng et al. [18], and Krebs et al. [19] utilized two types of SAEs to evaluate and measure local similarities in MRI and CT images. These networks pre-train through unsupervised patch reconstruction, followed by fine-tuning with prediction layers. Simonovsky et al. [20] adopted a comparable approach by employing Convolutional Neural Networks (CNNs) to calculate similarity costs between matches originating from various modalities.

One of the most critical tasks in modern medicine is surveying medical imaging. CNNs have rapidly evolved and gained prominence in the medical imaging research community due to their exceptional performance in computer vision and GPU parallelization. CNNs have found application in medical imaging classification scenarios, including the analysis of computed tomography, X-ray images, and color fundus images. Notably, training based on discriminative local appearance has exhibited higher accuracy compared to global image context-based training. Additionally, hybrid approaches that fuse CNNs with other deep learning methods have been proposed. An illustrative example involves the amalgamation of deep learning with deformable models to achieve automated segmentation of the left ventricle from cardiac MRI data. A comprehensive survey conducted by Havaei et al. [21] provides an extensive overview of various CNN configurations introduced in the domain of medical image analysis. Overall, deep learning, particularly CNNs, has revolutionized medical image analysis and holds immense potential for advancing healthcare diagnostics and treatment.

14.4.2 Disease Diagnosis and Prognosis

Deep Learning (DL) stands out as a powerful technology capable of autonomously learning patterns and features, making it a robust approach. Its potential has enabled the creation of predictive models for early disease detection. In comparison to traditional Machine Learning (ML) methods, DL algorithms often outperform due to their high precision, automatic feature extraction, and extensive data analysis capabilities. Especially in handling large datasets, DL demonstrates a notable edge over ML. Furthermore, DL's predictive performance often surpasses human abilities, making it a preferred choice for image-related tasks [22]. DL has gained significant traction in the medical realm, particularly in image processing, where diagnosis revolves around extracting crucial information from images. In disease diagnosis by using images such as -ray, CT scan, and MRI, various types of DL methods are employed, including Convolutional Neural Networks (CNN), Deep Neural Networks (DNN), Deep Belief Networks (DBN), RNN, Deep Automatic Encoders, and their variants like BLSTM and MDLATM [23].

A distinctive DL technique tailored for medical data analysis is the Region Aggregation Graph Convolutional Network (RAGCN). This method employs Graph Convolutional Networks (GCNs) to consolidate insights from different image regions. Developed specifically for medical images like MRI scans, which frequently encompass various regions of interest, RAGCN segments the image into distinct regions and employs GCNs for feature extraction and predictions. An example is an automatic bone age estimation where CNN and GCN work in tandem [24].

The Lesion-Attention Pyramid Network (LAPNet) represents another novel deep learning technique in medical data analysis. It is specifically designed for the detection and classification of lesions in medical images. LAPNet adopts a pyramid-style architecture, enabling the extraction of features across different scales. Additionally, it incorporates an attention mechanism to highlight regions that are more likely to contain lesions. An application of LAPNet was seen in grading diabetic retinopathy, where the network was trained on medical images to recognize lesion regions [25].

14.4.2.1 Diagnosis and Prognosis of the Coronavirus disease pandemic

COVID-19, a viral infection caused by the severe acute respiratory syndrome coronavirus-2, has emerged as a significant global health concern [26]. The rapid transmission of this pandemic has raised worldwide alarm [27], leading to a reevaluation of healthcare norms by the World Health Organization [28]. Abbas et al. [29] introduced a CNN called DeTraC, which employs a class decomposition method to classify COVID-19 patient chest X-rays. DeTraC can handle dataset irregularities by examining class boundaries. It achieved an 85.12% accuracy in detecting COVID-19 X-rays amid normal and severe respiratory cases. Wang et al. [30] developed COVID-Net, a deep CNN model, which achieved a 93.3% accuracy in identifying normal, COVID-19, and pneumonia-infected X-rays. COVIDX-Net by Hemdan et al. [31] X-ray images are utilized to detect COVID-19 infection. The approach employs seven deep learning classifiers, with VGG19 and DenseNet201 showing superior performance. Although MobileNetV2 offers quick computation, there is potential for improvement, such as its integration with smart devices.

14.4.2.2 Diagnosis and Prognosis of Alzheimer's Disease

Alzheimer's Disease (AD) [32] is the leading neurodegenerative disorder and a major cause of Dementia. Researchers are exploring neuro-imaging techniques like T1 weighted Magnetic Resonance Imaging and Positron Emission Tomography, along with deep learning methods, to develop automated diagnostic tools for early-stage AD detection. The primary reason behind Alzheimer's Disease (AD) is the disruption of brain proteins, leading to the degeneration or loss of neurons, primarily in the cortex area. Plaques and Tangles are commonly identified as significant contributors to its advancement [33]. Deep Learning (DL) enables the creation of models containing computational and multi-processing layers, which can learn a collection of features from input data and categorize the output based on the learned input [34].

When it comes to early Alzheimer's Disease (AD) diagnosis, DL is considered a cutting-edge approach due to its superior accuracy in image classification when compared to conventional Machine Learning (ML) techniques.

Shui et al. [35] utilized a Convolutional Neural Network (CNN) as a classifier on the OASIS dataset. The OASIS dataset is a renowned compilation of neuroimaging data, particularly Magnetic Resonance Imaging (MRI) scans. It is extensively employed in research and encompasses brain images from both healthy subjects and individuals with diverse neurological conditions, rendering it a valuable resource for investigating brain structure and function. The OASIS dataset comprises approximately 140,000 images of both healthy and afflicted individuals. A noteworthy feature of this study is its use of the Leaky Rectified Linear Unit (ReLU), which enables the neurons' weights to be trainable even when input values are below zero. Additionally, an eight-layered CNN is employed, and data augmentation is applied due to the limited number of available images. In another study, Khan et al. [36] employed the ADNI dataset and utilized a 16-layer CNN with Transfer Learning (TL). This model closely resembles VGG-19 architecture and exhibits a 6% improvement in accuracy compared to the compared technique [37]. For the purpose of diagnosing Alzheimer's Disease (AD) using 2D MR images, a novel lightweight neural network named Biceph-net was recently introduced[38]. This network is designed to differentiate between Control (CN) and AD cases by training on gray matter brain regions, achieving a classification accuracy of 100%. However, further enhancements in sensitivity and specificity are required to validate the claimed classification accuracy.

14.4.2.3   Diagnosis and Prognosis of Heart Disease

Cardiovascular diseases have emerged as a significant global cause of mortality, particularly impacting developing nations in Africa and Asia. The early prediction of heart diseases not only empowers patients to take preventive measures but also enables healthcare professionals to understand the key factors leading to heart attacks and avert them before they manifest. This study [39] introduces a novel approach called CardioHelp, which employs Deep Convolutional Neural Networks to estimate the likelihood of cardiovascular disease presence in patients. The focus of our [39] method, CardioHelp, lies in temporal data analysis, utilizing CNN to forecast Heart Failure (HF) at its nascent stage. In their work, Nguyen et al. [40] proposed a real-time deep learning framework tailored for the classification of heart diseases within a medical context utilizing the Internet of Things (IoT). Their approach involves capturing heartbeat signals from ECG devices and processing them through a Wavelet Packet Decomposition (WPD) algorithm to obtain wavelet coefficients. The subsequent step involves feature extraction through a wavelet-based kernel Principal Component Analysis (WPCA). For the classification task, a deep neural network utilizing backpropagation is employed. This neural network consists of three hidden layers with node counts of 80, 40, and 20, respectively, to effectively classify various heart diseases. Mehmood et al. [39] focused on predicting the likelihood of a potential heart attack by employing attributes extracted from a dataset sourced from the UCI repository. The authors underscored the significance of attribute extraction methods in extracting valuable information for predictive purposes. They highlighted the potential of deriving diverse patterns through attribute extraction techniques to enable early heart disease prediction.

The research delved into various techniques within the domain of Artificial Neural Networks (ANN). The findings of the chapter indicated that while ANN achieved an accuracy of 94.7%, the implementation of principal component analysis resulted in a notable accuracy enhancement, reaching 97.7%.

14.4.3   DRUG DISCOVERY AND DEVELOPMENT

The process of discovering and developing a new drug is an intricate, time-consuming, expensive, and often inefficient journey that spans approximately 10 to 15 years. Even with significant investments, failures are not uncommon, leading to substantial financial setbacks. Despite technological advancements and a deep understanding of biological systems, the pharmaceutical industry has faced declining research and development productivity over the past 20 years [41]. This decline can be attributed to escalating costs and a reduction in the number of newly approved drugs. Regulatory challenges have grown, making it increasingly difficult to introduce innovative drugs, whether in new therapeutic areas or as superior alternatives to existing treatments. Given these challenges, the pursuit of innovative pharmaceutical solutions has grown more intricate. Advances in automation and information technology have generated vast data that can unveil patterns, potentially lowering drug discovery costs, enhancing patient survival rates, and enabling personalized care development.

In 2015, Wallach and colleagues presented AtomNet, a pioneering deep learning (DL) model, for the prediction of binding affinity in the context of drug discovery [42]. AtomNet was distinctive as it was the first DL model to utilize Convolutional Neural Networks (CNN) for predicting the binding affinity of small molecules. This approach uniquely integrated information from both the ligand and target protein structures. However, it's important to note that AtomNet necessitated the availability of three-dimensional (3D) structures for both the ligand and the target protein. These structures included the precise atom locations involved in the interaction at the target's binding site.

14.4.4   PRECISION MEDICINE AND GENOMICS

The rise of biotechnology and high-throughput sequencing has enabled researchers to analyze extensive genomic data. Given the enormity of this data, machine learning and deep learning methods are employed to decipher its meaning. These techniques aid in disease prediction, diagnosis, and the development of precision medicine tailored to individual genomes. Urda and colleagues [43] introduced a preliminary approach to employ a multi-layer feed-forward artificial neural network for the analysis of RNA-Seq gene expression data. Their model exhibited superior performance compared to the LASSO method when applied to the analysis of RNA-Seq gene expression profiles. Yuan and coauthors [44] introduced a convolutional neural network for co-expression (CNNC) that represents an advancement over previous techniques in deducing gene relationships from single-cell expression data tasks. This method holds applicability across diverse -omics research inquiries, spanning from prognosticating transcription factor targets to pinpointing disease-related genes and even causal inference. Another computational approach, DeepCpG (57), employs a CNN model for analyzing low-coverage single-cell methylation data. DeepCpG excels in predicting missing methylation states and identifying sequence motifs linked to alterations in methylation levels and inter-cell variability, surpassing the performance of state-of-the-art machine learning methods. Yuan and coauthors [44] introduced a convolutional neural network for co-expression (CNNC) that represents an advancement over previous techniques in deducing gene relationships from single-cell expression data tasks. This method holds applicability across diverse -omics research inquiries, spanning from prognosticating transcription factor targets to pinpointing disease-related genes and even causal inference. Another computational approach, DeepCpG [45], employs a CNN model for analyzing low-coverage single-cell methylation data. DeepCpG excels in predicting missing methylation states and identifying sequence motifs linked to alterations in methylation levels and inter-cell variability, surpassing the performance of state-of-the-art machine learning methods.

14.4.5 Medical Robotics and Surgical Assistance

Medical robotics and surgical assistance encompass a broad spectrum of technologies designed to assist surgeons and medical professionals in various aspects of patient care. These technologies encompass robotic systems assisting in surgery, and devices enhancing diagnostics and rehabilitation. These systems gather extensive data from diverse sensors, necessitating analysis to gauge practitioner skill levels. To accomplish this, ML and deep learning methods are utilized. These robots are able to perform the complex task of operating on humans or provide surgical assistance to doctors. Computer vision techniques based on DEEP CNN are employed in detecting surgical instruments, segmentation of instruments, tissue detection, action recognition, and physician skill assessment [46].

14.5 ETHICAL IMPLICATIONS OF DEEP CNN

The utilization of Deep Convolutional Neural Networks (CNNs) within the healthcare sector presents a range of ethical considerations that warrant thorough examination. As these robust AI-driven systems become increasingly prevalent in medical diagnoses, treatment strategies, and decision-making processes, it is imperative to address these ethical dilemmas to safeguard patient well-being, and privacy, and ensure equal access to high-quality healthcare. The following are some noteworthy ethical considerations linked to the implementation of deep CNNs in healthcare:

14.5.1 Safeguarding Patient Privacy and Data Security

The deployment of deep CNNs necessitates access to extensive patient data, encompassing medical records and images. Ensuring the confidentiality and security of this sensitive data is paramount to prevent unauthorized access, data breaches, and potential misuse.

14.5.2 Mitigating Bias and Ensuring Fairness

Inadequately trained and validated deep CNNs could inherit biases inherent in the training data, potentially leading to inaccurate diagnoses or treatment recommendations, especially for specific demographic groups. Ensuring impartial and equitable outcomes across diverse patient populations is a significant ethical concern.

14.5.3 Enhancing Transparency and Interpretability

Deep CNNs often operate as "black box" systems, rendering it challenging for healthcare practitioners to comprehend the rationale behind AI-generated decisions. Transparent and interpretable AI models are vital to foster trust and facilitate effective collaboration between AI systems and medical professionals.

14.5.4 Clarifying Clinical Responsibility and Accountability

Assigning liability and accountability when AI-generated recommendations deviate from human expert opinions is a complex issue. Clearly defining guidelines for the roles and responsibilities of healthcare practitioners and AI systems in patient care is crucial.

14.5.5 Informed Consent and Patient Autonomy

Patients should have the right to be informed when AI is involved in their diagnosis and treatment. Obtaining informed consent becomes more intricate when AI contributes to decision-making. Patients should retain autonomy in choosing between AI-driven approaches and traditional methods.

14.5.6 Preventing Overreliance on AI

Overreliance on AI-based diagnoses or treatment plans may potentially undermine the clinical judgment and expertise of healthcare professionals. Ensuring that AI serves as a supplementary tool rather than a complete substitute is of utmost importance.

14.5.7 Equitable Resource Allocation

The integration of deep CNNs demands substantial investments in terms of infrastructure, training, and upkeep. Ensuring equitable distribution of these resources, and avoiding contributions to healthcare inequalities, is an ethical consideration.

14.5.8 Balancing Intellectual Property and Accessibility

Ownership of AI algorithms and models employed in healthcare raises questions about intellectual property rights. Striking a balance between proprietary interests and the imperative of widespread access to life-saving technologies poses a challenge.

14.5.9 ANTICIPATING UNINTENDED CONSEQUENCES

The incorporation of AI in healthcare may lead to unanticipated outcomes, such as reduced human interaction in patient care, displacement of certain healthcare professionals' roles, and potential economic repercussions.

14.5.10 ESTABLISHING REGULATORY OVERSIGHT

Formulating appropriate regulations and standards for AI-driven healthcare technologies is crucial to ensuring patient safety and upholding the quality of care. Addressing these ethical implications necessitates collaborative efforts involving healthcare experts, AI specialists, policymakers, and regulatory entities. A well-balanced approach that prioritizes patient welfare, equity, and transparency is pivotal to harnessing the potential advantages of deep CNNs in healthcare while mitigating associated ethical challenges.

14.6 CONCLUSION

In summary, the integration of Deep Convolutional Neural Networks (CNNs) into healthcare presents a remarkable and transformative opportunity. These sophisticated AI-driven systems have exhibited exceptional capabilities in tasks such as medical diagnostics, treatment planning, and decision-making. As we venture into this dynamic realm, it is crucial to conscientiously address the ethical considerations that accompany these technological advancements. Protecting patient privacy and ensuring the security of medical data must be of utmost importance, safeguarding sensitive information from unauthorized access. Vigilance is essential to mitigate bias and uphold fairness, ensuring that AI-generated diagnoses and recommendations remain accurate and just across diverse patient groups.

Transparency and comprehensibility are pivotal to establishing trust between AI systems and healthcare professionals. Encouraging cooperation and mutual understanding necessitates AI models that can be intelligibly interpreted by medical experts. Navigating the intricate landscape of clinical responsibility and accountability is challenging as AI systems progressively impact patient care. Clearly defining the roles of healthcare practitioners and AI technologies is vital to prevent confusion and prioritize patient safety. The concept of informed consent becomes multifaceted when AI contributes to medical decision-making. Respecting patients' autonomy to choose between AI-assisted and traditional approaches becomes paramount. Guarding against overreliance on AI calls for strategic integration, placing AI as an adjunct tool to enhance the proficiency of healthcare professionals rather than replace it. Balancing resource allocation, intellectual property rights, and unintended consequences are essential to ensure equitable access to AI technologies and preclude unforeseen negative outcomes.

The establishment of robust regulatory frameworks becomes imperative to guide the responsible development, deployment, and utilization of deep CNNs in healthcare. These frameworks play a pivotal role in safeguarding patient well-being and upholding the highest standards of quality care. In this evolving healthcare landscape shaped by deep CNNs, successful navigation of ethical complexities requires a collaborative effort involving healthcare practitioners, AI specialists, policymakers, and regulatory bodies. Embracing a patient-centric, transparent, and equitable approach empowers us to harness the transformative potential of deep CNNs, revolutionizing healthcare while upholding ethical values, integrity, and the overall well-being of humanity.

REFERENCES

[1] Y. LeCun, Y. Bengio, G. Hinton, Deep learning, Nature 521 (7553) (2015) 436–444. doi:10.1038/nature14539.

[2] A. Esteva, A. Robicquet, B. Ramsundar, V. Kuleshov, M. DePristo, K. Chou, C. Cui, G. Corrado, S. Thrun, J. Dean, A guide to deep learning in healthcare, Nature Medicine 25 (1) (2019) 24–29. doi:10.1038/s41591-018-0316-z.

[3] A. Krizhevsky, I. Sutskever, G. E. Hinton, Imagenet classification with deep convolutional neural networks, in: Advances in Neural Information Processing Systems (NIPS), Springer, 2012, pp. 1097–1105.

[4] S. K. Pandey, R. R. Janghel, Recent deep learning techniques, challenges and its applications for medical healthcare system: A review, Neural Processing Letters 50 (2) (2019) 1907–1935. doi:10.1007/s11063-018-09976-2.

[5] M. M. Najafabadi, F. Villanustre, T. M. Khoshgoftaar, N. Seliya, R. Wald, E. Muharemagic, Deep learning applications and challenges in big data analytics, Journal of Big Data 2 (1) (2015) 1–21.

[6] S. Suthaharan, Big data classification: Problems and challenges in network intrusion prediction with machine learning, ACM SIGMETRICS Performance Evaluation Review 41 (4) (2014) 70–73.

[7] X. Glorot, A. Bordes, Y. Bengio, Domain adaptation for large-scale sentiment classification: A deep learning approach, in: Proceedings of the 28th International Conference on Machine Learning (ICML-11), Springer, 2011, pp. 513–520.

[8] X.-W. Chen, X. Lin, Big data deep learning: Challenges and perspectives, IEEE Access 2 (2014) 514–525.

[9] H.-I. Suk, D. Shen, Deep learning-based feature representation for ad/mci classification, in: Medical Image Computing and Computer-Assisted Intervention–MICCAI 2013: 16th International Conference, Nagoya, Japan, September 22–26, 2013, Proceedings, Part II 16, Springer, 2013, pp. 583–590.

[10] T. Brosch, R. Tam, A. D. N. Initiative, Manifold learning of brain MRIS by deep learning, in: Medical Image Computing and Computer-Assisted Intervention–MICCAI 2013: 16th International Conference, Nagoya, Japan, September 22–26, 2013, Proceedings, Part II 16, Springer, 2013, pp. 633–640.

[11] S. M. Plis, D. R. Hjelm, R. Salakhutdinov, E. A. Allen, H. J. Bockholt, J. D. Long, H. J. Johnson, J. S. Paulsen, J. A. Turner, V. D. Calhoun, Deep learning for neuroimaging: A validation study, Frontiers in Neuroscience 8 (2014) 229.

[12] D. Yang, S. Zhang, Z. Yan, C. Tan, K. Li, D. Metaxas, Automated anatomical landmark detection on distal femur surface using convolutional neural network, in: 2015 IEEE 12th International Symposium on Biomedical Imaging (ISBI), IEEE, 2015, pp. 17–21.

[13] Y. Zheng, D. Liu, B. Georgescu, H. Nguyen, D. Comaniciu, 3d deep learning for efficient and robust landmark detection in volumetric data, in: Medical Image Computing and Computer-Assisted Intervention–MICCAI 2015: 18th International Conference, Munich, Germany, October 5–9, 2015, Proceedings, Part I 18, Springer, 2015, pp. 565–572.

[14] F. C. Ghesu, B. Georgescu, T. Mansi, D. Neumann, J. Hornegger, D. Comaniciu, An artificial agent for anatomical landmark detection in medical images, in: Medical Image Computing and Computer-Assisted Intervention-MICCAI 2016: 19th International Conference, Athens, Greece, October 17–21, 2016, Proceedings, Part III 19, Springer, 2016, pp. 229–237.

[15] C. F. Baumgartner, K. Kamnitsas, J. Matthew, S. Smith, B. Kainz, D. Rueckert, Real-time standard scan plane detection and localisation in fetal ultrasound using fully convolutional neural networks, in: Medical Image Computing and Computer-Assisted Intervention–MICCAI 2016: 19th International Conference, Athens, Greece, October 17–21, 2016, Proceedings, Part II 19, Springer, 2016, pp. 203–211.

[16] Y. Xie, Z. Zhang, M. Sapkota, L. Yang, Spatial clockwork recurrent neural network for muscle perimysium segmentation, in: Medical Image Computing and Computer-Assisted Intervention–MICCAI 2016: 19th International Conference, Athens, Greece, October 17–21, 2016, Proceedings, Part II 19, Springer, 2016, pp. 185–193.

[17] G. Wu, M. Kim, Q. Wang, Y. Gao, S. Liao, D. Shen, Unsupervised deep feature learning for deformable registration of mr brain images, in: Medical Image Computing and Computer-Assisted Intervention–MICCAI 2013: 16th International Conference, Nagoya, Japan, September 22–26, 2013, Proceedings, Part II 16, Springer, 2013, pp. 649–656.

[18] X. Cheng, L. Zhang, Y. Zheng, Deep similarity learning for multimodal medical images, Computer Methods in Biomechanics and Biomedical Engineering: Imaging & Visualization 6 (3) (2018) 248–252.

[19] J. Krebs, T. Mansi, H. Delingette, L. Zhang, F. C. Ghesu, S. Miao, A. K. Maier, N. Ayache, R. Liao, A. Kamen, Robust non-rigid registration through agent-based action learning, in: Medical Image Computing and Computer Assisted Intervention- MICCAI 2017: 20th International Conference, Quebec City, QC, Canada, September 11–13, 2017, Proceedings, Part I 20, Springer, 2017, pp. 344–352.

[20] M. Simonovsky, B. Gutie´rrez-Becker, D. Mateus, N. Navab, N. Komodakis, A deep metric for multimodal registration, in: Medical Im- age Computing and Computer-Assisted Intervention-MICCAI 2016: 19th International Conference, Athens, Greece, October 17–21, 2016, Proceedings, Part III 19, Springer, 2016, pp. 10–18.

[21] M. Havaei, N. Guizard, H. Larochelle, P.-M. Jodoin, Deep learning trends for focal brain pathology segmentation in MRI, Machine Learning for Health Informatics: State-of-the-Art and Future Challenges (2016) 125–148.

[22] C. G. Chee, Y. Kim, Y. Kang, K. J. Lee, H.-D. Chae, J. Cho, C.-M. Nam, D. Choi, F. Lee, J. W. Lee, et al., Performance of a deep learning algorithm in detecting osteonecrosis of the femoral head on digital radiography: A comparison with assessments by radiologists, American Journal of Roentgenology 213 (1) (2019) 155–162.

[23] C. C. Aggarwal, et al., Neural networks and deep learning, Springer 10 (978) (2018) 3.

[24] X. Li, Y. Jiang, Y. Liu, J. Zhang, S. Yin, H. Luo, Ragcn: Region aggregation graph convolutional network for bone age assessment from x-ray images, IEEE Transactions on Instrumentation and Measurement 71 (2022) 1–12.

[25] X. Li, Y. Jiang, J. Zhang, M. Li, H. Luo, S. Yin, Lesion-attention pyramid network for diabetic retinopathy grading, Artificial Intelligence in Medicine 126 (2022) 102259.

[26] R. Suman, M. Javaid, A. Haleem, R. Vaishya, S. Bahl, D. Nandan, Sustainability of coronavirus on different surfaces, Journal of Clinical and Experimental Hepatology 10 (4) (2020) 386–390.

[27] World Health Organization, et al., Coronavirus disease 2019 (COVID-19): Situation report, 73 (2020).

[28] A. Haleem, M. Javaid, R. Vaishya, Effects of COVID-19 pandemic in daily life, Current Medicine Research and Practice, 10 (2) (2020) 78–79.

[29] A. Abbas, M. M. Abdelsamea, M. M. Gaber, Classification of covid-19 in chest x-ray images using detrac deep convolutional neural network, Applied Intelligence 51 (2021) 854–864.

[30] L. Wang, Z. Q. Lin, A. Wong, Covid-net: A tailored deep convolutional neural network design for detection of covid-19 cases from chest x-ray images, Scientific Reports 10 (1) (2020) 19549.

[31] E. E.-D. Hemdan, M. A. Shouman, M. E. Karar, Covidx-net: A framework of deep learning classifiers to diagnose covid-19 in x-ray images, arXiv preprint arXiv:2003.11055 (2020).

[32] R. Sharma, T. Goel, M. Tanveer, C. T. Lin, R. Murugan, Deep learning based diagnosis and prognosis of Alzheimer's disease: A comprehensive review, IEEE Transactions on Cognitive and Developmental Systems (2023) 1–1. doi:10.1109/TCDS.2023.3254209.

[33] X. Wang, M. L Michaelis, E. K Michaelis, Functional genomics of brain aging and Alzheimer's disease: Focus on selective neuronal vulnerability, Current Genomics 11 (8) (2010) 618–633.

[34] Y. LeCun, Y. Bengio, G. Hinton, Deep learning, Nature 521 (7553) (2015) 436–444.

[35] S.-H. Wang, P. Phillips, Y. Sui, B. Liu, M. Yang, H. Cheng, Classification of Alzheimer's disease based on eight-layer convolutional neural network with leaky rectified linear unit and max pooling, Journal of Medical Systems 42 (2018) 1–11.

[36] N. M. Khan, N. Abraham, M. Hon, Transfer learning with intelligent training data selection for prediction of Alzheimer's disease, IEEE Access 7 (2019) 72726–72735.

[37] E. Hosseini-Asl, G. Gimel'farb, A. El-Baz, Alzheimer's disease diagnostics by a deeply supervised adaptable 3d convolutional network, arXiv preprint arXiv:1607.00556 (2016).

[38] A. H. Rashid, A. Gupta, J. Gupta, M. Tanveer, Biceph-net: A robust and lightweight framework for the diagnosis of Alzheimer's disease using 2d-MRI scans and deep similarity learning, IEEE Journal of Biomedical and Health Informatics 27 (3) (2022) 1205–1213.

[39] A. Mehmood, M. Iqbal, Z. Mehmood, A. Irtaza, M. Nawaz, T. Nazir, M. Masood, Prediction of heart disease using deep convolutional neural networks, Arabian Journal for Science and Engineering 46 (4) (2021) 3409–3422.

[40] T.-H. Nguyen, T.-N. Nguyen, T.-T. Nguyen, A deep learning framework for heart disease classification in an IoTs-based system, A Handbook of Internet of Things in Biomedical and Cyber Physical System (2020) 217–244.

[41] A. Lavecchia, Deep learning in drug discovery: Opportunities, challenges and future prospects, Drug Discovery Today 24 (10) (2019) 2017–2032.

[42] I. Wallach, M. Dzamba, A. Heifets, Atomnet: A deep convolutional neural network for bioactivity prediction in structure-based drug discovery, arXiv preprint arXiv:1510.02855 (2015).

[43] D. Urda, J. Montes-Torres, F. Moreno, L. Franco, J. M. Jerez, Deep learning to analyze rna-seq gene expression data, in: Advances in Computational Intelligence: 14th International Work-Conference on Artificial Neural Networks, IWANN 2017, Cadiz, Spain, June 14–16, 2017, Proceedings, Part II 14, Springer, 2017, pp. 50–59.

[44] Y. Yuan, Z. Bar-Joseph, Deep learning for inferring gene relationships from single-cell expression data, Proceedings of the National Academy of Sciences 116 (52) (2019) 27151–27158.

[45] C. Angermueller, H. J. Lee, W. Reik, O. Stegle, Deepcpg: Accurate prediction of single-cell DNA methylation states using deep learning, Genome Biology 18 (1) (2017) 1–13.

[46] S. M. Hussain, A. Brunetti, G. Lucarelli, R. Memeo, V. Bevilacqua, D. Buongiorno, Deep learning based image processing for robot assisted surgery: A systematic literature survey, IEEE Access 10 (2022) 122627–122657. doi:10.1109/ACCESS.2022.3223704.

15 An Improved Multi-Class Breast Cancer Classification and Abnormality Detection Based on Modified Deep Learning Neural Network Principles

Jullie Josephine D.C., Sudhakar J.,
Helan Vidhya T., Anusuya R., and Ramkumar G.

15.1 INTRODUCTION

When it comes to diagnosing medical conditions and evaluating the results of clinical trials, medical imaging is a crucial tool. Cancer therapy that takes advantage of biomedical imaging is essential. Today, cancer represents a huge threat to global health. In 2018, cancer was responsible for 9.6 million deaths, and it is expected to cause 10 million fatalities worldwide in 2020, as reported by the WHO. Breast cancer tumors result from cellular proliferation that is out of control [1]. Also, as life expectancy, development, and Western habits spread throughout the developing globe, so does the prevalence of breast cancer there. While there is some promise in reducing risk through avoidance, early identification remains critical to enhancing breast cancer prognosis and survival.

Among females, breast cancer is the second-greatest cause of mortality. When a cluster of cancerous cells grows abnormally in the breast, it is called breast cancer. The mammary glands of the breast are the original source of these cells. The pace at which these abnormal cells multiply and their impact on surrounding normal cells, which can spread throughout the body, are key factors in determining their categorization. The most common kind of cancer among females is breast cancer. But 42% of NHS trusts say they don't have enough employees to assign patients because they have so little professional nursing expertise in breast cancer, according to a poll by Breast Cancer Care (BCC). Detection methods for breast cancer were developed so

DOI: 10.1201/9781032635149-15

that anomalies in breast tissue could be identified and the disease could be classified. The purpose of doing so is to aid in the detection of breast cancer [2].

The standard method of breast cancer detection is mammography. Ultrasound, MRI, X-ray, and recent developments like molecular breast imaging and digital breast tomosynthesis (DBT) are just a few of the methods that may be used to examine the breast. Mammography, an imaging modality that examines the breast using low-dose X-ray equipment, is the gold standard for detecting anomalies in the breast before they can be clinically palpable [3]. It has been shown that roughly 50% of pre-existing lesions on mammograms are now detectable using retrospective imaging due to improved screening and follow-up throughout the diagnostic phase. Figure 15.1 displays several breast cancer pictures. Therefore, it caused radiologists to speculate that even mammograms taken a few years ago that showed no obvious

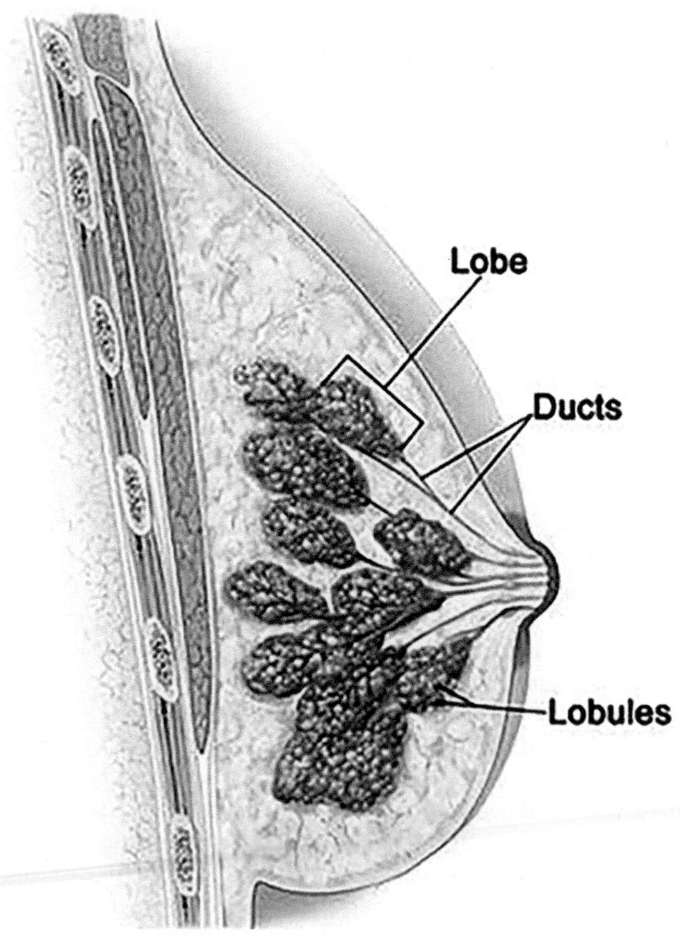

FIGURE 15.1 Breast cancer dataset.

abnormalities could really carry information about the patient's future risk of tumor development. Using databases of ultrasound images, a very effective computer-aided device for early breast cancer diagnosis may be created. These real-time, inexpensive, non-invasive screening and diagnostic tools are highly convenient. An agreed-upon naming system radiologists often utilize the Breast Imaging Reporting and Data System (BI-RADS) to categorize the many image-based elements typically described in breast imaging.

Psychologically, computer-aided detection (CAD) techniques for breast cancer are essential because they reduce radiologists' workload and improve detection accuracy. The standard approach to identifying and labeling medical abnormalities such as breast masses, skin lesions, and brain tumors relies on pattern identification. Breast cancer detection often begins with a human operator manually extracting information from a mammogram before feeding those features into a machine learning classifier. Still, various imaging difficulties and differences in the tumor locations make it difficult to get an appropriate categorization. This means that over the past decade, AI has played an increasingly important role in the diagnosis and classification of medical infections, most notably breast cancer. The development of CAD methods for identifying anomalies has received a lot of attention because of the critical nature of breast cancer screening. Detecting small but critical abnormalities in mammograms has always been a task for CAD methods that relied on manually created picture characteristics [4]. With the advent of deep neural networks, it is now possible to automatically learn features from massive amounts of training data, allowing for a comprehensive solution that encompasses everything from feature extraction to classifier development. This learning system is also well-suited to abnormality detection in mammography since it is resistant to noise in training data.

Mammography abnormality detection as well as computer-aided diagnosis have recently been developed and are crucial in screening for breast cancer. New developments in machine learning and deep learning (DL) systems have emerged as potent tools, allowing for automatic feature extraction and identification across many domains, including medical pictures. Recent research employing DL techniques, in particular convolutional neural networks with supervised learning, has enhanced radiologists' capacity to detect even the tiniest breast tumors in the early stages, therefore notifying radiologists when additional study is required. While supervised approaches have a better track record overall, they are susceptible to failure when assessing data that is vastly dissimilar to what the model was trained on. Supervised learning also necessitates massive investments of time and people to label massive volumes of training information.

Recent developments in image processing, and notably in medical image processing, have sparked optimism that effective automated systems for detecting and classifying breast cancer could one day be developed. Computer algorithms are becoming increasingly valuable in the medical industry, and those that are utilized in deep learning can leverage the layers of neural networks to identify patterns [5]. Although there has been a lot of progress made in automating breast cancer applications, it is still difficult to correctly identify or classify breast abnormalities. Moreover, deep learning needs huge training data, which is notoriously hard to come by in the medical arena. Consequently, there is room for improvement in the precision of cancer screening through the study of automated applications for breast cancer detection.

To locate and diagnose breast cancers with the same or greater effectiveness as human interpretation, machine learning has recently shown enthusiasm for adopting modern algorithms that can extract sophisticated information. To help radiologists save time and effort in interpreting and evaluating mammogram pictures, deep learning techniques have been devised, made possible by the ever-increasing availability of mammography data and the existence of huge computing machines.

In this study, researchers used a sophisticated neural network technique called differential evolution to classify breast cancer into its several subtypes. A Deep Neural Network (DNN) was used as the basis for the technique's classification model. Variable values were optimized with the help of Mayfly Optimization, and feature vectors were created with the help of an EfficientNet feature extractor. As a result, the study utilized deep learning to successfully categorize hyper-spectral data. In this chapter, we looked at how DNN may be used to shed light on hidden data properties, ultimately allowing for the more accurate categorization of breast cancer data using DNN at every level of its processing.

15.2 RELATED WORKS

Subtyping cancer is a critical first step toward individualized therapy, providing important insights into the study of cancer heterogeneity. Molecular subgroups of cancer have been established in breast cancer research to correlate with distinct patient outcomes and treatment strategies. Recent research, however, has shown inconsistencies in subtype classifications of breast cancer using various methodologies, indicating that the present methods have not been optimized. Besides being inefficient in dealing with high-dimensional data beyond gene expression, the current crop of computation-based approaches is constrained by their reliance on insufficient previous information. Moanna is a revolutionary deep learning-based system that can include multi-omics data for subtyping breast cancer. To facilitate generalization, Moanna is built on a semi-supervised Autoencoder and a multi-task learning system for analyzing gene expression, copy number, and somatic mutation data simultaneously. To evaluate Moanna's performance, we first employed a subset of the METABRIC breast cancer dataset for training purposes, before testing it on the full dataset and an independent collection of TCGA samples. We utilized Autoencoder to identify breast cancer subtype-related patterns; the author in [6] showed that it outperformed other dimensionality reduction techniques. The whole Moanna model also performed exceptionally well when predicting ER status (96%), differentiating basal-like samples (98%), and classifying samples into PAM50 subtypes (85%). More so than the initial PAM50 subtypes, Moanna's projected subtypes are significantly correlated with patient survival.

The chances of recovery are considerably improved by prompt diagnosis and therapy. Long-term death rates from breast cancer can also be drastically reduced with early detection. The highest chance of survival can be achieved by detecting cancer cells as soon as possible. Mammography, ultrasonography, positron emission tomography, and biopsies are only some of the diagnostic methods for breast cancer that have been studied [7]. However, these approaches aren't ideal because of their high price tag, lengthy procedure duration, and inapplicability to younger ladies. There must be an immediate and sensitive method for diagnosing breast cancer in its earliest stages. Research into nanoparticles, particularly those with potential medicinal applications, has expanded recently due to the exponential development of nanotechnology. Research into gold nanoparticles (AuNPs) and their application as research instruments yields new insights that push the limits of nanotechnology forward at a rapid pace. The potential of AuNPs in all stages of cancer care, from detection and monitoring to therapy, is attracting more and more attention. Since cancer is a complex disease with many potential causes, these initiatives seek to completely revamp the way the disease is currently treated.

In order to combat cancer, one of the most pressing health issues of the modern day, applications of artificial intelligence are crucial. Skin cancer constitutes one of the most common types of cancer, and a study in [8] looked into deep learning methods that might be beneficial in the diagnosis of breast cancer at its earliest stages. Investigators were capable of telling if cases of breast cancers, as well as skin cancers, were benign or malignant by using deep learning algorithms. The classifications were made using the Convolutional Neural Network (CNN) algorithm, which is part of the deep learning methodology. Based on the type of cancer being investigated, the data sets are classified as either benign or malignant. With the help of the outcomes from the logistic regression method, we compared the two types of success charts we created from the data we analyzed. The results may be seen in the accuracy and loss graphs for both cancer kinds. The research's stated goal is to use deep learning to evaluate the similarities and differences between breast and skin cancers. And sometimes, doctors mistake breast cancer for skin cancer. This study established a framework for distinguishing between these two cancer forms in future research.

The current imaging methods for breast cancer have some restrictions. As an alternative to or perhaps a replacement for traditional imaging modalities, diffuse optical imaging has demonstrated promising results in the diagnosis and tracking of therapy responses in breast cancer. Diffuse optical breast-scanning (DOB-Scan) probe may distinguish between healthy and cancerous breast tissue using a machine learning algorithm, as demonstrated by the author in [9]. We have used our model to predict the optical parameters of malignant and normal breasts in a dataset containing information from 15 individuals with breast cancer. In order to estimate the scattering coefficients for individual patients, a regression model is used that takes into account the relationship between radial reflectance as well as optical tissue qualities. Due to the model's classification capabilities, researchers have discovered substantial disparities in the scattering coefficients of healthy and cancerous cells. Scattering results for the longitudinal information have also been computed, allowing for a more nuanced evaluation of patients' reactions to chemotherapy. To conclude, the diffuse optical scattering coefficient showed promise as an early predictor of breast cancer in our study.

Cancer's increasing prevalence and status as a major killer make it a pressing public health concern. In recent years, research has demonstrated that breast cancer has become one of the most common types of cancer among women. Individuals with breast cancer have a better chance of survival and can save money on treatment if it is caught early. Nevertheless, there are limitations to the current healthcare systems' emphasis on early identification. All people have a hard time gaining access to these services, and they require a lot of human resources and have lasting impacts. Technologies that are easy to use, corroborated by scientific methods, and universally accessible are needed for early breast cancer diagnosis. Breast cancer can now be detected and treated earlier, thanks to advances in artificial intelligence. The purpose of [10] is to identify characteristics that distinguish between benign and malignant breast cancers in images. We employed the ANN, SVM, and RF classifiers to categorize the characteristics extracted from the photos. The Wisconsin Breast Cancer dataset was used for the experiments. The Artificial Neural Network technique was shown to be responsible for 99% of the best results in experimental evaluations.

15.3 METHODOLOGY

15.3.1 DATASETS

In these fields, researchers often use Figure 15.2's Wisconsin Breast Cancer Dataset (WBCD). Features are derived from digitalized pictures of breast mass cells obtained by fine needle aspiration (FNA) biopsy. Investigators want to use this information to develop models for forecasting that can indicate, given a set of characteristics, which tumors have a greater probability of being benign and those that are more probable to be malignant. The 699 cases in the dataset come in for a single biopsy. The diagnosis determines whether or not these cases are classified as benign (non-cancerous) or malignant (cancerous). The WBCD is a small, well-defined dataset that is ideal for

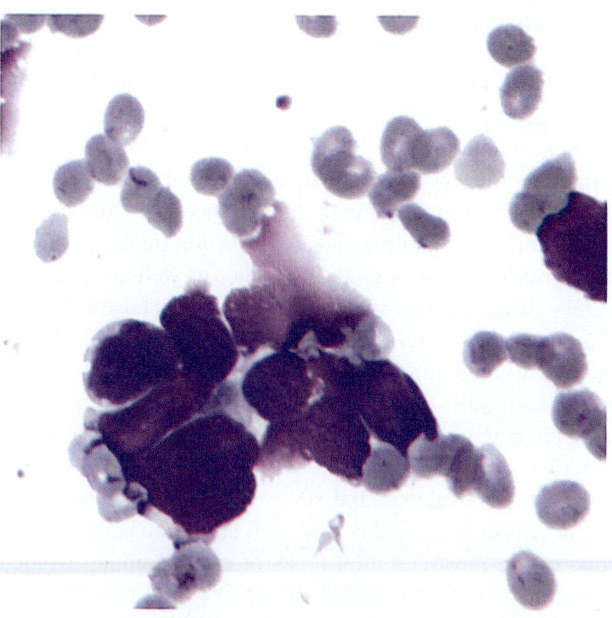

FIGURE 15.2 Wisconsin breast cancer dataset.

use as a starting point when learning about and experimenting using techniques for categorization in the field of machine learning.

15.3.2 DATA PREPROCESSING

In order to elevate the quality of raw pictures, eliminate unwanted noise, and increase the precision of analysis prior to additional analysis or processing using methods like computer vision, image recognition, as well as machine learning, a set of techniques known as "image preprocessing" must be done to them. Figure 15.3 demonstrates the importance of image preprocessing in addressing differences in lighting circumstances, noise, and other defects that might hinder algorithmic effectiveness. The input dimensions must be constant across the whole dataset for training models, thus resizing photographs to a fixed size is a must. The computational burden of training and inference can be lightened by resizing pictures to lower size. Models may be trained more effectively and delivered on devices with limited resources if pictures are scaled down.

15.3.3 DATA AUGMENTATION

The purpose of data augmentation is to fortify models against input data fluctuations, enhance generalization, and broaden the scope of training instances. When there is a scarcity of training data, this method shines. Resizing works well in tandem with other methods of enhancing data. To create augmented copies of the same picture that may be used to expand the training dataset, photos are resized to bigger dimensions before being cropped or padded to the required input size. Image data is effectively doubled when flipped horizontally or vertically. This is especially helpful for jobs in which the orientation of an item doesn't make a difference to its properties.

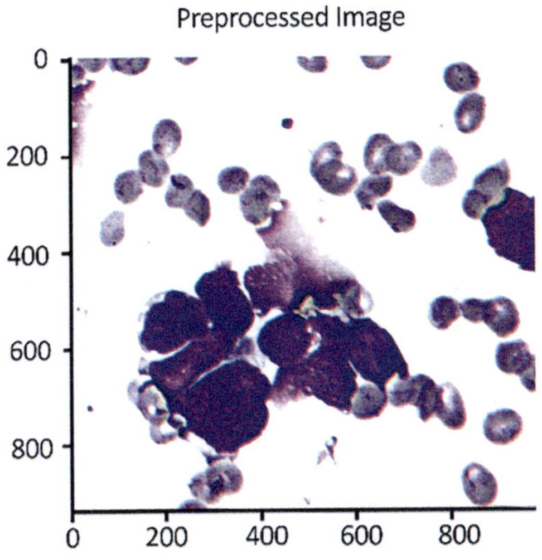

FIGURE 15.3 Pre-processed image.

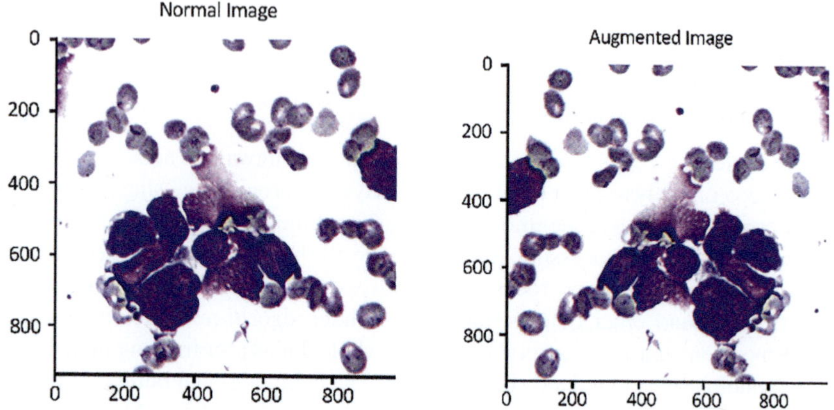

FIGURE 15.4　Normal and augmented image.

Image perspective and orientation changes can be simulated by rotating them over a range of angles. Data augmentation is typically incorporated into the deep learning framework's information loading pipeline. While being input into the model, every set of information undergoes real-time enhancement throughout the training phase. This saves us from having to implicitly save every upgraded version of the data. In Figure 15.4, we see both the original and the modified picture.

15.3.4　EfficientNet Feature Extractor

With the goal of striking a balance among model size, computational effectiveness, and effectiveness on a variety of computer vision applications, EfficientNet is a family of convolutional neural network (CNN) structures. To maximize the neural network's performance in both depth and breadth, the EfficientNet design makes use of a revolutionary compound scaling approach. This method paves the way for the creation of more accurate and efficient models that can be used with a wide variety of available resources. Different iterations of the EfficientNet model (EfficientNet-B0, EfficientNet-B1, . . . , EfficientNet-B7) exist. Different scaling parameters in these variants establish the network's depth, breadth, and total amount of layers. Varieties with higher version numbers tend to be bigger and more powerful, but they may also be more resource intensive to run. The suggested model's architecture is depicted in Figure 15.5.

The weights that were previously trained in an EfficientNet network, which has been learned on a large dataset, often ImageNet, can be used in the context of employing EfficientNet as a method for extracting features. Develop a feature extractor that reliably extracts informative visual features from photos by skipping the last categorization layer and instead utilizing the ones that came before it as features. After gathering these characteristics, they may be used in further processing for things like categorization, object identification, and segmentation.

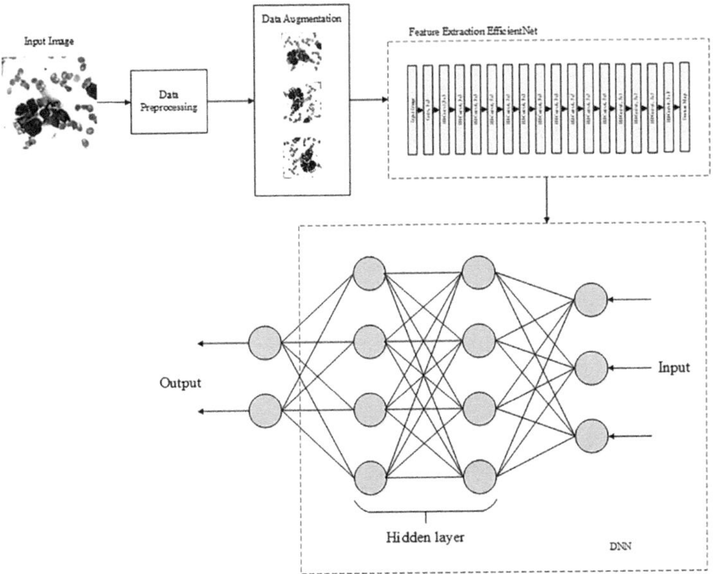

FIGURE 15.5 Architecture of proposed model.

15.3.5 Benefits of Using EfficientNet as a Feature Extractor

In order to capture important characteristics from pictures while minimizing computing costs, the EfficientNet model was developed. It is possible to transfer the robust features that pre-trained EfficientNet models have learned on big datasets to smaller tasks with fewer data points. For many image classification applications, EfficientNet's compound scaling method provides satisfactory results.

These are the standard procedures for employing EfficientNet as a feature extractor:

1. Load a pre-trained EfficientNet model.
2. Remove the classification layers (usually the final dense layers).
3. Extract features from your dataset using the modified model.
4. Use the extracted features as input for your downstream tasks or models.

Extracting useful features from breast cancer pictures using a pre-trained EfficientNet model is the goal of using an EfficientNet feature extractor for classification. When fed into a classifier, these traits can help determine whether a tumor shown in a biopsy picture is benign or malignant. Without having to train a whole CNN from start, an EfficientNet feature extractor can help you access the potential of deep learning for breast cancer categorization. A smaller collection of breast cancer photos can nevertheless yield respectable results with careful attention paid to feature extraction and fine-tuning. The benefits of deep learning may be utilized for a wide range of computer vision applications while considerable training time and computing resources are saved using this method.

15.3.6   Deep Neural Network

Artificial neural networks having several hidden layers between the input and output layers are known as Deep Neural Networks (DNNs). Digital neural networks (DNNs) are built to learn hierarchical representations of input, which allows them to deal with complicated patterns and jobs. Here is an excellent breakdown of what goes into constructing a Deep Neural Network.

15.3.7   Input Layer

Information in any form (pictures, text, audio, etc.) is sent into the system at the input layer. This layer's neuron count is proportional to the total amount of dimensions included in the input data.

15.3.8   Hidden Layers

Among the input as well as output levels, there are hidden layers that serve as intermediaries. There are many neurons within every buried layer, and they all work together to process data and pass it on to the layer below. The extent to which the network has these undiscovered levels is what gives it its "deep" character.

15.3.9   Neurons

In a DNN, the neurons use an activation function to compute utilizing the information that they receive. The output of one neuron feeds into the input of the next neuron in the same layer. With proper training, neurons can detect and extract characteristics from a variety of data sources.

15.3.10   Weights and Biases

There are biases and weights associated with each neuronal connection. These weights are modified throughout the training process in order to reduce the deviation from the desired output. Optimization methods, including gradient descent, are used to make these modifications.

15.3.11   Activation Functions

Networks may learn intricate correlations in the data when non-linearity is introduced via activation functions. Rectified Linear Unit (ReLU), sigmoid, as well as tanh activation functions are typical examples.

15.3.12   Output Layer

Final forecasts or categorizations are generated at the output layer using the characteristics learned in the previous levels. Whether this layer has a small number of neurons or a large number of neurons depends on the job at hand (binary classification, multi-class classification, regression, etc.).

15.3.13 Loss Function

The loss function is a metric that evaluates how far the model is from the desired output. The objective of training is to use optimization methods to find the minimum value of this loss function.

In order to determine if a particular breast cancer biopsy picture represents a benign or malignant tumor, a Deep Neural Network (DNN) can be built and trained. Collect a database of photos depicting breast cancer, together with labels indicating whether the tumors seen are benign or malignant. The photos should be preprocessed by scaling them all to the same input size and adjusting the brightness and contrast. The size of the input layer should correspond to the size of the photos before processing. The data that is fed to the system is going to be a matrix containing the pixel values for every picture. Convolutional layers downsample the dimension of the picture to minimize computation, while pooling layers learn local characteristics from the pictures. To learn hierarchical features, we can combine several convolutional and pooling layers. Following the convolutional and dense layers, add non-linearity with activation functions like ReLU (Rectified Linear Unit). A sigmoid activation function applied to a single neuron in the output layer can calculate the likelihood of cancer. The effectiveness of the DNN may be improved by experimenting with alternative values for the hyperparameters that control its learning rate, number of layers, number of neurons, and dropout rates.

15.3.14 Mayfly Optimization

The mating rituals of the Ephemeroptera insects, which include mayflies, serve as the inspiration for the Mayfly Optimization method. The purpose of this method is to locate optimum or near-optimal solutions to optimization problems. In the realm of optimization algorithms, Mayfly Optimization ranks lower in popularity than its more well-known counterparts such as Genetic Algorithms and Particle Swarm Optimization.

A brief summary of Mayfly Optimization is as follows:

1. The average life span of a mayfly is only a few hours. Mayflies spend their short time as adults flying about in search of mates. Mayfly Optimization is based on this mating behavior, which combines exploration and selection.
2. Mayfly Population: The method keeps track of a group of hypothetical insects that each stand in for a different possible answer to the optimization issue.
3. Mating and Selection: Each mayfly is given a fitness score that reflects how well it solved the optimization issue. More likely to reproduce and pass on their characteristics to offspring are mayflies who have greater fitness scores.
4. Exploration and Exploitation: The mayfly does exploration by hopping to uncharted areas of the search space. The process of exploitation entails focusing the investigation on the most promising options.
5. Mating and Reproduction: Mayflies are paired off in Mayfly Optimization depending on their fitness scores. These matings help generate novel possibilities by mixing and matching characteristics of the parent mayflies.

6. Movement and Adaptation: Members of the mayfly population probe the search space by shifting places according to predetermined norms. The physical condition of the individual mayfly, the optimal solution discovered so far, and the behavior of neighboring mayflies all play a role in motivating their own movement.

7. Termination Criterion: The method repeats its steps until some condition is fulfilled, such as the maximum amount of iterations, a fixed degree of convergence, or the achievement of a desired result.

Depending on the issue area, issue characteristics, as well as variable settings, Mayfly Optimization's effectiveness might vary, hence it has not been as widely accepted as similar well-established techniques for optimization. Tuning technique parameters, picking suitable fitness functions, and comprehending the nature of the issue at hand are all necessary for the successful implementation of any optimization technique.

15.4   RESULTS AND DISCUSSION

Training, validation, and testing sets were created from the datasets for the purpose of model evaluation. To do this, we utilize what is called a "training set," which is just a representation of the sample data. This information is used by the latter to learn, and it accounts for 80% of the data it uses. Forty percent from each group was taken into account to guarantee diversity. Tuning the parameters necessitates the selection of a validation set to prevent bias in the evaluation of the training set. The remaining 20% was split evenly between the test set and the evaluation set. Selecting optimal values for our model's variables is the primary function of the validation set. The model is being thoroughly assessed with the help of the test set. Test accuracy, validation accuracy, and training accuracy are therefore used as measures.

The preliminary findings demonstrate that the model is overfitting and does poorly on extended datasets. Dropout regularization was explored as a potential solution to this issue. During training, dropout regularization is known to disregard a random subset of neurons regardless of whether or not they are hidden. Layer activation and picture characteristics are two examples of inputs that may be removed using this method. The model is eventually forced to learn more robust features due to this change in network architecture, which improves the model's generalizability. Using the original data and the enhanced pictures, the datasets were rebuilt. At first, it wasn't considered important to keep track of how many photographs fell into each category. While testing out several combinations of classes, it became apparent that one class had too few photos, which might be affecting the validation performance. More photographs were evaluated in each category, and existing ones were enhanced. The effectiveness of several models is compared in Table 15.1. Figures 15.6, 15.7, 15.8, and 15.9. compare the various models with regard to precision, sensitivity, specificity, and accuracy.

The model is improved much more by playing about with the learning rate. Several tests led to the conclusion that the model could accurately represent the underlying primitives. However, more training was shown to be necessary when attempting to master higher-level features. Indeed, we modified the network's weights during

TABLE 15.1

Performance Evaluation of Various Models

Model	Precision	Sensitivity	Specificity	Accuracy
SVM	0.88	0.89	0.86	0.87
RF	0.90	0.92	0.93	0.93
Inception	0.91	0.88	0.89	0.92
MobileNet	0.94	0.93	0.92	0.93
AlexNet	0.95	0.94	0.93	0.94
Proposed	0.98	0.97	0.98	0.96

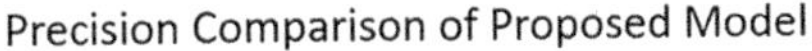
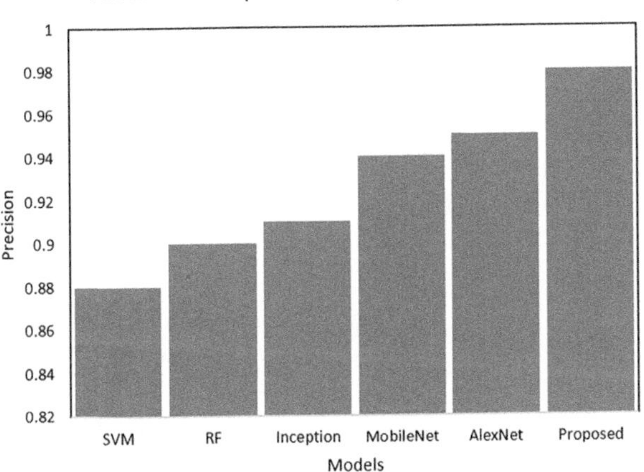

FIGURE 15.6 Accurate model comparisons.

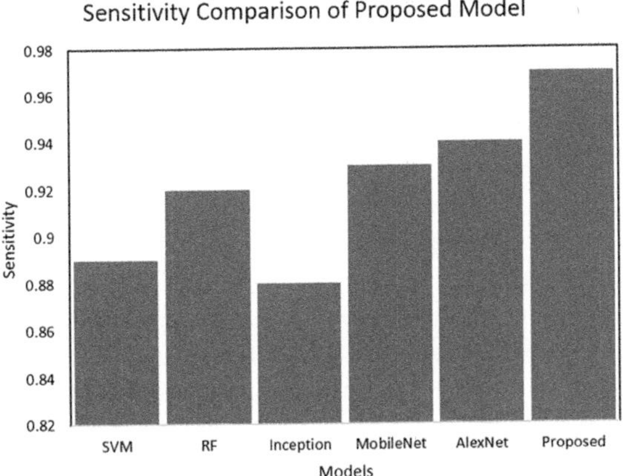

FIGURE 15.7 The sensitivity of different models.

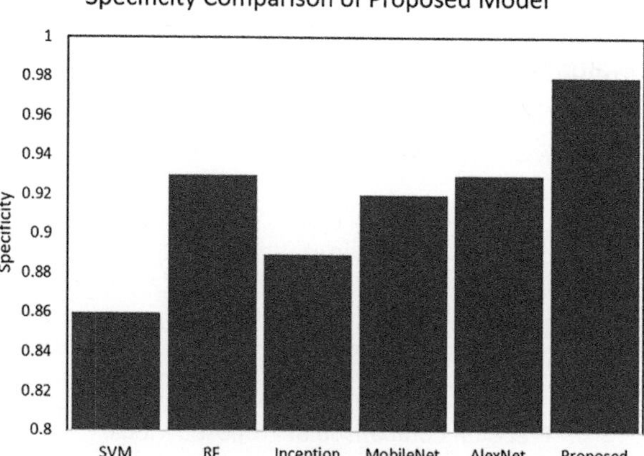

FIGURE 15.8 Model specificity evaluation.

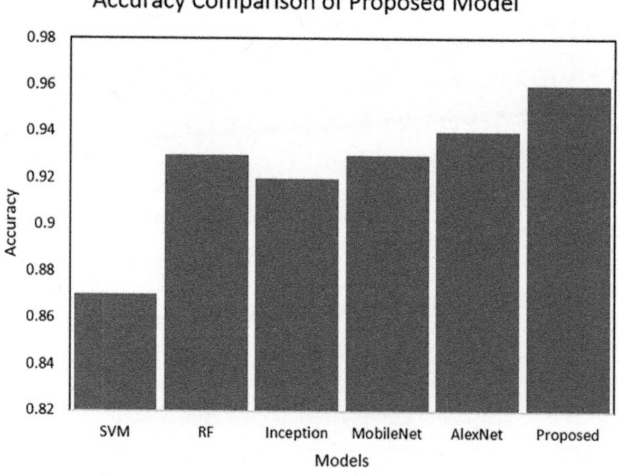

FIGURE 15.9 Evaluation of model accuracy.

training at regular intervals (per epoch) and at a fixed learning rate. To achieve the lowest possible error, selecting the best possible learning rate is crucial. Setting a fixed pace of learning is one option. However, if the value is more than the ideal value, the system will still create curve fluctuations. If, on the other hand, the chosen value is suboptimal, the model will slow the pace of convergence. In addition, we have employed two methods to make the learning rate adaptable in every stage of training during the testing phase since picking the ideal value of the learning rate is a difficult assignment. The first method takes into account the learning curve, which is evaluated after each stage of implementation. If an upward trend is seen, the learning rate is slowed by a multiplicative factor determined by a variable coefficient whose value is less than one. Support Vector Machine (SVM), Random Forest (RF), Inception (IN), MobileNet (MNET), AlexNet (AltNet), and the proposed model (proposed) are the models tested. The SVM model attained a precision of 0.88, sensitivity of 0.89, specificity of 0.86, and accuracy of 0.87. A precision of 0.90, sensitivity of 0.92, specificity of 0.93, and accuracy of 0.93 are all very respectable results for the RF model. The Inception model has a sensitivity of 0.88, specificity of 0.89, and precision of 0.91. The MobileNet model did quite well, with a sensitivity of 0.93, a specificity of 0.92, and a precision of 0.94. High precision was demonstrated by the AlexNet model, which had a value of 0.95, sensitivity of 0.94, specificity of 0.93, and accuracy of 0.94. The suggested model has superior performance to all previous models, with a remarkable 0.96 accuracy rate, sensitivity of 0.97, and specificity of 0.98.

With each successive rise, the learning rate is multiplied by a variable coefficient with a value greater than one. The improved model was then put to the test on the validation data. With the improved model, the training accuracy is 96.7% on the training set and 95.3% on the validation set (Figure 15.10). This demonstrates how the improved CNN achieves better results and can pick up on more generic characteristics for accurate breast abnormality classification. Loss on both the training and validation sets converges toward zero, as seen in Figure 15.11.

Accuracy, precision, recall, and F1-score were only a few of the assessment criteria used to contrast the model's recommendations with those of others. A confusion matrix was used for the assessment of these features. Figure 15.12 shows how this matrix was used in the study to get at the details. Using 20% of the training data for the test data helps to shed light on discrepancies caused by overfitting. The suggested model is more trustworthy than competing ones since it has fewer instances of incorrect data classification.

Earlier, in Table 15.2 and Figure 15.13, we can see the temporal complexity of several models in seconds (s). Every model's execution time is shown under "Time Complexity (s)." This data is useful for contrasting the computational effectiveness of different models' execution times. Time complexity is lowest for the SVM, coming in at just 36.49 seconds. After that comes the RF, which takes 57.848 seconds to calculate. It takes 93.451 seconds to complete Inception. MobileNet takes 117.83

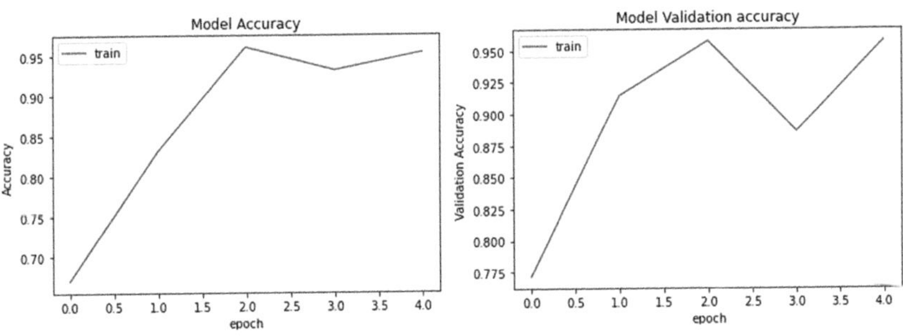

FIGURE 15.10 The validity and precision of several models.

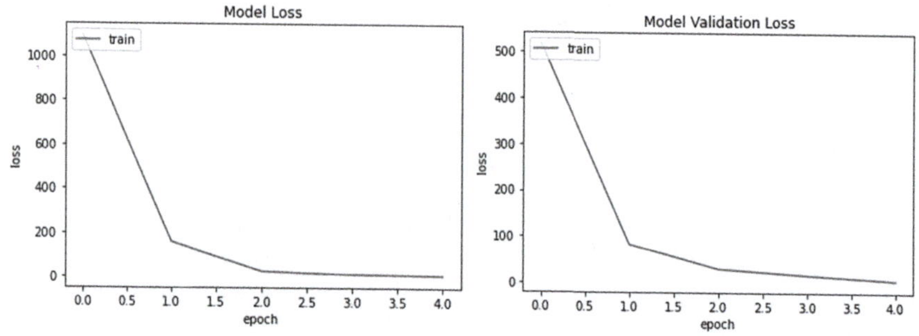

FIGURE 15.11 Comparison of model and validation error rates.

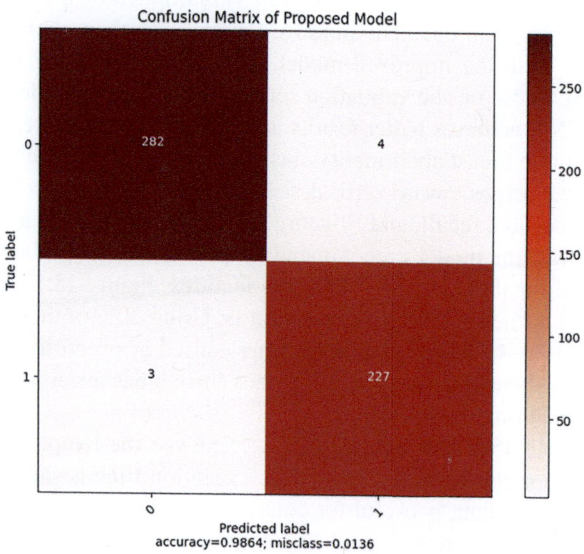

FIGURE 15.12 Confusion matrix of proposed model.

TABLE 15.2

Time Complexity of Various Models

Model	Time Complexity (s)
SVM	36.49
RF	57.848
Inception	93.451
MobileNet	117.83
AlexNet	189.767
Proposed	102.909

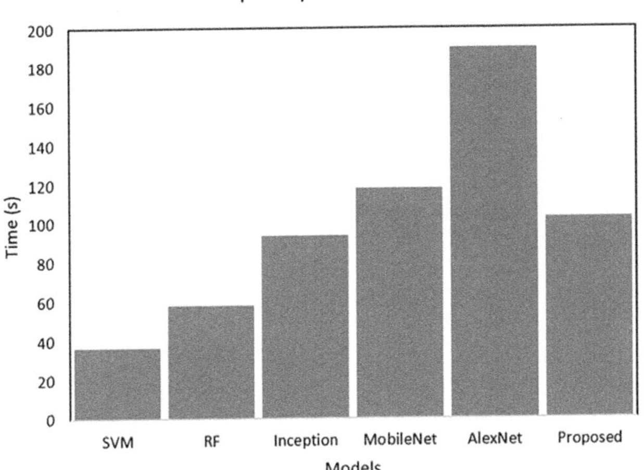

FIGURE 15.13 Different models' time complexities.

seconds. For comparison, AlexNet's time complexity is 189.767 seconds. The temporal complexity of the suggested model is 102.909 seconds, putting it between the two extremes.

15.5 CONCLUSION AND FUTURE SCOPE

In this research, breast cancer subtypes were identified using a cutting-edge neural network method called differential evolution modeling (DEM). The DEM method's classifier was a Deep Neural Network (DNN). An EfficientNet feature extractor was used to create the feature vectors, with the parameters being tuned via Mayfly Optimization. To properly categorize hyper-spectral data pertaining to breast cancer, the researchers turned to deep learning methods. In order to reveal subtle facets of the data, this research made use of the DNN model in particular. Using the DNN model, breast cancer data has to be processed on various levels for categorization. The UCI repository's Wisconsin Breast Cancer Dataset (WBCD) was utilized to measure the system's efficacy. For the sake of experimentation, the dataset was partitioned into many train-test splits. Accuracy, sensitivity, specificity, precision, and recall were among the measures used to evaluate the system's efficacy. The results showed that the system was able to outperform other state-of-the-art methods with an excellent accuracy rate of 98.72%. This demonstrates the efficacy of the proposed DEM method, which employs DNN with efficient feature extraction and parameter optimization, in correctly categorizing various breast cancers. In conclusion, this research shows that deep learning approaches may be effectively used for breast cancer categorization, with the suggested DEM methodology being shown to be superior in terms of accuracy to existing current techniques. In the future, a Bayesian optimization approach will be chosen for the initialization of the hyperparameters, and an optimal feature fusion approach will be explored for fixing the computational time problem.

REFERENCES

[1] M. Akhil and P. V. S. Kumar, "Breast Cancer Prognosis using Machine Learning Applications," in 2022 4th International Conference on Advances in Computing, Communication Control and Networking (ICAC3N), Greater Noida, India, 2022, pp. 488–493, doi: 10.1109/ICAC3N56670.2022.10074517.

[2] B. Bılgıç, "Comparison of Breast Cancer and Skin Cancer Diagnoses Using Deep Learning Method," in 2021 29th Signal Processing and Communications Applications Conference (SIU), Istanbul, Turkey, 2021, pp. 1–4, doi: 10.1109/SIU53274.2021.9477992.

[3] X. Jia, W. Meng, S. Li, Z. Tong and Y. Jia, "A Rare Case of Intracystic Her-2 Positive Young Breast Cancer," in 2021 IEEE International Conference on Bioinformatics and Biomedicine (BIBM), Houston, TX, USA, 2021, pp. 2598–2602, doi: 10.1109/BIBM52615.2021.9669897.

[4] J. Khan, N. A. Golilarz, J. P. Li, P. Kuzeli, A. Addeh and A. U. Haq, "Breast Cancer Diagnosis using Digitized Images of FNA Breast Biopsy and Optimized Neurofuzzy System," in 2020 17th International Computer Conference on Wavelet Active Media Technology and Information Processing (ICCWAMTIP), Chengdu, China, 2020, pp. 286–290, doi: 10.1109/ICCWAMTIP51612.2020.9317387.

[5] R. Lupat, R. Perera, S. Loi and J. Li, "Moanna: Multi-Omics Autoencoder-Based Neural Network Algorithm for Predicting Breast Cancer Subtypes," IEEE Access, vol. 11, 2023, pp. 10912–10924, doi: 10.1109/ACCESS.2023.3240515.

[6] S. Momtahen, M. Momtahen, R. Ramaseshan and F. Golnaraghi, "A Machine Learning Approach: NIR Scattering Data Analysis for Breast Cancer Detection and Classification," in 2022 IEEE 1st Industrial Electronics Society Annual On-Line Conference (ONCON), Kharagpur, India, 2022, pp. 1–6, doi: 10.1109/ONCON56984.2022.10127055.

[7] S. Nelli and B. Kezia Rani, "Prediction of Early Stage Breast Cancer by Injection of Gold Nano Particles and Analyzing Images using Data Analytics," in 2022 IEEE 2nd International Conference on Mobile Networks and Wireless Communications (ICMNWC), Tumkur, Karnataka, India, 2022, pp. 1–5, doi: 10.1109/ICMNWC56175.2022.10031956.

[8] A. Rovshenov and S. Peker, "Performance Comparison of Different Machine Learning Techniques for Early Prediction of Breast Cancer using Wisconsin Breast Cancer Dataset," in 2022 3rd International Informatics and Software Engineering Conference (IISEC), Ankara, Turkey, 2022, pp. 1–6, doi: 10.1109/IISEC56263.2022.9998248.

[9] G. Sajiv and G. Ramkumar, "Automated Breast Cancer Classification based on Modified Deep Learning Convolutional Neural Network following Dual Segmentation," in 2022 3rd International Conference on Electronics and Sustainable Communication Systems (ICESC), Coimbatore, India, 2022, pp. 1562–1569, doi: 10.1109/ICESC54411.2022.9885299.

[10] G. Sajiv, et al, "Multiple Class Breast Cancer Detection Method Based on Deep Learning and MIRRCNN Model," in 2022 International Conference on Inventive Computation Technologies (ICICT), Nepal, 2022, pp. 981–987, doi: 10.1109/ICICT54344.2022.9850707.

Index